Lippincott's
CONCISE ILLUSTRATED ANATOMY:
Thorax, Abdomen & Pelvis

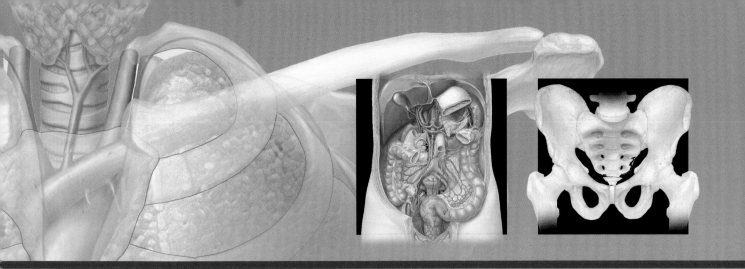

Lippincott's CONCISE ILLUSTRATED ANATOMY:
Thorax, Abdomen & Pelvis

VOLUME 2

Ben Pansky, PhD, MD

Professor Emeritus
Department of Surgery
University of Toledo College of Medicine
and Life Sciences
Toledo, Ohio

Thomas R. Gest, PhD

Professor of Anatomy
Division of Clinical Anatomy
Department of Radiology
University of South Florida Morsani College of Medicine
Tampa, Florida

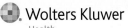

Wolters Kluwer | Lippincott Williams & Wilkins
Health

Philadelphia • Baltimore • New York • London
Buenos Aires • Hong Kong • Sydney • Tokyo

Acquisitions Editor: Crystal Taylor
Product Manager: Julie Montalbano
Marketing Manager: Joy Fisher Williams
Designer: Steve Druding
Compositor: SPi Global

Library of Congress Cataloging-in-Publication Data

Pansky, Ben.
  Lippincott's concise illustrated anatomy. Vol. 2, Thorax, abdomen & pelvis / Ben Pansky, Thomas R. Gest.
    p. ; cm.
  Concise illustrated anatomy
  Thorax, abdomen & pelvis
  ISBN 978-1-60913-028-2
 I. Gest, Thomas R. II. Title. III. Title: Concise illustrated anatomy. IV. Title: Thorax, abdomen & pelvis.
  [DNLM: 1. Thorax—anatomy & histology—Atlases. 2. Abdomen—anatomy & histology—Atlases.
3. Pelvis—anatomy & histology—Atlases. 4. Perineum—anatomy & histology—Atlases. WE 17]
  612.9′4—dc23

                                                                    2012009842

To purchase additional copies of this book, call our customer service department at (800) 638–3030 or fax orders to (301) 223–2320. International customers should call (301) 223–2300.

Visit Lippincott Williams & Wilkins on the Internet: http://www.lww.com. Lippincott Williams & Wilkins customer service representatives are available from 8:30 am to 6:00 pm, EST.

                                                9 8 7 6 5 4 3 2 1

CCS0612

I dedicate this new endeavor to my dearly beloved wife **JULIE**, who will live in my loving memory forever, after our more than 50 years together, whose love, patience, understanding, encouragement and constant inspiration, supported me through the seasons of my maturation and productive life.

And to my loving son, **JONATHAN**, who grew up and matured along with me, my writings, illustrations, and stories. He is ever present by my side with love and encouragement helping me maintain the "Spark of Life and Creativity," which has forever glowed brightly within me.

—Ben Pansky

For my students, past, present, and future, who make teaching so enjoyable, and to all of the courageous body donors, past, present, and future, who teach me and my students so much more than gross anatomy through their amazingly brave and charitable gift.

—Tom Gest

Medical education continues to be in a constant state of change. Dedicated teachers experiment with teaching methods and curricula, always striving to refine, to define, to update, and to narrow the gap between the what, the how, and the why of what is being taught and the state of our present knowledge. Academic traditions are often quite rigid, cemented into place by a "yardstick of established time (hours)," so any effort to change becomes formidable and medical, clinical, and scientific relevance may receive secondary consideration. What the art of medicine always requires, no matter how much manipulating is done, is a strong foundation in the basic sciences. To fully appreciate and understand the complexities and nuances of variation in us all, Anatomy is the keystone in that foundation.

Lippincott's Concise Illustrated Anatomy series presents human gross anatomy in more than a synopsis form and far less than one encounters in a massive traditional text. Each title in the series is a highly illustrated, complete, functionally oriented, clinically informative text, concerned with "living" anatomy and stressing the importance of the relationship between structure and function. Repetition only occurs as needed to emphasize particular points or to demonstrate continuity between regions.

Terminology adheres to the *Terminologia Anatomica* (1998) approved by the Federative Committee on Anatomical Nomenclature (FCAT) of the International Federation of Associations of Anatomists (IFAA). Official English-equivalent terms are used throughout this edition.

Anatomy requires one to think three-dimensionally, which is often a new concept for students and a difficult one for practitioners desiring to review. Studying and palpating a body at a dissection table may be the best way to comprehend the three-dimensional fundamentals of anatomy and the relationships of many of its parts. However, lacking the physical body, this text maintains a tradition utilized in six editions of *Review of Gross Anatomy* by Ben Pansky of being planned and written around its illustrations, which come predominantly from the highly acclaimed *Lippincott Williams & Wilkins Atlas of Anatomy* by Drs. Tank and Gest, together with a reworking of a number of illustrations from Dr. Pansky's 6th edition of *Review of Gross Anatomy*, into beautiful, full-color illustrations closely coordinated with those of the *Atlas*.

The illustrations present anatomical images concisely in a logical sequence, making them easier and faster to use, a critical and essential need in this era of compressed anatomical curricula.

The hundreds of illustrations in full color combined with an abbreviated, outlined, but comprehensive and detailed text convey a simplified, multi-faceted, 3-dimensional aspect of the beauty and function of the human body not found in other texts.

Because the overall volume of material (in text and illustration) needed to present the true, complete reality of the human body is so massive, many texts have become larger and larger over the years. It was felt that a huge "tome" of 1,000 or more pages would be too overwhelming and formidable as well as difficult for students to tackle without great trepidation. Thus, we have decided to present 3 volumes for the 9 chapters or units of associated areas of the body—namely, Volume 1: Back, Upper Limb & Lower Limb; Volume 2: Thorax, Abdomen, & Pelvis; and Volume 3: Head & Neck. Each volume is approximately 300 pages. Thus, as one studies a respective body region, one needs to essentially carry, transport and study from a single volume at a time. Furthermore, if a student or practitioner is predominantly involved only in one or two major body areas, they may be able to concentrate on the essentials of her/his study or review (i.e., general practitioner, physical therapy, occupational therapy, nursing, orthopedics, dentistry, ophthalmology, surgery, etc.) without carrying around a large tome. They would still have the other volume(s) for reference since the body functions as a unit and one part depends on or is related to the other.

Progression from region to region, from the Back to the Upper and Lower Limbs, to the Thorax, Abdomen, and Pelvis, and to the Head and Neck, allows one to fully appreciate the continuity between the regions. The regional approach duplicates that used in many human anatomy courses and laboratories of dissection as well as in surgical areas of concentration. However, the illustrations show some overlapping of structures to allow the student to move easily from one region to the next.

The body is discussed from its superficial layers to its deep structures, except for the osteology. Because the bones form the framework of the body and lend themselves to the attachment of soft parts, they tend to appear early in the text and are also to be studied early in most courses. This makes understanding of the relationships of the soft body parts more easily and clearly understood.

By extracting information from within the living organism, the student and practitioner are better able to describe and define both normal and abnormal states. Increasingly, sophisticated tools help them understand that continuum. At first, students of the medical arts used only observations and palpation, then they undertook dissection, and now "tools" have gained momentum, moving quickly from the stethoscopes and ophthalmoscopes to powerful X-rays and imaging technologies. To put this in perspective, X-rays were discovered at the close of the 19th century; nuclear medicine and ultrasonography were introduced in the 1950s; computed tomography (CT), positron emission tomography (PET), single-photon emission computed tomography (SPECT), digital radiography, and nuclear magnetic resonance (NMR) became available in the 1970s.

Thus, an anatomy text would be incomplete without some discussion and illustration of radiography, CT, NMR, PET, SPECT, and cross-sectional anatomy, which provide a good clinical introduction to the current state of the patient's health. This has been included in our books since the sooner one learns to identify normal anatomy on X-ray film and computer imaging, the easier it becomes to locate and understand the changes brought on by genetics, disease, or trauma and thus, anatomy becomes a "keystone" to all of medicine and its many related fields.

Although much basic and essential clinical consideration has been presented in many areas of our texts, all clinically relevant material cannot be fully discussed for each anatomical region. However, its importance in one's understanding of basic anatomy and how that can be altered is essential for truly appreciating what is generally "normal" before it becomes altered and creates clinical signs and symptoms.

The functional anatomy of the thorax, abdomen, and pelvis is presented in a concise manner, together with correlated clinical material, so that the student can appreciate the relevance of the anatomy to clinical practice. Special functional summaries, especially for autonomic innervation, should help the student to grasp this difficult material.

We, as educators in the Anatomical Sciences, are aware of the fact that gross anatomy is a subject quickly memorized and just as easily forgotten, unless the student or practitioner constantly reviews the material. Time can be an adversary and multiple duties are often overwhelming. It is our hope that in this series we have been concise, direct, and meaningful, without "running on and on" with excessive non-essentials, and that we have been able to create books that will guide the reader easily and thoughtfully through the very complex detail that makes up the human body and its many parts.

Many thanks to those at Lippincott Williams and Wilkins who participated in the development of this textbook, including Acquisitions Editor Crystal Taylor, Product Manager Julie Montalbano, Art Director Jennifer Clements, and Designer Steve Druding. Additional thanks goes to Kelly Horvath for her editorial guidance and copyediting.

Marcelo Oliver and Body Scientific International did a superb job of converting many of Dr. Pansky's original black-and-white illustrations into full color, managing to duplicate the tone, color, and beauty of the illustrations from the *Lippincott Williams & Wilkins Atlas of Anatomy* by Drs. Tank and Gest.

Much gratitude is extended to Danelle Mooi, Secretary, Department of Surgery, and Nick Andrew Bell, Secretary, Departments of Nursing, Emergency Medicine and Staff Development, both at The University of Toledo Medical Center for their persistent encouragement, understanding, and great help to Dr. Pansky with their knowledge of the computer and digital world, which made his transgression into the realm of computers and wireless connections possible and a great learning experience.

Thanks goes to Summer Decker, PhD, Assistant Professor of Radiology, University of South Florida Morsani College of Medicine for her help in obtaining CT scans of the abdominopelvic cavity to match the cross sectional illustrations of this region.

And special thanks goes to Patrick Tank, PhD, Professor of Neurobiology and Developmental Sciences, University of Arkansas for Medical Sciences. His inspiration and hard work on the initial chapter of the initial volume of this series helped to get this project underway.

Ben Pansky
Thomas Gest

CONTENTS

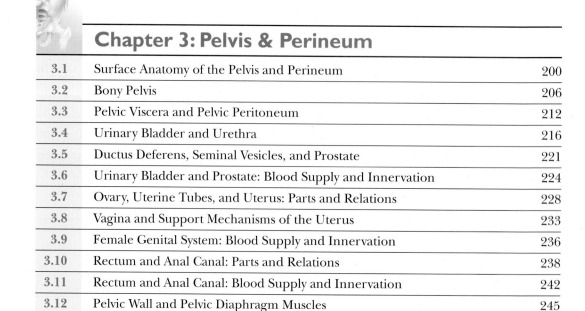

Chapter 3: Pelvis & Perineum

Thorax

Surface Anatomy of the Thoracic Wall

I. Introduction to the Thorax (Fig. 1.1A)

A. Thorax represents superior part of trunk
   1. Located between neck superiorly and abdomen inferiorly
   2. Upper limbs attach to chest wall where thorax meets neck via pectoral girdles (clavicle and scapula)
B. Thorax boundaries
   1. Superior: 1st rib (not palpable), jugular notch of manubrium, and T1 vertebra
   2. Inferior: costal margins (arch or angle) of rib cage
C. Palpable features of the thorax
   1. Except for 1st rib, most ribs can be palpated
   2. Sternum and its parts (manubrium, body, and xiphoid process) readily palpated
   3. Sternal angle felt as elevation between manubrium and body
      a. Lies at level of costal cartilage of 2nd rib
      b. Can be used as guide for counting ribs

II. Landmark Lines of the Thorax: Vertical Lines for Orientation and Description (Fig. 1.1B–D)

A. Midclavicular line: through midpoint of clavicle and nipple
B. Anterior axillary line: through anterior axillary fold (pectoralis major)
C. Midaxillary line: through axilla
D. Posterior axillary line: through posterior axillary fold (latissimus dorsi)
E. Scapular line: through inferior angle of scapula
F. Paravertebral line: through transverse processes of vertebrae

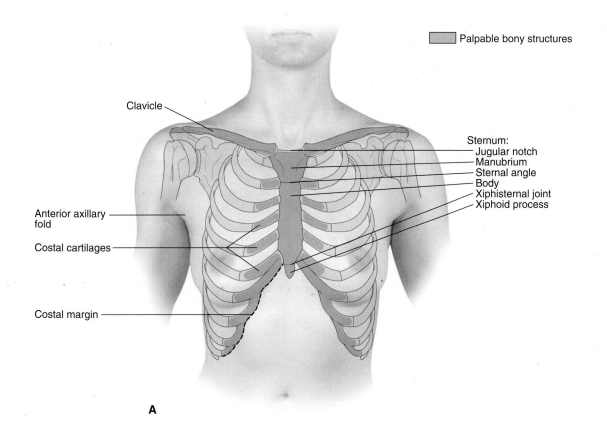

Palpable bony structures

Clavicle

Sternum:
Jugular notch
Manubrium
Sternal angle
Body
Xiphisternal joint
Xiphoid process

Anterior axillary fold

Costal cartilages

Costal margin

A

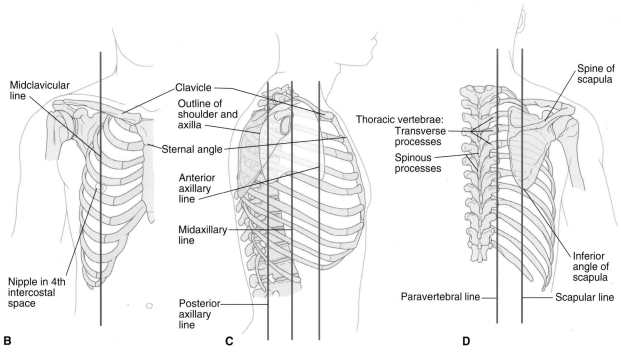

Midclavicular line

Clavicle

Outline of shoulder and axilla

Sternal angle

Anterior axillary line

Midaxillary line

Nipple in 4th intercostal space

Posterior axillary line

B

C

Spine of scapula

Thoracic vertebrae:
Transverse processes

Spinous processes

Inferior angle of scapula

Paravertebral line

Scapular line

D

FIG. 1.1A–D. **A.** Palpable Features of the Thorax, Anterior View. **B.** Landmark Lines of the Thorax, Anterior View. **C.** Lateral View. **D.** Posterior View.

III. Thoracic Dermatomes: Segmental Innervation of the Thoracic Wall (Fig. 1.1E,F)

A. C6–C8: found on back and upper limb but not represented on anterior body wall

B. T2–T12: not involved in formation of plexuses; best segmental distributions of spinal nerves in the body

C. T7–T12: represent thoracoabdominal innervation, distributing onto anterior abdominal wall

D. T4: crosses the nipple location

E. T7: crosses the xiphoid process

F. T10: crosses the umbilicus

IV. Clinical Considerations: Herpes Zoster (Shingles)

A. Adulthood reactivation and proliferation of childhood chickenpox infection

B. Called "shingles" because, during initial infection, chickenpox virus (varicella zoster) leaves the skin and invades the spinal ganglia, where it remains latent until adult reactivation, then travels through sensory axons to dermatome

C. Virus continues to proliferate in dermatome, forming a rash and/or blisters accompanied by intense burning or tingling pain (dermatological pain may persist even after skin changes have resolved)

D. Patients are contagious as long as they have blisters

E. Approximately 10% of adults develop shingles in their lifetime, most after age 50 years

F. Usually self-limiting but can recur

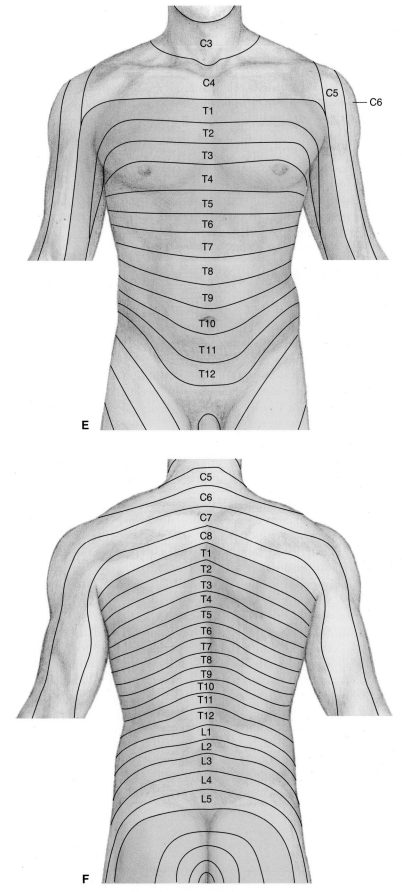

FIG. 1.1E,F. Dermatomes of the Thorax. **E.** Anterior View. **F.** Posterior View.

Thoracic Cage as a Whole

I. Thoracic Wall Topography (Fig. 1.2A)

A. Shaped like a truncated cone; flattened anteroposteriorly
B. Anterior wall: sternum and 1st 10 pairs of ribs with their costal cartilages
C. Lateral walls: formed by ribs that slope obliquely downward and forward
D. Posterior wall: made up of 12 thoracic vertebrae and ribs as far as their angles
E. Superior aperture (inlet): kidney shaped
   1. Slopes down and forward
   2. Formed by body of 1st thoracic vertebra, 1st ribs and cartilages, and manubrium sterni
F. Inferior aperture (outlet): large, irregular
   1. Formed by costal margin (7th to 12th costal cartilages, ribs 11 and 12), 12th thoracic vertebra, and xiphisternal joint
   2. Occupied by diaphragm

II. Sternum (Breast Bone)

A. Elongated flat bone
B. Parts
   1. Manubrium: at level with 3rd and 4th thoracic vertebrae; roughly quadrangular
      a. Has 2 surfaces (anterior and posterior); both are smooth and concave
      b. Has 4 borders (superior, inferior, and 2 lateral)
         i. Superior border: jugular (suprasternal) notch in middle; flanked by oval articular surfaces for clavicles (clavicular notches)
         ii. Inferior border: rough; normally covered with cartilage for articulation with body (at sternal symphysis)
         iii. Lateral borders: marked above by depression for 1st costal cartilage and below by small articular facet at the sternal symphysis, which, together with similar one on body, forms a joint with 2nd costal cartilage
   2. Body: long and narrow
      a. Lies opposite 5th to 9th thoracic vertebrae
      b. Has 2 surfaces (anterior and posterior) and 4 borders (superior, inferior, and 2 lateral)
         i. Anterior surface has 3 transverse ridges at the level of the articular depressions for the 3rd, 4th, and 5th costal cartilages
         ii. Superior border: oval; articulates with manubrium at the sternal symphysis or **sternal angle** (of Louis), which lies at level of disk between vertebrae T4–T5 and about 5 cm below jugular notch
         iii. Each lateral border: at superior angle, small notch for 2nd costal cartilage; below this, 4 costal notches for cartilages of rib 3 to 6; at inferior angle, small facet in xiphoid holds 7th costal cartilage with adjoining costal cartilage
         iv. Inferior border: narrow, for articulation with xiphoid
   3. Xiphoid process: smallest, most variable and most caudal
      a. May be bifid
      b. Has 2 surfaces (anterior and posterior) and 3 borders (superior and 2 lateral)
      c. At superior end, has small depression for part of 7th costal cartilage
      d. Cartilaginous until early childhood
C. Ossification from 6 centers: 1 manubrium, 4 body, and 1 xiphoid

Location	Appears	Fuses
Manubrium	6th fetal month	25th year
1st body	6th fetal month	25th year
2nd and 3rd body	7th fetal month	25th year
4th body	1st postnatal year	Puberty
Xiphoid	5th–18th year	30 to >40 years

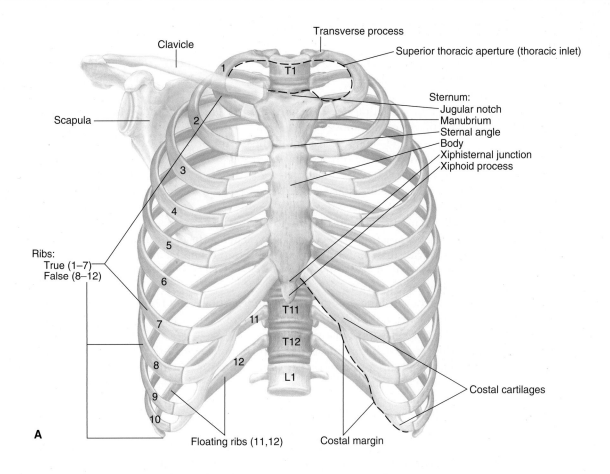

Clavicle

Transverse process

Superior thoracic aperture (thoracic inlet)

Scapula

T1

Sternum:
Jugular notch
Manubrium
Sternal angle
Body
Xiphisternal junction
Xiphoid process

Ribs:
True (1–7)
False (8–12)

T11

T12

L1

Costal cartilages

Floating ribs (11,12)

Costal margin

A

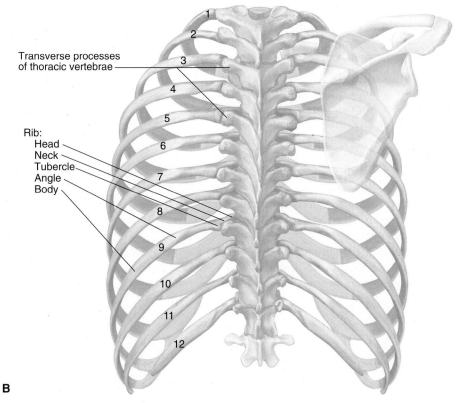

Transverse processes
of thoracic vertebrae

Rib:
Head
Neck
Tubercle
Angle
Body

B

FIG. 1.2A,B. Thoracic Skeleton. **A.** Anterior View. **B.** Posterior View.

III. Ribs (Fig. 1.2B)

A. Classification

   1. True ribs (1–7): articulate behind with vertebrae and in front, through cartilages, with sternum

   2. False ribs

      a. Vertebrochondral (8–10): join the vertebrae behind, but ventrally join costal cartilages of ribs above

      b. Floating (11–12): anterolateral ends of the ribs are capped with cartilage, which does not join with other costal cartilages

B. General characteristics of typical ribs (Fig. 1.2C)

   1. Head: has articular surface divided into 2 parts by a ridge; articulates with intervertebral disc and edges of adjacent vertebral bodies

   2. Neck: ≈2cm in length, just lateral to head

   3. Tubercle: at junction of neck and body; articular facet for transverse process of vertebra

   4. Angle of rib: anteroinferior bend just beyond tubercle

   5. Body (shaft): thin, flat, and curved with 2 surfaces (external and internal) and 2 borders (superior and inferior)

   6. Costal groove: along inner aspect of inferior border of body

   7. Anterior extremity ends in oval concavity for costal cartilage

C. General characteristics of atypical ribs

   1. 1st rib (Fig. 1.2D): has greatest curvature and is shortest

      a. Flattened superoinferiorly, providing superior and inferior surfaces with lateral and medial borders

      b. Head has single articular facet for T1 vertebral body

      c. Tubercle: thick and prominent

      d. No angle

      e. Upper surface shows 2 shallow grooves (for subclavian artery and vein), separated by **scalene tubercle** for attachment of anterior scalene muscle

      f. No costal groove

      g. Anterior extremity is larger and thicker than other ribs

   2. 2nd rib: longer than 1st and intermediate in form between 1st rib and typical rib

      a. Curvature similar to the 1st rib, but is not as flattened superoinferiorly

      b. Angle is slight and close to tubercle

   3. 10th rib: like a typical rib except with single articular facet on head

   4. 11th and 12th ribs (Fig. 1.2E)

      a. Have a single articular facet on head

      b. Have neither neck nor tubercle

      c. Anterolateral ends are pointed

      d. 11th has very shallow costal groove; 12th has none

D. Ossification

   1. Ribs 1 to 10 ossify from 4 centers: body, head, and articular and nonarticular parts of tubercle

      a. Centers appear in body near angle in 8th fetal week (seen first in ribs 6 and 7)

      b. Centers for head and tubercles appear between 16th and 20th years and unite with body in 25th year

E. Costovertebral articulations: most ribs have 2 costovertebral joints, 1 between head of rib and intervertebral disc and adjacent vertebral bodies, other between tubercle and transverse process (costotransverse joints)

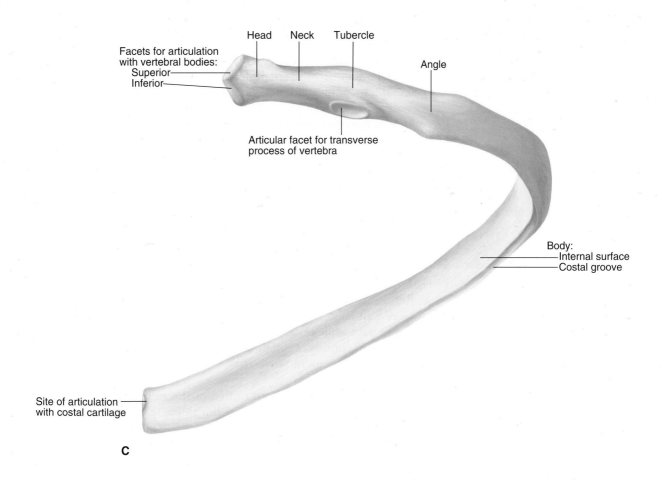

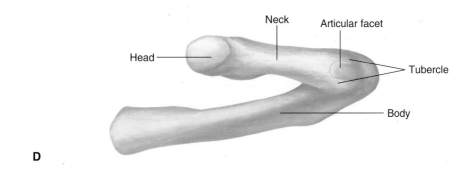

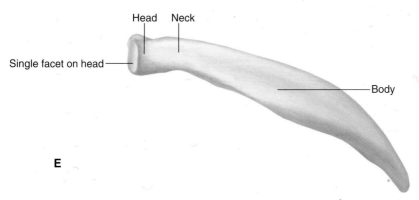

FIG. I.2C–E. Ribs. **C.** 6th Rib, Posterior View. **D.** 1st Rib, Posterior View. **E.** 12th Rib, Posterior View.

IV. Clinical Considerations

A. Age changes in chest shape
1. Circular for first 2 years of life, so that breathing is abdominal (diaphragmatic) because circumference remains constant
2. Oval shaped in adult (flattened anteroposteriorly) with breathing becoming intercostal (thoracic)
B. Pigeon breast (pectus carinatum): sternum projects forward in keel shape
C. Funnel chest (pectus excavatum): chest concave anteriorly due to rib overgrowth
D. Serious chest deformities are predominantly congenital and associated with rib overgrowth; slight deformities and asymmetries are common, cause no disability
E. Rib fractures: weakest area of rib is located anterior to angle
1. Fractures are usually result of direct blows or crushing injuries
2. Middle ribs most vulnerable
3. Internal organs may be injured by broken rib end
4. Flail chest
   a. Results from multiple rib fractures leading to relatively freely moveable section of chest wall, which moves in and out with respiration, causing severe pain while breathing
   b. Treatment consists of stabilizing loose section with wires or other means to prevent movement
F. Sternal fracture
1. Uncommon but may occur most often at the sternal angle as a result of crush injury that compresses the anterior thoracic wall
2. Frequently comminuted, creating multiple bone pieces
G. Needle biopsies of sternum: for examination of bone marrow for transplantation as well as for detection of metastatic cancer
H. Rib separation: dislocation; seen in contact sports, usually at junction of costal cartilage with sternum, producing a "lump" deformity at the dislocation and pain in deep breathing
I. Extra (supernumerary) ribs: typically extra cervical or lumbar ribs
1. Cervical ribs tend to articulate with the C7 vertebra and may compress spinal nerves C8 and T1 or the inferior trunk of the brachial plexus; may also compress the subclavian artery leading to ischemic muscle pain
2. Extra lumbar ribs are relatively rare

Articulations of the Thoracic Wall

I. Intrasternal (Fig. 1.3A)

A. Between manubrium and body of sternum
1. Type: symphysis (secondary cartilaginous joint) with fibrocartilage between edges of bone, strengthened by fibrous tissue
   a. Articulating surfaces covered with hyaline cartilage
   b. Synovial cavity may be present
   c. In old age, ossification may occur (synostosis)
2. **Sternal angle:** bony ridge at the manubriosternal joint
   a. Clinically important because it marks inferior border of superior mediastinum
   b. Costal cartilage of 2nd rib (highest palpable rib) articulates at sternal angle
3. In most people, joint moves slightly during respiration
B. Between xiphoid and body of sternum
1. Type: synarthrosis (synchondrosis); bones are united by hyaline cartilage
2. After 40th year, bone usually replaces cartilage (synostosis)

II. Sternocostal Articulations

A. Between sternum and 1st rib
1. Type: synchondrosis (synarthrosis): bones firmly united by cartilage
B. Between sternum and costal cartilages of ribs 2 to 7
1. Type: synovial (arthrodial)
2. Movements: gliding
3. Ligaments
   a. Articular capsule
   b. Radiate sternocostal: from anterior and posterior surfaces of cartilages to anterior and posterior surface of sternum
   c. Intraarticular sternocostal: usually found with 2nd rib only, where ligament runs from end of cartilage to fibrocartilage between manubrium and body of sternum

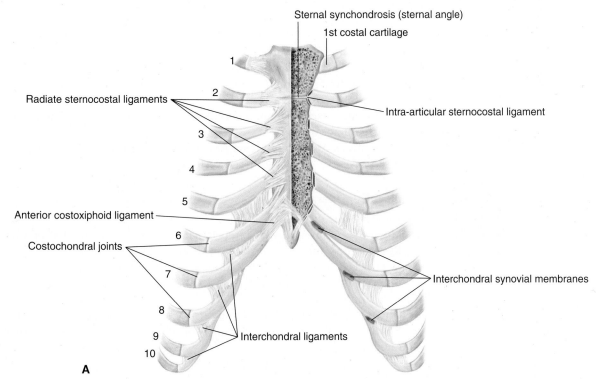

FIG. 1.3A. Articulations of the Anterior Thoracic Wall.

    d. Costoxiphoid: join anterior and posterior surfaces of 7th costal cartilage to anterior and posterior sides of xiphoid process

C. Interchondral
1. Between costal cartilages of ribs 6 to 8 (sometimes through 10), joined together at adjacent articular facets
   a. Articulations between adjacent borders of 6th and 7th, 7th and 8th, and 8th and 9th costal cartilages are plane synovial joints
   b. Each articulation enclosed in fibrous capsule lined with synovial membrane
2. Between 9th and 10th costal cartilages is a fibrous joint in which cartilages are joined by fibrous tissue
3. Ligaments
   a. Articular capsules
   b. Interchondral, running from 1 cartilage to another

D. Costochondral
1. Between depression in medial end of rib and lateral end of costal cartilage
2. These are synarthroses, surrounded by fibrous tissue continuous with periosteum/ perichondrium

III. Costovertebral Articulations (Fig. 1.3B,C)

A. Costovertebral joint
1. Between head of rib and vertebral bodies
2. Type: plane synovial joint
3. Movements: gliding
4. Bones: head of rib and superior and inferior costal facets on side of 2 adjacent vertebral bodies
   a. Ribs 1, 10, 11, 12 articulate with only 1 vertebra
5. Articular capsule reinforced by ligaments
   a. **Radiate ligament**: from anterior part of head of rib to bodies and intervertebral disc
   b. **Intraarticular ligament**
      i. From interarticular crest of rib to fibrocartilage
      ii. Located within joint and divides synovial cavity into 2 cavities

B. **Costotransverse joint**
1. Between rib and transverse process
2. Type: plane synovial joint
3. Movements: gliding
4. Bones: tubercle of rib with transverse process
5. Articular capsule reinforced by ligaments
   a. **Costotransverse ligament**: from posterior surface of neck of rib to anterior surface of adjacent transverse process
   b. **Superior costotransverse ligament**: from superior border of neck of rib to transverse process of vertebra above
   c. **Lateral costotransverse ligament**: from nonarticulated part of tubercle of rib to tip of transverse process of same numbered vertebra

IV. Clinical Considerations

A. Sternoclavicular dislocation
1. Much less common than acromioclavicular dislocation (shoulder separation)
2. Results from violent fall or blow to shoulder
3. Sternoclavicular ligaments rupture, and intraarticular fibrocartilage remains attached to clavicle

B. Thoracic outlet syndrome
1. Due to compression of subclavian artery between clavicle and 1st rib
2. Results in coldness and pallor of skin of upper extremity and a drop in radial pulse

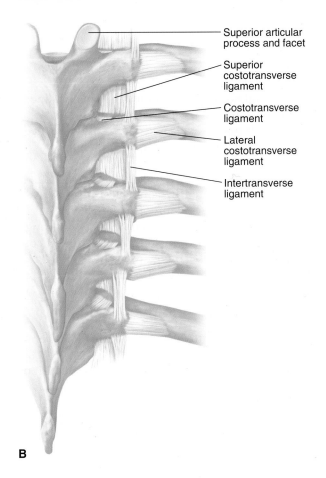

Superior articular
process and facet

Superior
costotransverse
ligament

Costotransverse
ligament

Lateral
costotransverse
ligament

Intertransverse
ligament

B

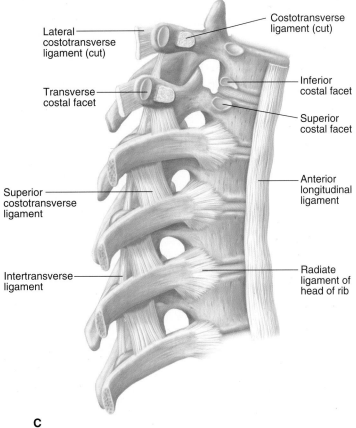

Lateral
costotransverse
ligament (cut)

Costotransverse
ligament (cut)

Transverse
costal facet

Inferior
costal facet

Superior
costal facet

Superior
costotransverse
ligament

Anterior
longitudinal
ligament

Intertransverse
ligament

Radiate
ligament of
head of rib

C

FIG. 1.3B,C. Articulations of the Posterior Thoracic Wall. **B.** Posterior View. **C.** Lateral View.

Mammary Gland

I. Topography (Fig. 1.4A)

A. From 2nd to 6th or 7th rib and lateral border of sternum to midaxillary line
B. Nipple is just below center of gland at 4th intercostal space in men
C. Superolateral part frequently projects toward axilla as **axillary tail** (of Spence) in relation to pectoralis major muscle and pectoral (anterior axillary) lymph nodes

II. Structure (Fig. 1.4B,C)

A. Made up of 15 to 20 separate lobes, separated by connective tissue septa and further divided into lobules and acini, arranged like segments of a citrus fruit
B. Type of gland: compound tubuloalveolar gland, with multiple ducts emptying onto nipple
C. Entire gland lies in superficial fascia with lobes embedded in fat (round contour); deep surface is separated from muscle fascia by loose connective tissue
D. **Suspensory ligaments** (of Cooper) run from pectoral fascia to skin; well developed in upper breast

III. Ducts

A. **Lactiferous duct** drains each lobe and leads into dilated **lactiferous sinus** (or ampulla) just deep to areola
B. At base of nipple, ducts narrow down, change direction, and run to summit of nipple

IV. Nipple

A. Skin wrinkled
B. Contains smooth muscle fibers that contract on tactile stimulation, inducing firmness and prominence

V. Areola

A. Pigmented 1–2-cm area surrounding nipple that is pink before pregnancy but turns permanently brown after pregnancy
B. **Areolar glands** (of Montgomery)
　1. Sebaceous glands that enlarge in pregnancy and secrete an oily substance to provide a protective lubricant for areola and nipple
　2. Produce little irregularities or small projections in areolae

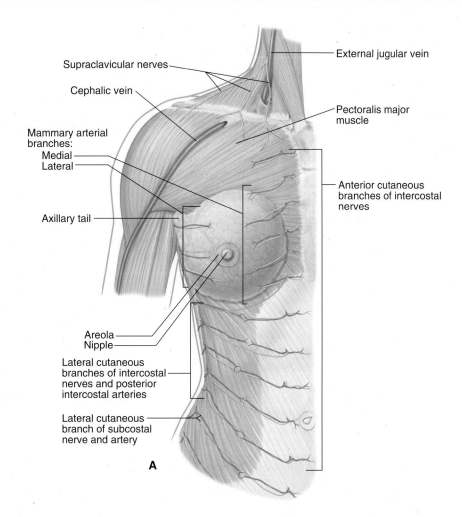

External jugular vein

Supraclavicular nerves

Cephalic vein

Pectoralis major muscle

Mammary arterial branches:
Medial
Lateral

Anterior cutaneous branches of intercostal nerves

Axillary tail

Areola
Nipple

Lateral cutaneous branches of intercostal nerves and posterior intercostal arteries

Lateral cutaneous branch of subcostal nerve and artery

A

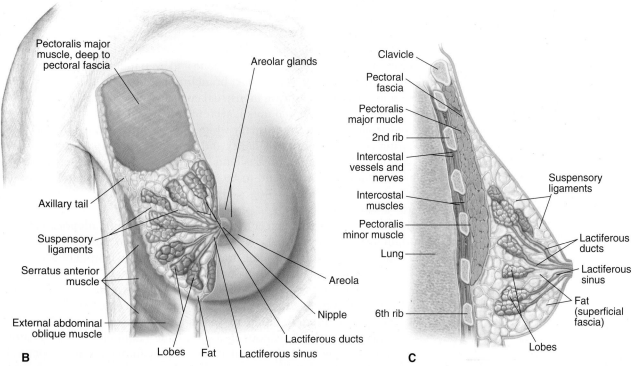

Pectoralis major muscle, deep to pectoral fascia

Areolar glands

Axillary tail

Suspensory ligaments

Serratus anterior muscle

External abdominal oblique muscle

Lobes   Fat   Lactiferous sinus

Areola

Nipple

Lactiferous ducts

B

Clavicle

Pectoral fascia

Pectoralis major mucle

2nd rib

Intercostal vessels and nerves

Intercostal muscles

Pectoralis minor muscle

Lung

6th rib

Suspensory ligaments

Lactiferous ducts

Lactiferous sinus

Fat (superficial fascia)

Lobes

C

FIG. 1.4A–C. A. Cutaneous Nerves and Superficial Vessels of the Anterior Thoracic Wall, Anterior View. **B.** Breast, Anterior View. **C.** Breast, Sagittal View.

VI. Blood Supply (Fig. 1.4D)

A. Arteries

  1. From axillary artery: lateral thoracic artery, which gives rise to lateral mammary branches

  2. From posterior intercostal arteries: anterior branches (lateral mammary branches) of lateral cutaneous branches in 3rd, 4th, and 5th intercostal spaces

  3. From internal thoracic artery: perforating branches (medial mammary branches) in 2nd to 4th intercostal spaces

B. Veins: from anastomotic circle around nipple, drain to axillary, internal thoracic, lateral thoracic, and upper posterior intercostal veins

VII. Nerves

A. From anterior and lateral cutaneous branches of 2nd to 6th intercostal nerves

B. Intercostal nerves convey sensory fibers from skin of breast and sympathetic fibers to blood vessels in the breast and smooth muscle and sweat glands in skin and nipple

VIII. Lymphatic Drainage (Fig. 1.4E)

A. Principal

  1. Originates from extensive perilobular plexus

  2. Follows lactiferous ducts to areola to form subareolar plexus

  3. Drains into pectoral (anterior axillary) group of axillary nodes deep to lateral edge of pectoralis major muscle

B. Secondary

  1. From medial side of gland to parasternal nodes; some channels cross to opposite gland

  2. From upper gland to apical axillary nodes or to supraclavicular nodes

  3. From inferior portion of gland, vessels may pass to diaphragmatic lymph nodes

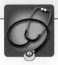

IX. Clinical Considerations

A. **Polymastia** (supernumerary breasts) and **polythelia** (more than 2 nipples)

  1. May develop above or below (most common) normal breasts

  2. Seen in ≈1% of female population and usually genetic

  3. Extra breast usually consists of rudimentary breast and areola, along mammary ridges (crests) and found from axilla to groin

  4. Polythelia uncommon, but may be seen in males

  5. Accessory breasts may have normal tissue and even function during lactation

B. Breast changes (i.e., lactiferous duct branching)

  1. Seen in breast tissue during menstrual cycle and pregnancy for secretion in midpregnancy, but actual milk is secreted after birth

  2. **Colostrum**: premilk fluid usually white or yellow that tends to be secreted during last trimester of pregnancy and into early nursing

  3. In multiparous women, breasts tend to enlarge and become pendulous

  4. In older adults, breasts tend to be small because of fat loss and glandular atrophy

C. Breast cancer

  1. Most common form of cancer in women; most commonly adenocarcinomas originating from epithelial cells of lactiferous ducts in gland lobules

    a. Interference with lymphatic drainage may result in **lymphedema** (excess fluid in the subcutaneous tissue)

    b. Thickened, leather-like skin with "orange-peel" appearance (**peau d'orange sign**) is seen from skin dimpling due to tension on connective tissue septa

    c. If ducts are invaded, nipple may invaginate or invert

    d. Cancer spreads via venous and lymphatic channels as well as along fibrous tissue to deeper structures (retromammary space, pectoralis fascia, etc.) to a wide variety of lymph nodes (i.e., anterior axillary or pectoral, parasternal, abdominal, and supraclavicular and to the opposite nodes across sternum)

Continued

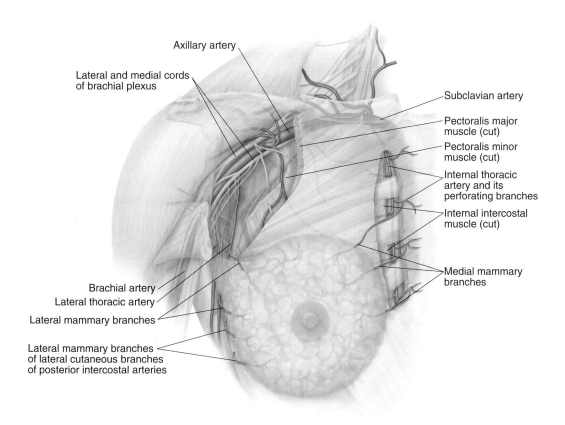

Axillary artery

Lateral and medial cords
of brachial plexus

Subclavian artery

Pectoralis major
muscle (cut)

Pectoralis minor
muscle (cut)

Internal thoracic
artery and its
perforating branches

Internal intercostal
muscle (cut)

Medial mammary
branches

Brachial artery

Lateral thoracic artery

Lateral mammary branches

Lateral mammary branches
of lateral cutaneous branches
of posterior intercostal arteries

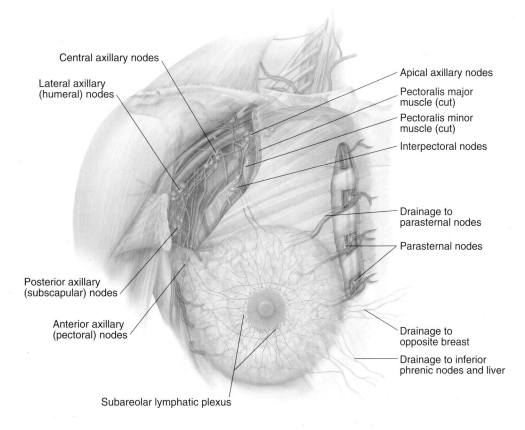

Central axillary nodes

Lateral axillary
(humeral) nodes

Apical axillary nodes

Pectoralis major
muscle (cut)

Pectoralis minor
muscle (cut)

Interpectoral nodes

Drainage to
parasternal nodes

Parasternal nodes

Posterior axillary
(subscapular) nodes

Anterior axillary
(pectoral) nodes

Drainage to
opposite breast

Drainage to inferior
phrenic nodes and liver

Subareolar lymphatic plexus

FIG. 1.4D,E. D. Arterial Supply of the Breast, Anterior View. **E.** Lymphatic Drainage of the Breast,
Anterior View.

2. Treatment
   a. Mammography: radiographic examination of breasts that can serve as guide in surgical removal of tumors, cysts, abscesses, etc. and in treatment by radiation or chemotherapy
   b. Mastectomy (excision of breast): not as common as previously
      i. Simple mastectomy: breast is removed down to the retromammary space
      ii. Radical mastectomy: removal of the breast, pectoral muscles, fat, fascia, and lymph nodes in the axilla and pectoral region
   c. Newer, less-radical therapy
      i. Removes only lymph nodes directly involved and others nearby (as necessary), while conserving others, followed by radiation and chemotherapy
      ii. Prevents excessive edema in region as well as in upper extremity

Muscles and Neurovasculature of the Thoracic Wall

I. Muscles: 3 Layers with Accessory Muscles, Innervated by Local Intercostal Nerves

A. External intercostal (Fig. 1.5A)
   1. Between adjacent ribs (11 pairs)
   2. Origin: lower border of rib
   3. Insertion: in upper border of rib below; extend from tubercle of rib to costal cartilage
   4. External intercostal membrane replaces muscle from costal cartilages to sternum

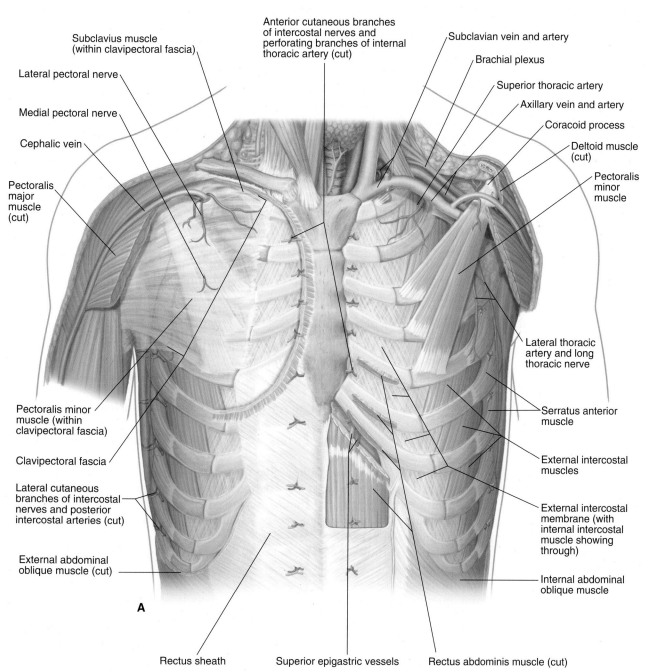

Subclavius muscle (within clavipectoral fascia)

Lateral pectoral nerve

Medial pectoral nerve

Cephalic vein

Pectoralis major muscle (cut)

Pectoralis minor muscle (within clavipectoral fascia)

Clavipectoral fascia

Lateral cutaneous branches of intercostal nerves and posterior intercostal arteries (cut)

External abdominal oblique muscle (cut)

Anterior cutaneous branches of intercostal nerves and perforating branches of internal thoracic artery (cut)

Subclavian vein and artery

Brachial plexus

Superior thoracic artery

Axillary vein and artery

Coracoid process

Deltoid muscle (cut)

Pectoralis minor muscle

Lateral thoracic artery and long thoracic nerve

Serratus anterior muscle

External intercostal muscles

External intercostal membrane (with internal intercostal muscle showing through)

Internal abdominal oblique muscle

A

Rectus sheath

Superior epigastric vessels

Rectus abdominis muscle (cut)

FIG. 1.5A. Intercostal Muscles, Superficial Dissection, Anterior View.

B. Internal intercostal (Fig. 1.5B)
   1. Between adjacent ribs (11 pairs)
   2. Origin: from inner surface of lower border of rib
   3. Insertion: in upper border of rib below; extend from sternum to angles of rib
   4. Internal intercostal membrane replaces muscle between angle of rib and vertebrae
C. Innermost intercostal muscle layer: 3 muscles
   1. Transversus thoracis (Fig. 1.5C): on inner chest wall
      a. Origin: from posterior body and xiphoid process of sternum and sternal ends of costal cartilages of ribs 4 to 6
      b. Insertion: on lower border and costal cartilages of ribs 2 to 6
      c. Action: draws ribs down
   2. Innermost intercostal
      a. Origin: from inner surface of rib; insertion: in upper border of rib below
      b. Extends from midclavicular line (approximately) to subcostalis at angles of ribs
   3. Subcostalis (Fig. 1.5D)
      a. Origin: from inner surface of rib near angle
      b. Insertion: 2 ribs below
      c. Action: when last rib is fixed by quadratus lumborum muscle, it lowers ribs
D. Accessory respiratory muscles
   1. Levatores costarum (12 pairs): on posterior thorax
      a. Origin: from ends and transverse processes of vertebrae C7–T11
      b. Insertion: into outer surface of rib immediately below origin
      c. Action: raise ribs; extend, laterally flex, and rotate the vertebral column to opposite side
   2. Serratus posterior superior: on posterior of upper thorax
      a. Origin: from ligamentum nuchae, supraspinous ligament, and spines of vertebrae C7–T3
      b. Insertion: on upper borders of ribs 2 to 5, lateral to angles
      c. Action: raises ribs
   3. Serratus posterior inferior: on posterior of lower thorax
      a. Origin: from supraspinous ligament and spines of vertebrae T11–L3
      b. Insertion: on lower border of ribs 9 to 12, lateral to angles
      c. Action: lowers ribs

II. Intercostal Neurovascular Bundles

A. Run between the 2nd (internal intercostal) and 3rd (innermost intercostal) layers of intercostal muscles
B. Run in or near costal groove, with vein most superior, artery intermediate, and nerve below artery
C. Collateral branches (small) descend to run on upper border of rib below
D. Posterior intercostal arteries: 11 pairs
   1. First 2: branch from supreme intercostal artery, which is branch of costocervical trunk from subclavian
   2. 3rd to 11th: arise from posterolateral sides of aorta
      a. Right posterior intercostals cross vertebral bodies to reach intercostal spaces
      b. Branches: to muscles, lateral cutaneous, and collateral
      c. Anastomose with anterior intercostal branches of internal thoracic artery near midclavicular line
      d. Dorsal ramus: runs posteriorly between necks of ribs to supply spinal cord and tissues of back
E. Anterior intercostal arteries
   1. From internal thoracic (upper 6 intercostal spaces) and musculophrenic artery (spaces 7–10)
   2. 2 small arteries per space
   3. Anastomose with posterior intercostals near midclavicular line
   4. Perforating branches to muscle, skin, and mammary gland

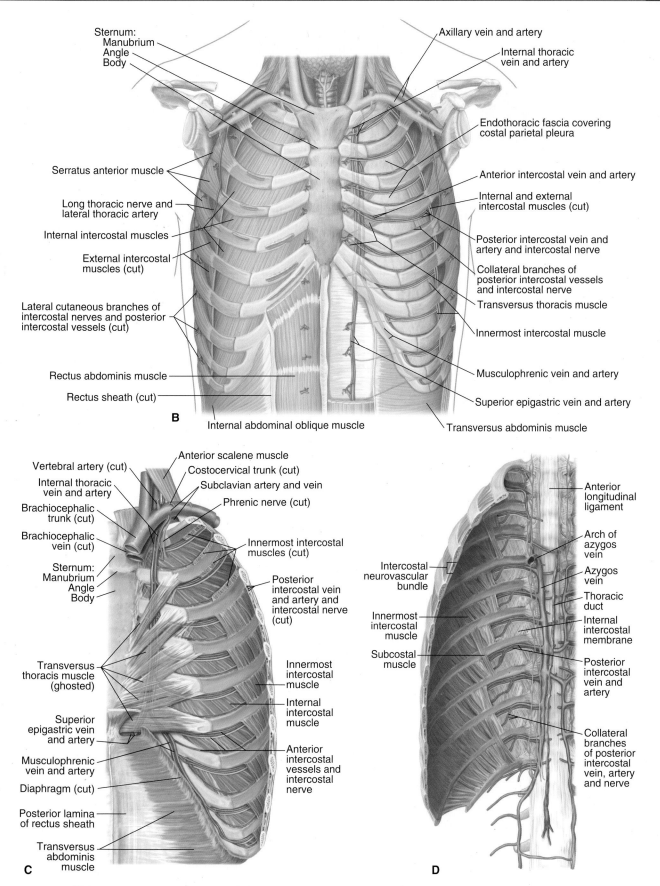

Sternum:
Manubrium
Angle
Body

Axillary vein and artery

Internal thoracic
vein and artery

Serratus anterior muscle

Endothoracic fascia covering
costal parietal pleura

Anterior intercostal vein and artery

Long thoracic nerve and
lateral thoracic artery

Internal and external
intercostal muscles (cut)

Internal intercostal muscles

Posterior intercostal vein and
artery and intercostal nerve

External intercostal
muscles (cut)

Collateral branches of
posterior intercostal vessels
and intercostal nerve

Transversus thoracis muscle

Lateral cutaneous branches of
intercostal nerves and posterior
intercostal vessels (cut)

Innermost intercostal muscle

Musculophrenic vein and artery

Rectus abdominis muscle

Rectus sheath (cut)

Superior epigastric vein and artery

B

Internal abdominal oblique muscle

Transversus abdominis muscle

Vertebral artery (cut)

Anterior scalene muscle

Costocervical trunk (cut)

Internal thoracic
vein and artery

Subclavian artery and vein

Brachiocephalic
trunk (cut)

Phrenic nerve (cut)

Brachiocephalic
vein (cut)

Innermost intercostal
muscles (cut)

Sternum:
Manubrium
Angle
Body

Posterior
intercostal vein
and artery and
intercostal nerve
(cut)

Transversus
thoracis muscle
(ghosted)

Innermost
intercostal
muscle

Superior
epigastric vein
and artery

Internal
intercostal
muscle

Musculophrenic
vein and artery

Diaphragm (cut)

Anterior
intercostal
vessels and
intercostal
nerve

Posterior lamina
of rectus sheath

Transversus
abdominis
muscle

C

Intercostal
neurovascular
bundle

Anterior
longitudinal
ligament

Arch of
azygos
vein

Azygos
vein

Thoracic
duct

Innermost
intercostal
muscle

Internal
intercostal
membrane

Subcostal
muscle

Posterior
intercostal
vein and
artery

Collateral
branches
of posterior
intercostal
vein, artery
and nerve

D

FIG. 1.5B–D. Intercostal Muscles. **B.** Deep Dissection, Anterior View. **C.** Anterior Thoracic Wall, Posterior View.
D. Deep Dissection, Anterior View.

III. Intercostal Nerves (11 Pairs) (Fig. 1.5E,F)

A. Anterior rami of T2–T11 and the intercostal part of T1 anterior ramus

B. Branches: muscular, lateral cutaneous and anterior cutaneous

IV. Clinical Considerations

A. **Thoracentesis** or **paracentesis**

   1. Because main intercostal vessels and nerves lie along or below lower borders of ribs, needle should be passed through thoracic wall close to upper border of lower rib in intercostal space

   2. Collateral branches there are relatively small

B. **Intercostal nerve block**

   1. Intended to anesthetize intercostal nerves prior to performing minor surgery on some part of thoracic wall (i.e., relief of pain in rib fracture or sewing up laceration)

   2. Note: several intercostal nerves must be blocked to accomplish true anesthesia in a single segment because of presence of collateral branches

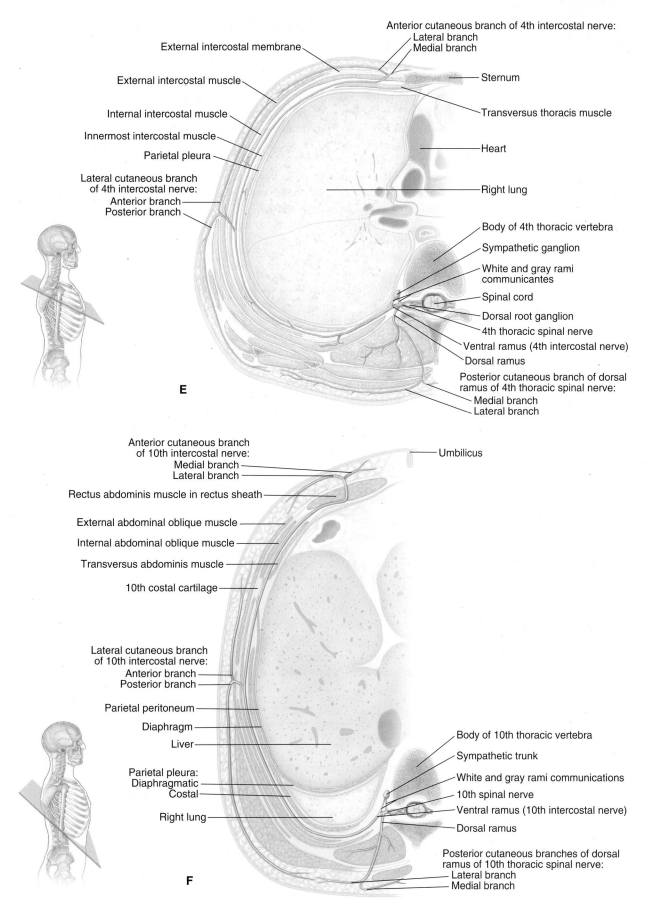

External intercostal membrane

Anterior cutaneous branch of 4th intercostal nerve:
Lateral branch
Medial branch

External intercostal muscle

Sternum

Internal intercostal muscle

Transversus thoracis muscle

Innermost intercostal muscle

Heart

Parietal pleura

Lateral cutaneous branch
of 4th intercostal nerve:
Anterior branch
Posterior branch

Right lung

Body of 4th thoracic vertebra

Sympathetic ganglion

White and gray rami
communicantes

Spinal cord

Dorsal root ganglion

4th thoracic spinal nerve

Ventral ramus (4th intercostal nerve)

Dorsal ramus

Posterior cutaneous branch of dorsal
ramus of 4th thoracic spinal nerve:
Medial branch
Lateral branch

E

Anterior cutaneous branch
of 10th intercostal nerve:
Medial branch
Lateral branch

Umbilicus

Rectus abdominis muscle in rectus sheath

External abdominal oblique muscle

Internal abdominal oblique muscle

Transversus abdominis muscle

10th costal cartilage

Lateral cutaneous branch
of 10th intercostal nerve:
Anterior branch
Posterior branch

Parietal peritoneum

Diaphragm

Liver

Parietal pleura:
Diaphragmatic
Costal

Right lung

Body of 10th thoracic vertebra

Sympathetic trunk

White and gray rami communications

10th spinal nerve

Ventral ramus (10th intercostal nerve)

Dorsal ramus

Posterior cutaneous branches of dorsal
ramus of 10th thoracic spinal nerve:
Lateral branch
Medial branch

F

FIG. 1.5E,F. Intercostal Nerves. **E.** T4, Sectional View. **F.** T10, Sectional View.

Movements of the Chest Wall in Respiration

I. Movements of Respiration

A. Anterior ends and bodies of ribs lie at more inferior level than posterior ends
B. Curve of each successive rib is greater than that of one above
   1. When ribs are pulled upward, diameters of thorax increase
   2. Results in increased volume and decreased pressure in thorax
C. Ribs 1 and 2 are less mobile than others and act as unit with manubrium
   1. When elevated, entire unit is raised, thus increasing diameter in superior portion
   2. Raising and fixing of ribs 1 and 2 make possible greater elevation of ribs below this level (important feature in forced inspiration)
D. Frequency of movement of joints of thorax is more often than any other joint combinations
E. Range of movement of any single thoracic joint is small, but any disorder that reduces joint mobility interferes with respiration
F. 2nd to 6th ribs: each moves around 2 axes
   1. At costovertebral joint in side-to-side axis, resulting in raising and lowering ribs' sternal ends, increases the anteroposterior diameter of thorax (elevates and moves sternum forward in a **pump-handle movement** (Fig. 1.6A)
   2. At same joint in front-to-back axis, resulting in depression or elevation of body of rib, increases transverse diameter of thorax (**bucket-handle movement**) (Fig. 1.6B)
G. 7th to 10th ribs
   1. Movements occur about similar axes
   2. Because their cartilages turn up, an elevation of anterior ends tends to be associated with anterior movement of sternum (pump-handle movement)

II. Action of Muscles in Respiration

A. Quiet respiration

Raise Ribs	Lower Ribs
External intercostal muscles (ribs 3–10)	No muscle, passive

B. Deep respiration

Raise Ribs	Lower Ribs
External intercostal muscles, scalenes, sternocleidomastoid, levator costarum, serratus posterior superior muscles	No muscle, passive

C. Forced respiration

Raise Ribs	Lower Ribs
All muscles listed above for deep respiration; levator scapulae, trapezius, and rhomboids raise and fix scapula so pectoral muscles and serratus anterior muscles can raise ribs	Quadratus lumborum, internal intercostals, subcostals, transversus thoracis, serratus posterior inferior, and rectus abdominis muscles

III. Thoracic Volume

A. Movement of only a few mm of bony cage forward, upward, or laterally can increase volume of cage by almost .5 L (volume of air entering or leaving lungs in quiet respiration)
B. Descent of diaphragm, which increases height of thoracic cavity, is other major factor in increasing thoracic volume

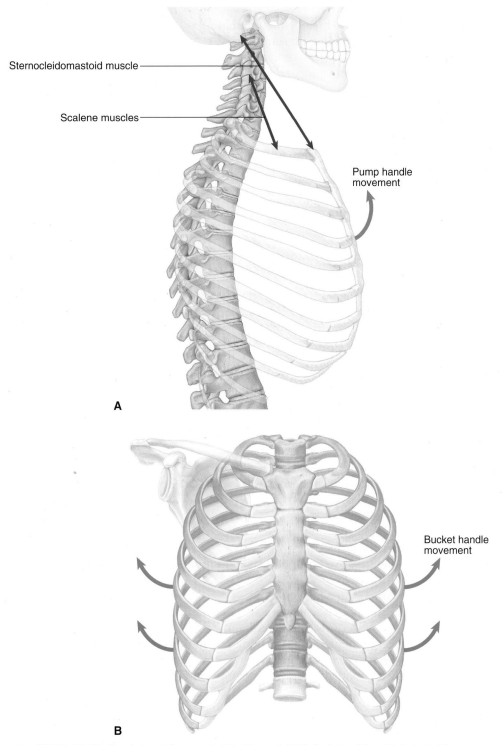

Sternocleidomastoid muscle

Scalene muscles

Pump handle movement

Bucket handle movement

A

B

FIG. 1.6A,B. Respiratory Movement of the Thoracic Wall. **A.** Lateral View. **B.** Anterior View.

Subdivisions of the Thoracic Cavity

I. Basic Subdivisions (Fig. 1.7A)

A. Pleural cavities (2)
  1. Surround but do not contain lungs
  2. Contain thin film of serous fluid
  3. Act as bursae to reduce friction of lung movements
  4. Lined by parietal pleura, a serous membrane
B. Lungs (2)
  1. Suspended from mediastinum by roots of lungs
  2. Surrounded by pleural cavities
  3. Covered by visceral pleura
C. Mediastinum ("middle standing")
  1. Represents thick middle partition in thorax
  2. Boundaries
    a. Laterally by pleurae and lungs
    b. Anteriorly by sternum
    c. Posteriorly by vertebral column

II. Mediastinum Subdivisions (Fig. 1.7B,C)

A. Superior mediastinum
  1. Boundaries
    a. Above by plane of 1st rib
    b. Below by horizontal line at level of sternal angle, which passes through intervertebral disc between 4th and 5th thoracic vertebrae
    c. Anteriorly by manubrium and origins of sternohyoid and sternothyroid muscles
    d. Laterally by pleura and upper lobes of lungs
    e. Posteriorly by vertebral bodies T1–T4
  2. Major contents (in anteroposterior order)
    a. Thymus gland or its fatty remnant in adult
    b. Brachiocephalic veins uniting to form superior vena cava, which receives azygos arch posteriorly
    c. Phrenic and vagus nerves
    d. Aortic arch and its branches: brachiocephalic trunk, left common carotid, left subclavian arteries
    e. Trachea
    f. Esophagus and thoracic duct
B. Inferior mediastinum
  1. Bounded above by superior mediastinum, below by diaphragm
  2. Further subdivided
    a. Anterior mediastinum
      i. Bounded anteriorly by body of sternum and transversus thoracis muscle, posteriorly by pericardium
      ii. Contents: lower portion of thymus, sternopericardial ligaments
    b. Middle mediastinum
      i. Bounded anteriorly and posteriorly by fibrous pericardium, laterally by hilum of each lung
      ii. Contents: phrenic nerves and pericardiacophrenic vessels, pericardial cavity and heart, great vessels (ascending aorta, pulmonary trunk, inferior end of superior vena cava, superior end of inferior vena cava), and roots of lungs (pulmonary arteries and veins, left and right primary bronchus)
    c. Posterior mediastinum
      i. Bounded anteriorly by pericardium, posteriorly by anterior longitudinal ligament on vertebral bodies T5–T12
      ii. Contents: esophagus and esophageal plexus, descending thoracic aorta and origins of its branches (posterior intercostals, bronchials, esophageals, superior phrenics), termination of azygos venous system, thoracic duct, thoracic splanchnic nerves

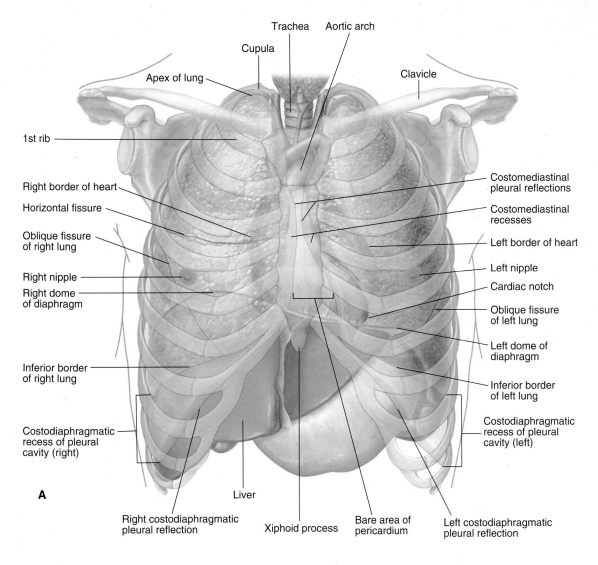

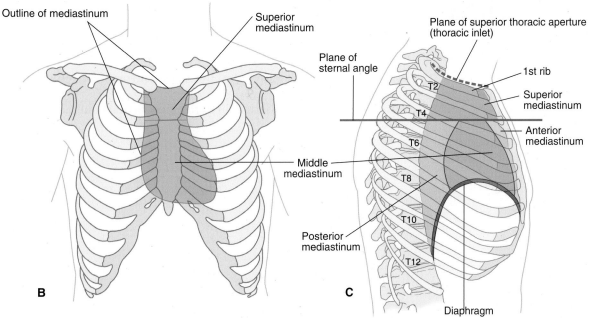

FIG. I.7A–C. **A.** Pleural Cavities, Lungs, and Mediastinum, Anterior View. **B.** Mediastinum, Anterior View. **C.** Lateral View.

Anterior Mediastinum and the Thymus Gland

I. Contents (Fig. 1.8)

A. Superior and inferior sternopericardial ligaments: fibrous bands connecting upper and lower body of sternum and xiphoid to anterior surface of pericardial sac
B. Lower portion of thymus gland
C. Small lymph nodes

II. Thymus Gland

A. Lymphoid organ
   1. Important in development and maintenance of immune system
   2. Active in T-cell production during infancy and childhood
   3. Undergoes gradual involution in adulthood, becoming replaced by fat
B. Childhood thymus
   1. Soft, flat, pinkish gray with 2 vertically ovoid lobes
   2. At birth, measures about 5 cm in length, 4 cm in width, and 0.5 cm in thickness
C. Location: primarily within anterior portion of superior mediastinum, although may extend from inferior border of thyroid to 4th costal cartilage posterior to sternum
   1. In neck: lies anterior to trachea and deep to sternohyoid and sternothyroid muscles
   2. In thorax: occupies anterior part of superior mediastinum and upper anterior mediastinum
      a. Anteriorly: manubrium of sternum
      b. Posteriorly: great vessels and upper part of fibrous pericardium
D. Arteries: from anterior mediastinal branches of internal thoracic arteries and possibly from inferior thyroid arteries
E. Veins: drain into left brachiocephalic vein and, possibly, internal thoracic and inferior thyroid veins
F. Lymphatic drainage: lymphatic vessels pass to parasternal, tracheobronchial, and anterior mediastinal lymph nodes
G. Innervation: very small; derived from both sympathetic and vagal branches

III. Clinical Considerations

A. Sternotomy
   1. Heart often accessed through midsagittal cut through sternum
   2. No other major structures or major vessels are in jeopardy, and heart sac is easy to access
B. Bone marrow harvest
   1. Although iliac crest is preferred site, bone marrow of sternum is sometimes harvested
   2. Large-gauge needle inserted through outer cortical bone, and marrow cells are aspirated

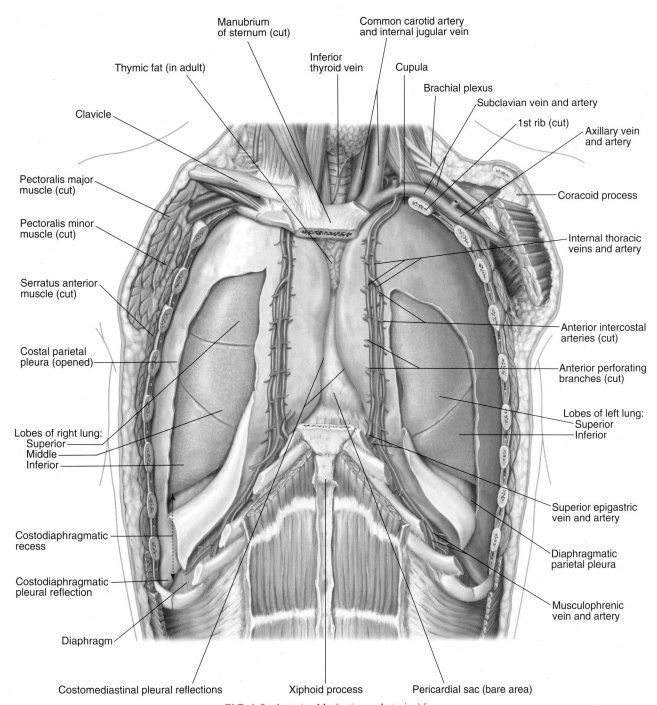

FIG. 1.8. Anterior Mediastinum, Anterior View.

Middle Mediastinum: Pericardial Sac and Heart

I. Surface Projections of the Heart (Fig. 1.9A,B)

A. Apex: in left 5th intercostal space, approximately 8 cm from midsternal line
B. Base: slightly oblique line at level of 3rd costal cartilage projecting 2 cm to left and 1 cm to right of lateral border of sternum
C. Inferior (diaphragmatic) border: slopes from level of 6th sternocostal junction on right, across xiphisternal junction to apex
D. Right border: begins at right end of base, curves slightly to right, reaching 2.5 cm from sternal margin in 4th intercostal space, ends at right end of inferior border
E. Left border: curves upward and medialward from apex to left end of base line

II. Pericardium (Fig. 1.9C)

A. Fibrous pericardium: tough, fibrous sac, closed above by attachments to great vessels
  1. Attached to sternum by superior and inferior sternopericardial ligaments
  2. Attached to central tendon of diaphragm
  3. Covered by mediastinal parietal pleura on either side
  4. Phrenic nerve and pericardiacophrenic vessels
    a. Run within 2 layers of fibrous pericardium (although appear to lie on pericardium)
    b. Pericardiacophrenic artery, from internal thoracic, supplies pericardium and small portion of central diaphragm
B. Serous pericardium: smooth membrane with mesothelial layer that lines fibrous sac and also covers surface of heart
  1. Parietal pericardium lines inner surface of fibrous pericardium, reflects onto great vessels of the heart to become visceral pericardium
  2. Visceral pericardium (epicardium) covers entire surface of heart and extends along its great vessels for 3 cm, where it is reflected onto inner surface of fibrous pericardium to become parietal pericardium

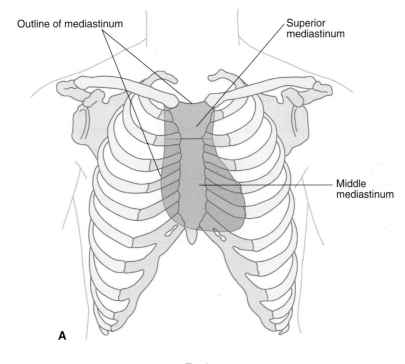

Outline of mediastinum

Superior mediastinum

Middle mediastinum

A

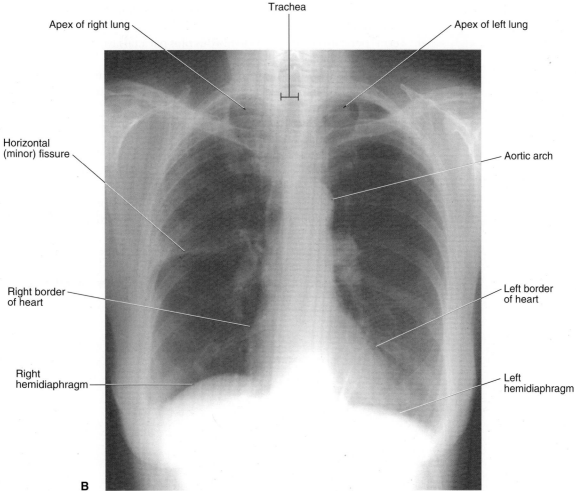

Trachea

Apex of right lung

Apex of left lung

Horizontal (minor) fissure

Aortic arch

Right border of heart

Left border of heart

Right hemidiaphragm

Left hemidiaphragm

B

FIG. 1.9A,B. A. Surface Projection of Middle Mediastinum, Anterior View. **B.** Radiograph of Thorax, PA View.

III. Pericardial Cavity (Fig. 1.9D)

A. Potential space between parietal and visceral pericardium

B. Acts as bursa to reduce friction of heart movements; pericardial surfaces are in contact, covered with watery fluid to allow for freedom of heart movement during contractions

C. Mesocardia: reflections of visceral pericardium along great vessels and onto fibrous pericardium, forming sinuses

    1. **Oblique pericardial sinus**: inverted U-shaped sinus framed by pulmonary veins and inferior vena cava

    2. **Transverse pericardial sinus**: behind ascending aorta and pulmonary trunk and anterior to superior vena cava

IV. Clinical Considerations

A. **Pericardial effusion**, or **hemopericardium**

    1. In injury or disease, fluid or blood may accumulate in pericardial cavity, which may compress veins entering heart and atria, inhibiting filling of heart (**cardiac tamponade**)

    2. Most commonly, fluid is withdrawn (**pericardiocentesis**) by abdominal approach, passing needle upward and to left between xiphoid process and left costal margin, directed toward nipple

        a. Anterior thoracic approach may also be used, passing needle just above 6th costal cartilage in 5th intercostal space, 1 fingerbreadth from left side of sternum

        b. Posterior thoracic approach: needle inserted over 8th rib, midway between inferior angle of scapula and midline, directed toward middle of chest

B. Term "pericardial sac" refers to fibrous plus parietal layer of serous pericardium surrounding heart

C. In severe pericarditis, pericardium becomes greatly thickened and adherent to heart (constrictive pericarditis), and pericardial friction rub is physical sign of acute pericarditis

D. **Bare area of pericardium**: due to cardiac notch in left lung, part of fibrous pericardium is uncovered by lung tissue

    1. This area of left chest is area of superficial cardiac dullness (with percussion)

    2. Also area of pericardial sac through which pericardiocentesis is normally performed

E. Percussion of heart: relays size and density of heart by creating vibration by tapping chest with finger and listening and feeling differences in conducted sound wave

    1. Usually tapped at 3rd, 4th, and 5th intercostal spaces from left anterior axillary line to right anterior axillary line

    2. Percussion sound goes from resonance to dullness, over heart, at about 6 cm to left border of sternum

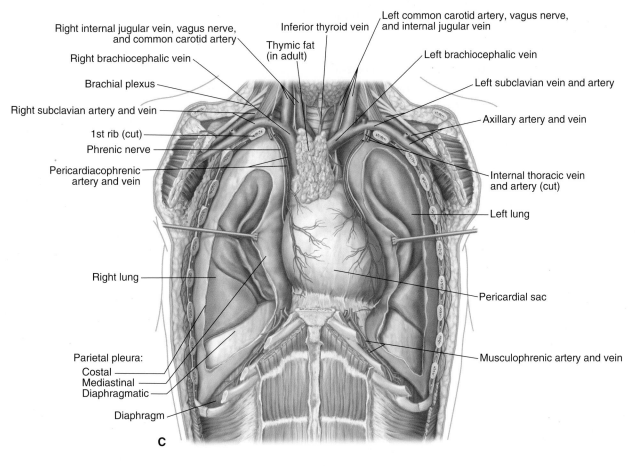

Right internal jugular vein, vagus nerve, and common carotid artery

Right brachiocephalic vein

Brachial plexus

Right subclavian artery and vein

1st rib (cut)

Phrenic nerve

Pericardiacophrenic artery and vein

Right lung

Parietal pleura:
Costal
Mediastinal
Diaphragmatic

Diaphragm

Inferior thyroid vein

Thymic fat (in adult)

Left common carotid artery, vagus nerve, and internal jugular vein

Left brachiocephalic vein

Left subclavian vein and artery

Axillary artery and vein

Internal thoracic vein and artery (cut)

Left lung

Pericardial sac

Musculophrenic artery and vein

C

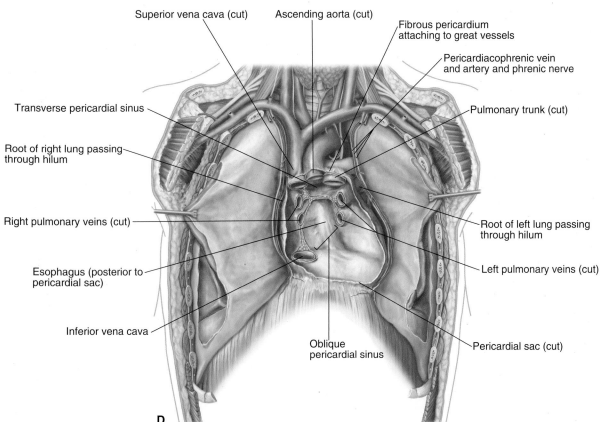

Superior vena cava (cut)

Ascending aorta (cut)

Fibrous pericardium attaching to great vessels

Pericardiacophrenic vein and artery and phrenic nerve

Transverse pericardial sinus

Root of right lung passing through hilum

Right pulmonary veins (cut)

Esophagus (posterior to pericardial sac)

Inferior vena cava

Pulmonary trunk (cut)

Root of left lung passing through hilum

Left pulmonary veins (cut)

Pericardial sac (cut)

Oblique pericardial sinus

D

FIG. I.9C,D. C. Pericardial Sac, Anterior View. **D.** Pericardial Sinuses, Anterior View.

Heart and its Blood Supply

I. Superficial Features of Heart (Fig. 1.10A–C)

A. Four chambers: right and left atria, right and left ventricles

B. Coronary sulcus: groove separating atria from ventricles

C. Anterior and posterior interventricular sulci: divide ventricles into right and left

D. Apex: points down and to left, located in left 5th intercostal space

E. Base: faces upward and backward toward right

F. Surfaces
   1. Anterior (sternocostal): beneath sternum and ribs, primarily right ventricle
   2. Diaphragmatic: against diaphragm, both ventricles

G. Margins
   1. Acute: sharp border where anterior surface meets diaphragmatic surface
   2. Obtuse (left): gently rounded border along left margin of left ventricle from apex to base

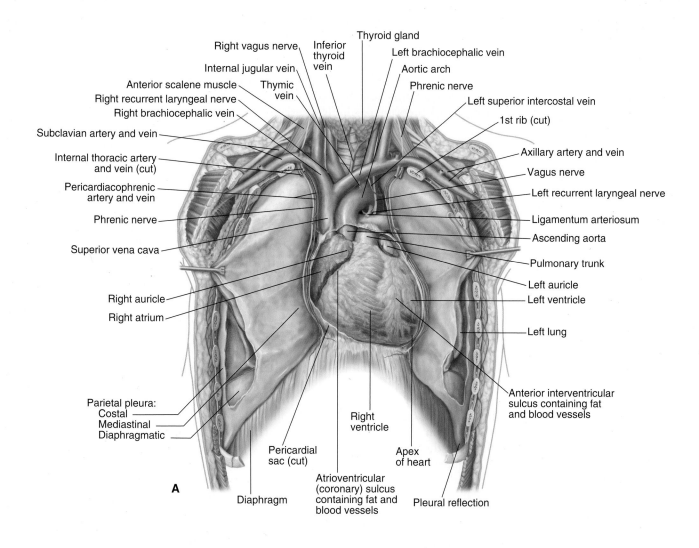

Thyroid gland
Right vagus nerve
Inferior thyroid vein
Left brachiocephalic vein
Internal jugular vein
Aortic arch
Anterior scalene muscle
Thymic vein
Phrenic nerve
Right recurrent laryngeal nerve
Left superior intercostal vein
Right brachiocephalic vein
1st rib (cut)
Subclavian artery and vein
Axillary artery and vein
Internal thoracic artery and vein (cut)
Vagus nerve
Left recurrent laryngeal nerve
Pericardiacophrenic artery and vein
Ligamentum arteriosum
Phrenic nerve
Ascending aorta
Superior vena cava
Pulmonary trunk
Left auricle
Right auricle
Left ventricle
Right atrium
Left lung
Parietal pleura:
Costal
Mediastinal
Diaphragmatic
Anterior interventricular sulcus containing fat and blood vessels
Right ventricle
Diaphragm
Pericardial sac (cut)
Apex of heart
Atrioventricular (coronary) sulcus containing fat and blood vessels
Pleural reflection

A

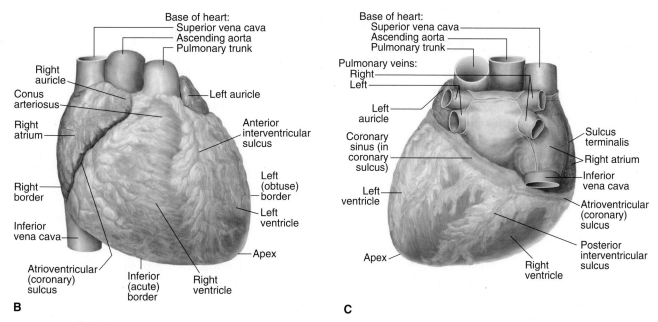

Base of heart:
Superior vena cava
Ascending aorta
Pulmonary trunk
Right auricle
Conus arteriosus
Left auricle
Right atrium
Anterior interventricular sulcus
Right border
Left (obtuse) border
Left ventricle
Inferior vena cava
Apex
Atrioventricular (coronary) sulcus
Inferior (acute) border
Right ventricle

B

Base of heart:
Superior vena cava
Ascending aorta
Pulmonary trunk
Pulmonary veins:
Right
Left
Left auricle
Sulcus terminalis
Coronary sinus (in coronary sulcus)
Right atrium
Inferior vena cava
Left ventricle
Atrioventricular (coronary) sulcus
Apex
Posterior interventricular sulcus
Right ventricle

C

FIG. 1.10A–C. A. Heart within the Pericardial Sac, Anterior View. **B.** Heart, Anterior View. **C.** Posterior View.

II. Coronary Arteries (Fig. 1.10D–G)

A. Introduction
1. Right and left coronary arteries supply heart and arise from right and left aortic sinuses, respectively
2. Supplied by autonomic and sensory fibers of cardiac plexus
3. No sharp demarcation line between distribution of arteries, and predominance of either right or left coronary supply is variable

B. Right coronary artery
1. Arises from right aortic sinus, superior to right cusp of aortic semilunar valve
2. Emerges between pulmonary trunk and right auricle, running in coronary sulcus to posterior of heart where it anastomoses with circumflex branch of left coronary
   a. Numerous branches to right atrium and right ventricle, with 1st branch supplying conus arteriosus
   b. Usually (55%), 1st part of right coronary gives off **sinuatrial (SA) nodal branch**, which runs upward and posteriorly to supply right atrium and circles superior vena cava to supply SA node within crista terminalis
   c. Right marginal branch: descends along acute margin of right ventricle toward apex
   d. Posterior interventricular branch: courses in posterior interventricular groove toward apex; supplies adjacent parts of both ventricles and sends septal branches 1/3 way into interventricular septum
   e. Atrioventricular (AV) nodal branch: passes into interatrial septum to supply AV node
   f. Anastomoses with circumflex branch of left coronary artery within coronary sulcus posteriorly

C. Left coronary artery
1. Arises from left aortic sinus behind pulmonary trunk
2. Courses between pulmonary trunk and left auricle to divide into anterior interventricular (left anterior descending, or LAD) branch and circumflex branch
3. Anterior interventricular branch
   a. Descends in anterior interventricular groove to apex of heart, turns around apex, and travels variable distance in posterior interventricular groove where it meets posterior interventricular artery
   b. Supplies both ventricles and is major blood supply to interventricular septum (its septal branches penetrate 2/3 distance of interventricular septum)
4. Circumflex branch
   a. Supplies adjacent parts of left ventricle (left marginal branch is relatively constant) and left atrium
   b. In 45% of people, SA nodal branch arises from beginning of circumflex branch, travels along upper border of left atrium and circles posteriorly around superior vena cava to reach SA node (Fig. 1.10H)
   c. In 15% of people, circumflex branch supplies posterior interventricular branch, which is termed **left heart dominance** because entire interventricular septum is supplied by branches of left coronary (Fig. 1.10I)

III. Cardiac Veins (Fig. 1.10J–M)

A. Coronary sinus: large vessel in posterior coronary sulcus; receives most veins of heart and ends in right atrium
1. Great cardiac vein: starts at apex, ascends in anterior interventricular sulcus, and meets oblique vein of left atrium to form coronary sinus
2. Posterior vein of left ventricle: on diaphragmatic surface, drains to sinus
3. Middle cardiac vein: ascends in posterior interventricular sulcus to coronary sinus
4. Small cardiac vein: on right side of coronary sulcus
   a. Begins as right marginal vein along acute margin
   b. Opens into end of sinus
5. Venae cordis minimae (smallest cardiac, or thebesian, veins): drain directly into heart chambers

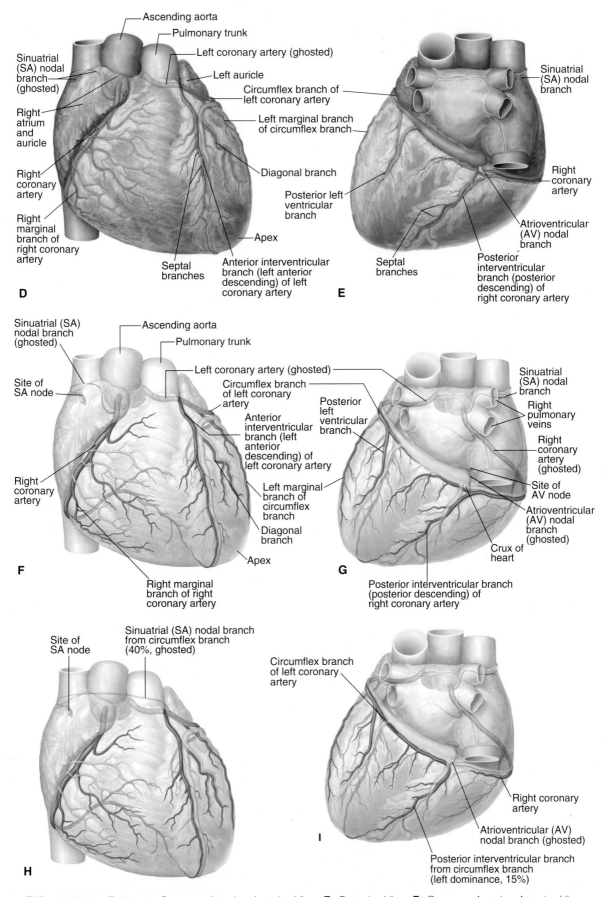

FIG. 1.10D–I. **D.** Heart, Coronary Arteries, Anterior View. **E.** Posterior View. **F.** Coronary Arteries, Anterior View. **G.** Posterior View. Coronary Arteries, Variation. **H.** Anterior View. **I.** Posterior View.

IV. Clinical Considerations

A. Numerous small arterial and precapillary anastomoses in most heart areas are inadequate to provide good collateral circulation if coronaries or major branches are occluded, but can enlarge if an occlusion develops slowly

B. Most common cause of ischemic heart disease is coronary insufficiency due to atherosclerosis leading to stenosis (narrowing)

C. Obstruction of coronary artery can lead to anoxia of heart area supplied, resulting in spasmodic contractions (heart attack), and eventually in death

D. Angina pectoris
   1. When coronary arteries narrow (atherosclerosis), blood supply to myocardium, sufficient at rest, may be inadequate when workload on heart increases; accumulation of metabolites in the hypoxic muscle activates afferent nerves that travel via sympathetic nerves to CNS and cause precordial pain relieved by rest
   2. Recurrent episodes of angina at rest, without changes in heart rate, blood pressure, or ventricular contractility, are due to constriction of coronary artery (vasospasm)

E. Myocardial infarction (MI): sudden occlusion of major artery by embolus results in infarction (bloodless area) of area supplied by artery and may lead to necrosis

F. Echocardiology (ultrasonic cardiography)
   1. Records position and motion of heart via beam of ultrasonic waves directed through thorax
   2. **Doppler echocardiography** records flow of blood through great vessels by Doppler ultrasonography

G. Coronary angioplasty
   1. Percutaneous, transluminal coronary angioplasty is surgical procedure (used selectively) in which coronary artery or branch is dilated by inserting catheter with small inflatable balloon attached to its tip through skin and lumen of vessel to site of narrowing
   2. When inflated, balloon flattens obstructing atherosclerotic plaque against vessel wall, and vessel is stretched to increase size of lumen
   3. In some cases, **thrombokinase** is injected via catheter to help dissolve blood clot
   4. **Stenting**: procedure used to treat restricted or blocked flow in blood vessels, bile ducts, or other tubular structures
      a. Structures can be held open to allow enhanced flow of blood, air, urine, or bile, foregoing more complicated invasive procedures to alleviate condition
      b. Stents may be simple base-metal, drug-eluted (drug-coated stent to limit scar tissue growth and avoid complications), or occasionally covered
      c. Most often used by vascular specialists when treating patients with carotid artery, peripheral artery, or coronary artery disease
      d. Commonly used in patients to hold arteries open, most often following angioplasty
         i. Specialist uses deflated balloon under stent to guide stent in place, where it is expanded to hold vessel open
         ii. Balloon is then deflated and removed with stent being held in place by blood vessel walls which grow around it

H. Coronary artery bypass graft (CABG) surgery
   1. Often undertaken in patients with severe angina or coronary artery obstruction
   2. Segment of artery or vein is connected to ascending aorta and distal to stenosis of coronary artery, bypassing obstruction
   3. Frequently used grafts are great saphenous vein (venous valves can be negated by reversing direction of implant), left internal thoracic artery, or radial artery

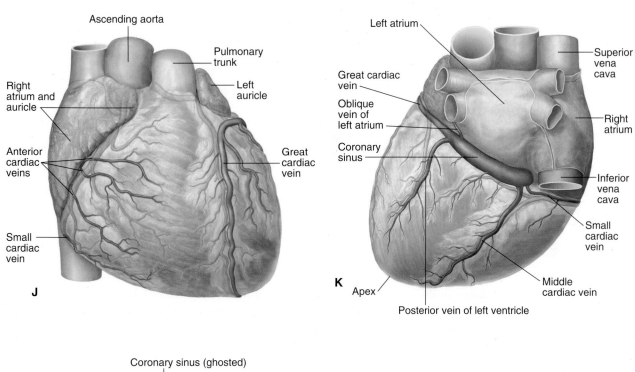

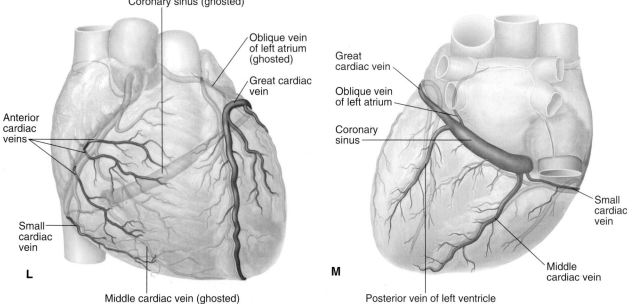

FIG. 1.10J–M. **J.** Heart, Cardiac Veins, Anterior View. **K.** Posterior View. **L.** Cardiac Veins, Anterior View. **M.** Posterior View.

Interior of the Heart

I. Right Atrium (Fig. 1.11A–D)

A. Auricle
1. Fleshy appendage lined by parallel ridges called **pectinate muscles**, which emanate from ridge, the crista terminalis
2. **Crista terminalis**
   a. Marked externally by **sulcus terminalis** between venae cavae
   b. Separates auricle anteriorly from sinus venarum posteriorly
   c. SA node lies within uppermost part of crista terminalis
B. Sinus venarum
1. Smooth walled, lying between venae cavae
2. Openings
   a. Superior vena cava: from above
   b. Inferior vena cava: from below; marked by valve of inferior vena cava, a crescent-shaped fold along anterior and left margin of cava (not functional valve, but embryological remnant)
   c. Coronary sinus: opens medial to orifice of inferior vena cava; marked by valve of coronary sinus
   d. Right AV orifice: oval-shaped opening into right ventricle; guarded by right AV (tricuspid) valve
C. Interatrial septum
1. Posteromedial wall of atrium
2. **Fossa ovalis**: oval depression, where septum is thin; marks location of fetal foramen ovale, which shunts blood from inferior vena cava into left atrium
3. Limbus of fossa ovalis: thick upper margin of fossa; directs inferior vena cava blood through foramen ovale in fetus
4. AV node: lies within interatrial septum superoposterior to septal cusp of tricuspid valve

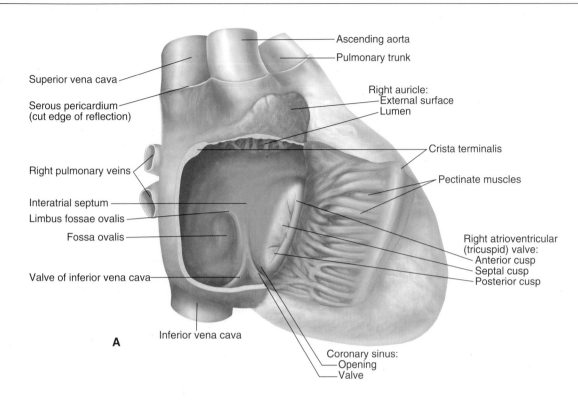

A. Ascending aorta
Pulmonary trunk
Superior vena cava
Serous pericardium
(cut edge of reflection)
Right auricle:
External surface
Lumen
Crista terminalis
Pectinate muscles
Right pulmonary veins
Interatrial septum
Limbus fossae ovalis
Fossa ovalis
Right atrioventricular
(tricuspid) valve:
Anterior cusp
Septal cusp
Posterior cusp
Valve of inferior vena cava
Inferior vena cava
Coronary sinus:
Opening
Valve

A

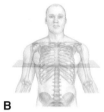

B

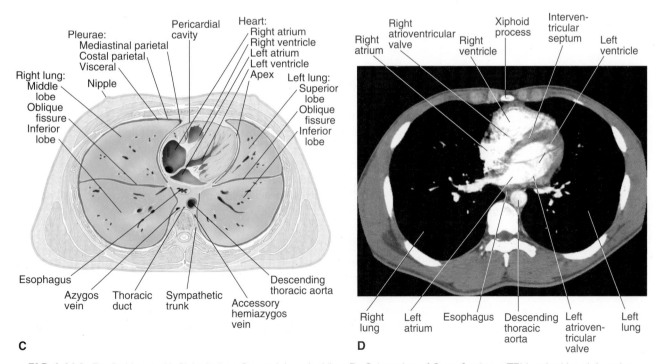

Pleurae:
Mediastinal parietal
Costal parietal
Visceral
Pericardial cavity
Heart:
Right atrium
Right ventricle
Left atrium
Left ventricle
Apex
Right lung:
Middle lobe
Oblique fissure
Inferior lobe
Nipple
Left lung:
Superior lobe
Oblique fissure
Inferior lobe
Esophagus
Azygos vein
Thoracic duct
Sympathetic trunk
Accessory hemiazygos vein
Descending thoracic aorta

C

Right atrium
Right atrioventricular valve
Right ventricle
Xiphoid process
Interventricular septum
Left ventricle
Right lung
Left atrium
Esophagus
Descending thoracic aorta
Left atrioventricular valve
Left lung

D

FIG. 1.11A–D. A. Heart with Right Atrium Opened, Anterior View. **B.** Orientation of Cross Section at T7 Vertebral Level, Anterior View. **C.** Cross Section of Thorax at T7 Vertebral Level. **D.** CT Image of Thorax at T7 Vertebral Level.

II. Right Ventricle (Fig. 1.11E)

A. Occupies most of anterior (sternocostal) surface from coronary to anterior interventricular sulcus; forms acute margin of heart and part of diaphragmatic surface

B. AV (tricuspid) valve

   1. Prevents backflow of blood into right atrium

   2. Anterior, posterior, and septal leaflets or cusps

C. Supraventricular crest: muscular ridge that separates ventricle into 2 parts

   1. Conus arteriosus (infundibulum): smooth superior part leading into pulmonary trunk (outflow tract); pulmonary semilunar valve prevents backflow

   2. Ventricle proper

     a. Trabeculae carneae: irregular bundles of muscle projecting on inner surface; **septomarginal trabecula** (moderator band), is enlarged bundle that connects interventricular septum with anterior papillary muscle

     b. Papillary muscles (3): conical projections into cavity, connected to inner margins of AV valve cusps by small tendinous strands called **chordae tendineae**

       i. Anterior: largest; partly from anterior and diaphragmatic walls

       ii. Posterior: from several attachments on diaphragmatic wall

       iii. Septal (frequently absent): from interventricular septum near septal end of supraventricular crest

     c. Interventricular septum: set obliquely; right convex side encroaches on right ventricle

       i. Muscular part: thickest part of septum; represents nearly 4/5 of anteroinferior portion of septum

       ii. Membranous part: thin upper part near atrium

III. Left Atrium (Fig. 1.11F)

A. Primarily smooth-walled portion with small muscular auricle

B. Pulmonary veins (4): right and left, superior and inferior; open into smooth-walled portion

C. Left AV orifice

   1. Leads to left ventricle

   2. Guarded by left AV (mitral, bicuspid) valve

IV. Left Ventricle (Fig. 1.11G)

A. Small part of anterior (sternocostal) surface, all of left (obtuse) border, and much of diaphragmatic surface

B. Left AV (mitral, bicuspid) valve

   1. Prevents backflow into left atrium

   2. Anterior and posterior leaflets, or cusps

C. Thicker walls and more dense trabeculae carneae than right ventricle

D. Papillary muscles (2)

   1. Anterior: attached to anterior wall

   2. Posterior: attached to diaphragmatic wall

E. Aortic vestibule: smooth-walled outflow tract leading to ascending aorta, guarded by semilunar valve

V. Clinical Considerations

A. Atrial septal defects: usually congenital anomalies due to failure of foramen ovale to close completely

B. Ventricular septal defects

   1. Membranous part is common site of defects that vary from 1–2.5 cm

   2. Result in left-to-right shunting of blood flow through deficit, increasing pulmonary blood flow and resulting in pulmonary hypertension

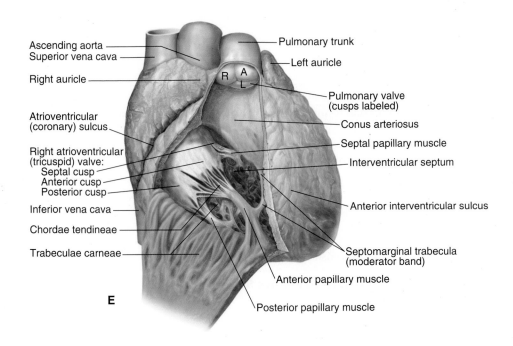

Ascending aorta
Superior vena cava
Right auricle
Atrioventricular (coronary) sulcus
Right atrioventricular (tricuspid) valve:
  Septal cusp
  Anterior cusp
  Posterior cusp
Inferior vena cava
Chordae tendineae
Trabeculae carneae

Pulmonary trunk
Left auricle
R A L
Pulmonary valve (cusps labeled)
Conus arteriosus
Septal papillary muscle
Interventricular septum
Anterior interventricular sulcus
Septomarginal trabecula (moderator band)
Anterior papillary muscle
Posterior papillary muscle

E

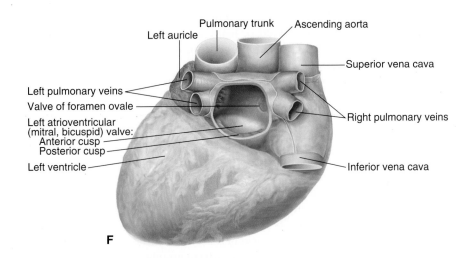

Left auricle
Pulmonary trunk
Ascending aorta
Superior vena cava
Left pulmonary veins
Valve of foramen ovale
Left atrioventricular (mitral, bicuspid) valve:
  Anterior cusp
  Posterior cusp
Left ventricle
Right pulmonary veins
Inferior vena cava

F

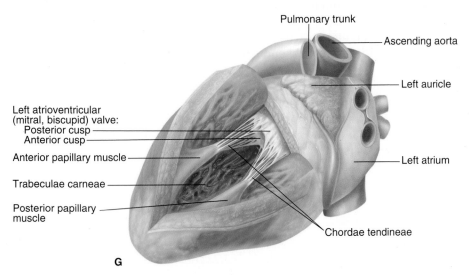

Pulmonary trunk
Ascending aorta
Left auricle
Left atrioventricular (mitral, biscuspid) valve:
  Posterior cusp
  Anterior cusp
Anterior papillary muscle
Trabeculae carneae
Posterior papillary muscle
Left atrium
Chordae tendineae

G

FIG. 1.11E–G. **E.** Heart with Right Ventricle Opened, Anterior View. **F.** Heart with Left Atrium Opened, Posterior View. **G.** Heart with Left Ventricle Opened, Lateral View.

Valves of the Heart

I. Surface Projections of Valves (Fig. 1.12A)

A. Pulmonary: left sternal border at 3rd sternocostal joint
B. Aortic: slightly below and medial to pulmonary, near left sternal border at 3rd intercostal space
C. Left AV (mitral, bicuspid): just to left of midline, opposite 4th sternocostal joint
D. Right AV (tricuspid): midsternal opposite 4th intercostal space

II. Auscultation of Valves

A. Pulmonary: left 2nd intercostal space lateral to sternal border
B. Aortic: right 2nd intercostal space lateral to sternal border
C. Left AV (mitral, bicuspid): left 5th intercostal space, 8 cm from midline
D. Right AV (tricuspid): left 4th intercostal space lateral to sternum

III. Structure: All Valve Leaflets Attach to Fibrous Skeleton of Heart (Anulus Fibrosus) (Fig. 1.12B)

A. AV
  1. Right (tricuspid): 3 fibrous cusps, thick near attached border, thin near free edges
    a. Anterior cusp: largest, attached to anterior wall near interventricular septum; receives chordae tendineae from anterior and septal papillary muscles
    b. Posterior cusp: from curved ventricular wall where anterior and diaphragmatic surfaces become continuous; receives chordae from both anterior and posterior papillary muscles
    c. Septal cusp: from interventricular septal wall; receives chordae from posterior and septal papillary muscles
  2. Left (bicuspid, mitral): 2 cusps
    a. Anterior: attached toward aortic vestibule; receives chordae from both papillary muscles
    b. Posterior: attached to posterolateral wall; receives chordae from both papillary muscles
B. Semilunar
  1. Each composed of 3 cusps attached along caudal convex curve
    a. Lunula: crescent-shaped, free edge of cusp
    b. Nodule: a thickened area in center of free margin of cusp
    c. Commissure: point where attachments of adjacent cusps come together
  2. Pulmonary: anterior, right, and left cusps
  3. Aortic: right, left, and posterior cusps
    a. Aortic sinuses: pockets above each cusp
    b. Coronary arteries arise from right and left aortic sinus

IV. Cardiac Skeleton

A. Fibrous tissue that surrounds AV and semilunar valves
B. Gives attachments to valve cusps and myocardium
C. Continuous with roots of aorta and pulmonary trunk as well as membranous part of interventricular septum

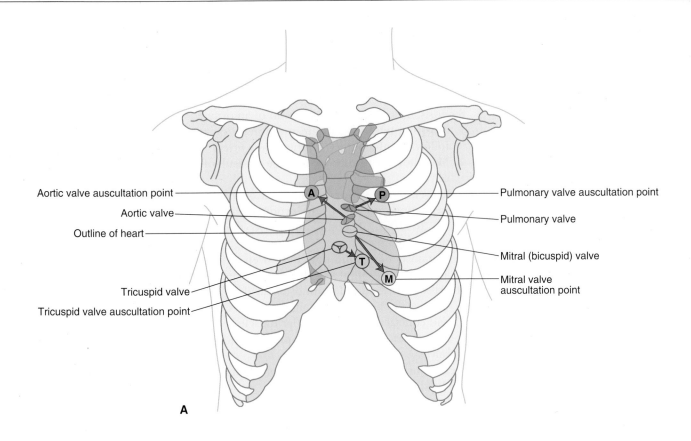

Aortic valve auscultation point

Aortic valve

Outline of heart

Tricuspid valve

Tricuspid valve auscultation point

Pulmonary valve auscultation point

Pulmonary valve

Mitral (bicuspid) valve

Mitral valve auscultation point

A

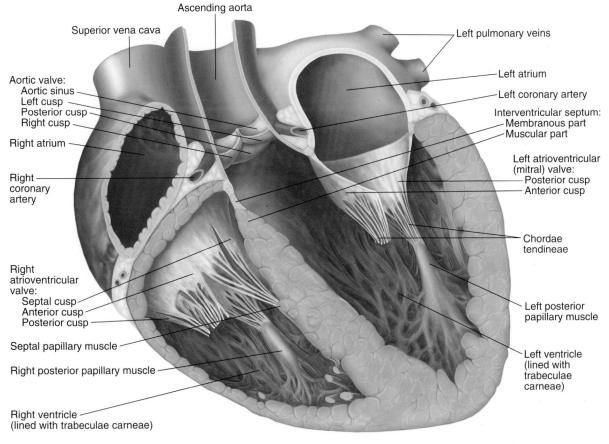

Superior vena cava

Ascending aorta

Left pulmonary veins

Aortic valve:
  Aortic sinus
  Left cusp
  Posterior cusp
  Right cusp

Right atrium

Right coronary artery

Right atrioventricular valve:
  Septal cusp
  Anterior cusp
  Posterior cusp

Septal papillary muscle

Right posterior papillary muscle

Right ventricle (lined with trabeculae carneae)

Left atrium

Left coronary artery

Interventricular septum:
  Membranous part
  Muscular part

Left atrioventricular (mitral) valve:
  Posterior cusp
  Anterior cusp

Chordae tendineae

Left posterior papillary muscle

Left ventricle (lined with trabeculae carneae)

B

FIG. 1.12A,B. A. Surface Projections of the Heart, Anterior View. **B.** Heart, Sectional View.

V. Clinical Considerations

A. Free margins (approximate when valves are closed) of valves are typically thin, but if thickened and inflexible or damaged through disease, close fit is no longer possible, enabling blood to flow back into chamber from which it has come

B. Stenosis: narrowing or constriction of an orifice

   1. Most frequently occurs in pulmonary or aortic opening due to scarring following infections (i.e., rheumatic fever)

   2. May allow for retrograde leakage as result of incompetence or insufficiency of valve

C. Prolapsed mitral valve: incompetent or insufficient valve can result in blood regurgitating into left atrium, producing murmur

   1. Up to 10% of population have this condition (with strong female predominance)

   2. Usually benign condition, but, when serious, produces shortness of breath and can develop into cardiac rhythm disturbances

D. Heart sounds: 2 audible sounds occur during each heartbeat: lubb-dupp

   1. 1st: low pitched and of long duration, caused by closure of both AV valves and contraction of ventricular muscle

   2. 2nd: short, sharp, and high pitched and is caused by closure of semilunar valves

E. Heart murmur or bruit (auscultatory sound at a valve) results from vibrations in blood due to turbulence

Conduction System of the Heart

I. Introduction

A. Cardiac muscle is inherently contractile; conduction system coordinates contractions
   1. Systole: wave of contraction begins at top of atria and proceeds toward AV orifices (systole)
   2. Diastole: contraction begins at bottom of ventricles and proceeds toward outflow tracts
B. Conduction system consists of specialized cardiac muscle fibers (nodal and Purkinje fibers); responsible for initiating and maintaining normal cardiac rhythm
C. Consists of SA and AV nodes, bundle (of His) and its two limbs (fasciculi, branches, or crura), and subendocardial plexuses of Purkinje fibers in ventricles where they terminate

II. SA Node (Fig. 1.13A)

A. Narrow, horseshoe shaped, and found in superior end of crista terminalis of right atrium
B. Bulk lies on sinus venarum side of crista terminalis and extends through atrial wall thickness from epicardium to endocardium
C. Because fusiform nodal fibers have higher rate of intrinsic rhythmic contraction than any cardiac muscle, cardiac cycle originates here
D. Called "pacemaker" of heart because normally other parts of heart contract at rate imposed on them
E. Because nodal fibers are in contact with cells of neighboring myocardial fibers, the impulse for cardiac contraction, beginning in node, is conducted throughout atria by ordinary atrial myocardial fibers, arriving eventually at AV node
   1. No Purkinje fibers in atrial walls
   2. Although previously believed that no specialized nodal pathways connected the nodes, now known that internodal cell-to-cell conduction takes place more rapidly along 3 functional interatrial pathways, or muscle fiber bundles
      a. Anterior pathway: via anterior interatrial band (Bachmann bundle), which passes directly between nodes (through interatrial septum) and synchronizes the 2 atria
      b. Middle and posterior internodal pathways: mixture of ordinary myocardial cells as well as some more specialized in conduction

III. AV Node

A. Smaller than SA node with broader, more cylindrical fibers
B. Lies above opening of coronary sinus, embedded in myocardial fibers of interatrial septum
C. Cells composing nodal fibers are contiguous with cells of atrial septal muscles and with those of AV bundle of His
D. Region of slow conductance for needed delay between atrial and ventricular contractions, allowing time for ventricles to fill

IV. AV Bundle (of His) (Fig. 1.13B)

A. Passes upward from AV node in right fibrous trigone beneath attachment of septal cusp of right AV valve to reach posterior margin of membranous interventricular septum, then turns forward below it, and divides into right and left limbs, or bundles, with division straddling upper end of muscular part of interventricular septum
B. Left limb descends as flattened band beneath endocardium on left side of septum and divides into 2 or more bundles (anterior and posterior) that descend to ventricular apex
   1. Bundles divide into variable number of branches, which pass into trabeculae carneae to reach papillary muscles
   2. Form plexus of Purkinje fibers from which branches pass beneath endocardium to all parts of left ventricle to become continuous with myocardial fibers at varying depths

C. Right limb is rounded and continuation of bundle
   1. Passes toward apex embedded in muscle near right surface of septum but later lies beneath endocardium
   2. One branch enters **septomarginal trabecula** (moderator band), which conveys it to base of anterior papillary muscle
   3. Forms Purkinje fiber plexus from which branches pass beneath endocardium to all parts of right ventricle and becomes continuous with myocardium fibers
D. AV node, bundle and limbs, and ventricular Purkinje plexuses are surrounded by delicate connective tissue sheath that insulates them from myocardium

V. Vascular Supply of Conducting System

A. SA nodal branch
   1. 55% from right coronary
   2. 45% from circumflex branch of left coronary
B. AV nodal branch
   1. 85% from right coronary
   2. 15% from circumflex branch of left coronary

VI. Clinical Considerations

A. Conduction system injury
   1. Often due to ischemia caused by coronary artery disease and results in disturbances of cardiac muscle contraction
   2. Because RCA supplies both SA and AV nodes, and anterior interventricular supplies AV bundle, if they are occluded, parts of conducting system are affected, and **heart block** can occur
   3. If patient survives, ventricles begin to contract independently at 25–30 times/min (slower than normal), whereas atria contract at normal rate of 40–45 times/min
   4. Damage to 1 bundle branch
      a. Leads to **bundle branch block**, and excitation passes only on unaffected branch, causing normally timed systole of that ventricle only
      b. Impulse spreads to other side via muscle propagation and produces late asynchronous contraction
      c. Cardiac pacemaker may be implanted to create predetermined more normal rate

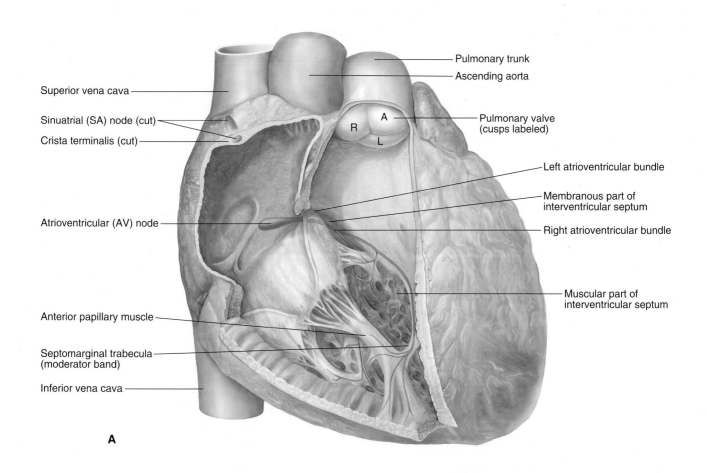

Pulmonary trunk

Ascending aorta

Superior vena cava

Sinuatrial (SA) node (cut)

Crista terminalis (cut)

Pulmonary valve (cusps labeled)

R   A   L

Left atrioventricular bundle

Membranous part of interventricular septum

Atrioventricular (AV) node

Right atrioventricular bundle

Muscular part of interventricular septum

Anterior papillary muscle

Septomarginal trabecula (moderator band)

Inferior vena cava

A

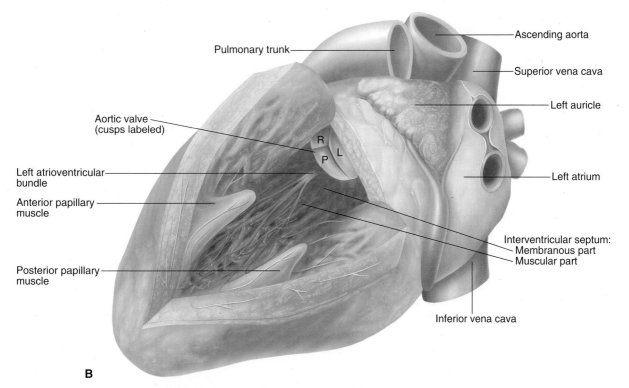

Pulmonary trunk

Ascending aorta

Superior vena cava

Left auricle

Aortic valve (cusps labeled)

R   P   L

Left atrioventricular bundle

Anterior papillary muscle

Left atrium

Interventricular septum:
Membranous part
Muscular part

Posterior papillary muscle

Inferior vena cava

B

FIG. 1.13A,B. Conduction System of the Heart. **A.** Anterior View. **B.** Lateral View.

Conduction System of the Heart and Electrocardiograms

I. Introduction (Fig. 1.14A)

A. Excitation spreading over heart and dissipating produces electrical field, changes in magnitude and direction of which, in time, can be sensed on body surface and reflected in changes in potential differences measured between various body surface sites

B. An **electrocardiogram** (ECG, or EKG) represents such potential differences as a function of time and is indicator of heart excitation, not contraction

C. Electrodes are attached to right arm and left leg to give bipolar recording from body surface in direction of long axis of heart

D. Positive and negative deflections, or waves, are seen

E. **Segment**: distance between 2 waves (e.g., PQ segment extends from end of P wave to beginning of QRS complex)

F. **Interval**: comprises both waves and segments (e.g., the PQ interval, from beginning of P wave to beginning of QRS wave)

　1. PQ interval: time from atrial excitation to ventricular excitation (less than 0.2 sec)

　2. QT interval depends on heart rate (as rate increases, interval decreases)

　3. RR interval, between peaks of two successive R waves, corresponds to period of beat cycle and is reciprocal of beat rate (60/RR interval(s) = beats/min)

II. P Wave (Fig. 1.14B)

A. 1st wave, represents spread of excitation over 2 atria (atrial depolarization)

B. During subsequent PQ segment, atria as whole are excited

C. As excitation in atria dies out, 1st deflection in ventricular part of curve begins (from beginning of Q to end of T wave)

III. QRS Complex

A. 2nd wave

B. Occurs about 0.1 to 0.2 sec after 1st wave and is expression of spread of excitation over both ventricles (ventricular depolarization)

IV. ST Segment

A. Analogous to PQ segment

B. Indicates excitation of ventricular myocardium

V. T Wave

A. Final wave: recovery in ventricles from excitation (ventricular repolarization)

B. No manifestation of atrial repolarization is seen because it occurs during ventricular depolarization and is masked by QRS complex

VI. From T to Next P Wave

A. Atria inactive

B. Ventricles inactive

VII. U Wave

A. May follow T wave

B. Corresponds to "dying out" of excitation in terminal branches of conducting system

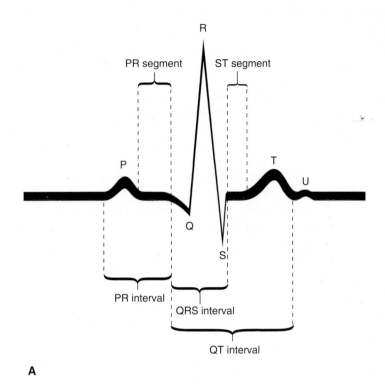

R

PR segment   ST segment

P

T

U

Q

S

PR interval

QRS interval

QT interval

A

Lead I

Lead aVF

Atrial Depolarization Vector

SA node

AV node

Common bundle of His

Right bundle branch

Left bundle branch

Lead I

Lead aVF

Late Ventricular Depolarization Vector

Lead I

Lead aVF

Repolarization Vector

Lead I

Lead aVF

Septal Depolarization Vector

Lead I

Lead aVF

Apical and Early Left Ventricular Depolarization Vector

B

FIG. 1.14.A,B. A. Electrocardiogram. **B.** Depolarization and Repolarization Vectors.

VIII. Clinical Considerations

A. Myocardial Infarction

1. Sudden insufficiency of arterial or venous blood supply due to emboli, thrombi, vessel torsion, or pressure that produces macroscopic area of necrosis

2. Complications

a. Most deaths in early hours after MI are due to ventricular fibrillation or cardiac arrest

b. Ventricular aneurysm can be due to continued bulging of fibrotic myocardium

c. Heart block may be due to impairment of blood supply of conducting tissue

B. **Tachycardia**: increased heart rate resulting from increased adrenergic activation of SA node (emotional stress or reflex response to fall in blood pressure)

C. **Bradycardia**: decreased heart rate, usually under 60 beats/min

Extrinsic Innervation of the Heart and the Cardiac Plexuses

I. Introduction (Fig. 1.15A)

A. Heart is influenced by autonomic control via the sympathetic and parasympathetic systems via cardiac plexuses

B. Presynaptic sympathetic fibers

 1. Arise in upper 4 or 5 thoracic segments of spinal cord and synapse in 3 cervical and upper 4 or 5 thoracic sympathetic ganglia

 2. Postsynaptic fibers form cardiac nerves in cervical region or thoracic visceral nerves in upper thorax

 3. Adrenergic sympathetic nerves increase heart rate (**chronotropic effect**) and force of cardiac contraction (**inotropic effect**)

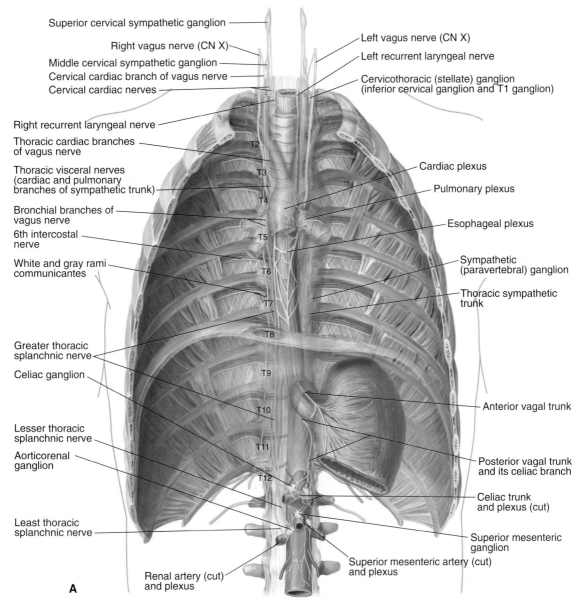

Superior cervical sympathetic ganglion

Right vagus nerve (CN X)

Middle cervical sympathetic ganglion

Cervical cardiac branch of vagus nerve

Cervical cardiac nerves

Right recurrent laryngeal nerve

Thoracic cardiac branches of vagus nerve

Thoracic visceral nerves (cardiac and pulmonary branches of sympathetic trunk)

Bronchial branches of vagus nerve

6th intercostal nerve

White and gray rami communicantes

Greater thoracic splanchnic nerve

Celiac ganglion

Lesser thoracic splanchnic nerve

Aorticorenal ganglion

Least thoracic splanchnic nerve

Renal artery (cut) and plexus

Left vagus nerve (CN X)

Left recurrent laryngeal nerve

Cervicothoracic (stellate) ganglion (inferior cervical ganglion and T1 ganglion)

Cardiac plexus

Pulmonary plexus

Esophageal plexus

Sympathetic (paravertebral) ganglion

Thoracic sympathetic trunk

Anterior vagal trunk

Posterior vagal trunk and its celiac branch

Celiac trunk and plexus (cut)

Superior mesenteric ganglion

Superior mesenteric artery (cut) and plexus

T2 T3 T4 T5 T6 T7 T8 T9 T10 T11 T12

A

FIG. 1.15A. Innervation of the Heart, Anterior View.

C. Presynaptic parasympathetic fibers are derived from dorsal nucleus of vagus and run in cardiac branches of vagus and recurrent laryngeal nerves to synapse in cells of cardiac plexuses and in atrial walls
   1. Postsynaptics supply the heart
   2. Cholinergic vagal cardiac fibers decrease heart rate
D. Significant component of sympathetic vasoconstrictor tone exists in coronary arterioles, and the release of this tone contributes to vasodilation under stress conditions
   1. Effects of antiadrenergic drugs and of chronic cardiac denervation suggest that sympathetic nerves augment coronary flow mainly by increasing metabolic demand
   2. Heart does not possess sympathetic vasodilator nerves as seen in skeletal muscle
   3. Cardiac parasympathetic vasodilator nerves exist, but their influence on resistance is small, and they have no known function

II. Cardiac Plexus (Fig. 1.15B,C)

A. Found at base of heart, divided into superficial and deep portions, which are closely connected; small ganglia are found in plexus, cardiac ganglion being largest and most consistent
B. **Superficial cardiac plexus** lies below aortic arch, anterior to right pulmonary artery and to right of ligamentum arteriosum
   1. Formation: left superior cervical cardiac nerve (from superior cervical ganglion), and left inferior cervical cardiac branch of vagus
   2. Distribution: to deep part of plexus, to right coronary plexus, and to left anterior pulmonary plexus
C. **Deep cardiac plexus**: lies on tracheal bifurcation above division of pulmonary trunk and posterior arch of aorta
   1. Formation: receives right superior, middle, and inferior and left middle and inferior cervical cardiac nerves from sympathetic trunk; thoracic visceral nerves from upper 4 or 5 thoracic sympathetic ganglia; superior and inferior cervical cardiac branches and thoracic branches of right vagus; and superior cervical cardiac and thoracic branches of left vagus

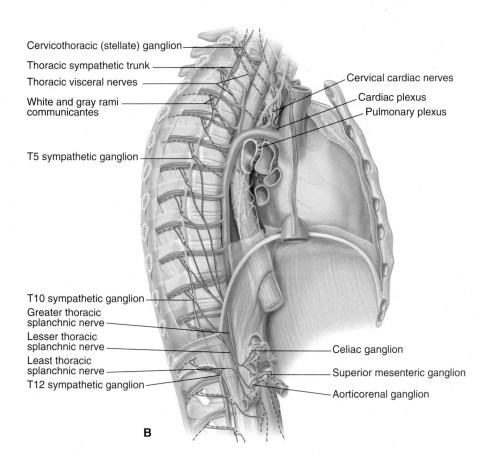

Cervicothoracic (stellate) ganglion

Thoracic sympathetic trunk

Thoracic visceral nerves

White and gray rami communicantes

T5 sympathetic ganglion

Cervical cardiac nerves

Cardiac plexus

Pulmonary plexus

T10 sympathetic ganglion

Greater thoracic splanchnic nerve

Lesser thoracic splanchnic nerve

Least thoracic splanchnic nerve

T12 sympathetic ganglion

Celiac ganglion

Superior mesenteric ganglion

Aorticorenal ganglion

B

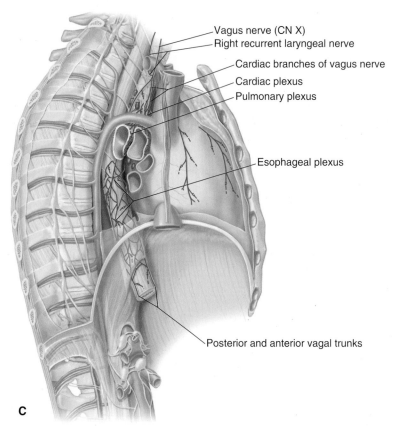

Vagus nerve (CN X)

Right recurrent laryngeal nerve

Cardiac branches of vagus nerve

Cardiac plexus

Pulmonary plexus

Esophageal plexus

Posterior and anterior vagal trunks

C

FIG. 1.15B,C. B. Sympathetic Innervation of the Heart, Lateral View. **C.** Parasympathetic Innervation of the Heart, Lateral View.

2. Distribution (Fig. 1.15D–F)
   a. Branches from right half of deep part
      i. Pass in front of right pulmonary artery, go to right anterior pulmonary plexus, and continue on to form right coronary plexus to supply right atrium and ventricle
      ii. Pass behind right pulmonary artery, to right atrium, and continue on to help form part of left coronary plexus
   b. Branches from left half of deep plexus connect with superficial part, give filaments to left atrium and to left anterior pulmonary plexus, and continue on to form greater part of left coronary plexus, which supplies left atrium and ventricle

III. Sensory Fibers

A. Cardiac branches of vagus and sympathetics contain afferent fibers, except for superior cervical cardiac nerve from superior cervical sympathetic ganglion, which contains efferent postganglionic fibers only
B. Pain
   1. Most pain from heart is carried in visceral afferent fibers contained in sympathetic nerves
   2. Pain is often referred to medial side of left arm, forearm, and hand because this area is covered by nerves from left 8th cervical and 1st thoracic spinal cord segments (those that receive afferents from heart)
C. Vagus carries visceral afferent fibers from aortic bodies for reflex control of respiration and from associated arteries for reflex control of heart output

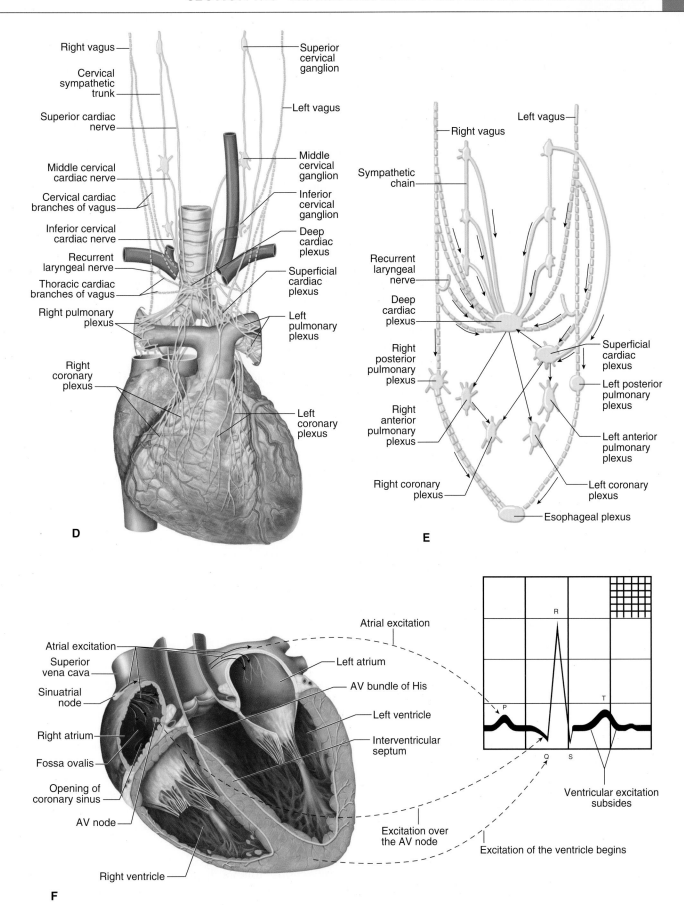

D.

Right vagus
Cervical sympathetic trunk
Superior cardiac nerve
Middle cervical cardiac nerve
Cervical cardiac branches of vagus
Inferior cervical cardiac nerve
Recurrent laryngeal nerve
Thoracic cardiac branches of vagus
Right pulmonary plexus
Right coronary plexus

Superior cervical ganglion
Left vagus
Middle cervical ganglion
Inferior cervical ganglion
Deep cardiac plexus
Superficial cardiac plexus
Left pulmonary plexus
Left coronary plexus

E.

Right vagus
Left vagus
Sympathetic chain
Recurrent laryngeal nerve
Deep cardiac plexus
Right posterior pulmonary plexus
Right anterior pulmonary plexus
Right coronary plexus

Superficial cardiac plexus
Left posterior pulmonary plexus
Left anterior pulmonary plexus
Left coronary plexus
Esophageal plexus

F.

Atrial excitation
Superior vena cava
Sinuatrial node
Right atrium
Fossa ovalis
Opening of coronary sinus
AV node
Right ventricle

Atrial excitation
Left atrium
AV bundle of His
Left ventricle
Interventricular septum
Excitation over the AV node
Excitation of the ventricle begins
Ventricular excitation subsides

R
P
Q   S
T

FIG. 1.15D–F. D. Summary of Innervation of the Heart, Anterior View. **E.** Schematic Summary of Innervation of the Heart. **F.** Innervation of Conduction System of the Heart, Anterior View.

Pleurae and the Surface Projections of Lungs and Pleura

I. Pleurae (Fig. 1.16A)

A. Pleura
1. Serous membrane forming a bursa-like sac (pleural cavity) for each lung
2. Pleural cavities
   a. Between visceral and parietal pleura
   b. Potential spaces filled with thin film of pleural fluid

B. Visceral pleura
1. Covers lungs and dips into fissures
2. Insensitive to pain due to autonomic innervation

C. Parietal pleura
1. Lines thoracic cavity; continuous with visceral pleura at hilum of lung
2. Sensitive to pain (especially its costal portion); innervated by branches of intercostal and phrenic nerves
3. Referred pain from parietal pleura
   a. Costal and peripheral parts of diaphragmatic pleura are referred along intercostal nerves to thorax and abdominal wall
   b. Mediastinal and central diaphragmatic pleural pain referred to root of neck and over shoulder (dermatomes C3–C5)
4. Named by location
   a. Costal: lines inner chest wall
   b. Diaphragmatic: lies on diaphragm
   c. Mediastinal: lies against structures within mediastinum
   d. Cervical (cupula): dome-like projection above anterior end of 1st rib, reinforced by scalene fascia

D. Reflections and recesses
1. Costodiaphragmatic reflection: where costal pleura turns to cover diaphragm, creating a potential space called **costodiaphragmatic recess**
2. Costomediastinal reflection: where costal pleura turns to cover mediastinum; anteriorly, this creates small potential space called **costomediastinal recess**
3. **Pulmonary ligament**: mediastinal pleura along lung root is prolonged inferiorly toward diaphragm as fold
4. Costodiaphragmatic recess: potential space between inferior borders of lungs and pleurae

E. Extent of pleura
1. Superiorly: cervical pleura reaches level of angle of 1st rib, which may be more than 1.5 cm above sternoclavicular joint
2. Anteriorly (costomediastinal reflection)
   a. Pleura of both sides descend medially from sternoclavicular joint to reach midline at sternal angle
   b. Pleurae of both sides remain in contact until level of 4th sternocostal junction
   c. Right side: deviates slightly to 7th sternocostal junction where it becomes costodiaphragmatic reflection
   d. Left side: deviates to left of sternal margin to cross 7th costal cartilage 1.5 cm from sternal margin
      i. Deviation creates **bare area of pericardium**, an area of pericardial sac not covered by pleura
      ii. Bare area used for pericardiocentesis
3. Inferiorly (costodiaphragmatic reflection): follows diaphragm attachment to costal margin
   a. At level of 8th costochondral junction in midclavicular line
   b. At 10th rib at midaxillary line
   c. At 12th rib at scapular line

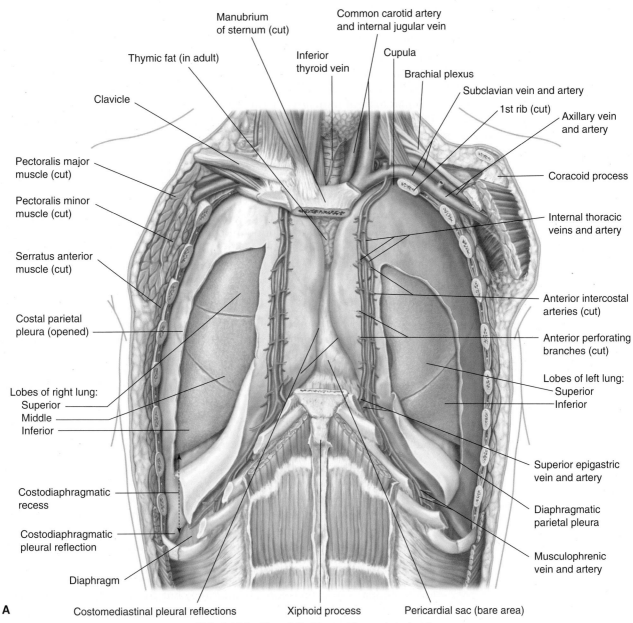

Manubrium of sternum (cut)

Common carotid artery and internal jugular vein

Thymic fat (in adult)

Inferior thyroid vein

Cupula

Brachial plexus

Clavicle

Subclavian vein and artery

1st rib (cut)

Axillary vein and artery

Pectoralis major muscle (cut)

Coracoid process

Pectoralis minor muscle (cut)

Internal thoracic veins and artery

Serratus anterior muscle (cut)

Costal parietal pleura (opened)

Anterior intercostal arteries (cut)

Anterior perforating branches (cut)

Lobes of left lung:
Superior
Inferior

Lobes of right lung:
Superior
Middle
Inferior

Superior epigastric vein and artery

Costodiaphragmatic recess

Diaphragmatic parietal pleura

Costodiaphragmatic pleural reflection

Musculophrenic vein and artery

Diaphragm

A

Costomediastinal pleural reflections

Xiphoid process

Pericardial sac (bare area)

FIG. 1.16A. Pleural Cavities and Lungs, Anterior View.

II. Lungs (Fig. 1.16B,C)

A. Respiration and lung borders

   1. Each year, an adult human inhales and exhales between 2 million and 5 million L of air (4–10 million breaths a year)

   2. Each breath consists of about .5 L of air

   3. In human lung, surface available for gas exchange is about 70 square meters (≈40× surface area of entire body)

B. Except for inferior limits and anterior limit on left side, extent of pleurae and lungs are similar

C. Apex: same for both lungs, about 1.5 cm above medial end of clavicle

D. Anterior border

   1. Right lung: descends in slight curve from sternoclavicular joint to near midline at sternal angle, descends near midline to 6th sternocostal junction

   2. Left lung: similar to right until level of 4th costal cartilage, then deviates to left to reach 6th costal cartilage near costochondral junction; this deviation is called **cardiac notch**

E. Inferior border

   1. Same for both lungs

   2. Extends along 6th cartilage, crosses 6th costochondral junction at midclavicular line, crosses 8th rib at midaxillary line, and 10th rib at scapular line

F. Fissures

   1. Oblique: starts posteriorly at level of spine of scapula or spine of T3, then passes obliquely around thorax to end near 6th costochondral junction

   2. Horizontal (right lung): starting at point where oblique fissure crosses midaxillary line (5th rib), this fissure runs nearly horizontally to anterior margin at level of 4th rib

III. Clinical Considerations

A. **Pleuritis**: result of inflammation of the pleurae (pleurisy)

   1. Lung surfaces become "rough" and result in "friction rub" (heard by auscultation using stethoscope)

   2. Symptoms tend to be sharp, with severe pain on exertion

B. **Thoracoscopy**: pleural cavity examined with thoracoscope via small incision in intercostal space

C. **Pneumothorax**: air within pleural cavity

   1. "Sucking chest wound": air can enter and exit pleural cavity as breathing occurs

   2. **Tension pneumothorax**

     a. Air is drawn into pleural cavity at inspiration, but due to tissue valve at the wound, it cannot escape

     b. Pressure builds within affected pleural cavity, pushing mediastinal structures to opposite side and compressing inferior vena cava

     c. Impeded venous return necessitates immediate release of pressure

   3. Spontaneous pneumothorax: rupture of lung tissue releases air into pleural cavity

D. Clinically, the base of the lung refers not to the anatomic base, which is related to diaphragm (and, therefore, is inferior), but to lower limit of posterior surface of lower lobe; therefore, to listen to base of lung, apply stethoscope to posterior chest wall about at level of 10th thoracic vertebra

E. Because pleural sacs are separate, it is possible to collapse lung on one side without collapsing lung on other side

F. **Thoracentesis**

   1. Introduction of needle or tube to drain blood or fluid from pleural cavity without endangering lungs

   2. Usually performed into costodiaphragmatic recess above 7th rib (midclavicular line), 9th rib (midaxillary line), or 11th rib (scapular line) to avoid lungs and intercostal vessels

   3. Direct needle upward to avoid puncturing diaphragm

G. Hydrothorax: accumulation of excess fluid in pleural cavity due to pleural effusion

H. Hemothorax: frequently result from injury to major intercostal vessel resulting in blood entering pleural cavity

I. Chylothorax: white or yellow fatty lymph fluid from torn thoracic duct is seen in thoracic cavity

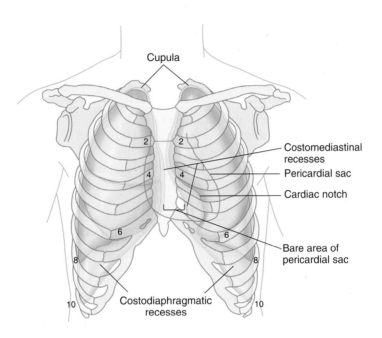

B

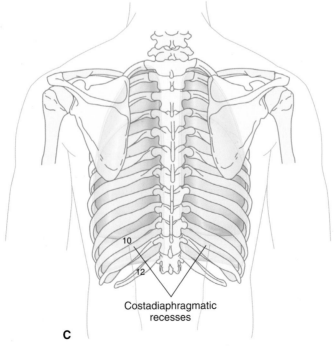

C

FIG. 1.16B,C. B. Surface Projection of Pleural Cavities and Lungs, Anterior View. **C.** Posterior View.

Lungs

I. Surfaces and Impressions (Fig. 1.17A–C)

A. Apex: rises 1.5–2.5 cm above sternoclavicular joint

B. Diaphragmatic surface (base): concave, rests on convexity of diaphragm

C. Costal surface: convex to conform to thoracic wall

D. Mediastinal surface
1. Cardiac impression for pericardial sac and heart, more pronounced on left lung
2. Hilum posterosuperior to cardiac impression
3. Above hilum on right lung
   a. Arched groove for azygos vein
   b. Groove for superior vena cava and right brachiocephalic vein
   c. Groove for right subclavian artery near apex
4. Posterior to hilum on right: groove for esophagus on right lung
5. Above hilum on left lung
   a. Groove for arch of aorta above hilum
   b. Groove for subclavian artery runs upward and lateralward from groove for aortic arch
   c. Groove for left brachiocephalic vein is anterior to groove for subclavian artery
6. Behind and below hilum of left lung: groove for descending thoracic aorta

II. Borders (Fig. 1.17D–F)

A. Inferior: sharp, where it separates base and costal surface; blunt at mediastinal border

B. Posterior (vertebral): broad and round to fit in groove lateral to vertebrae

C. Anterior: thin and sharp
   a. Overlaps pericardium on right; almost straight
   b. On left, cardiac notch marks lower anterior border of superior lobe

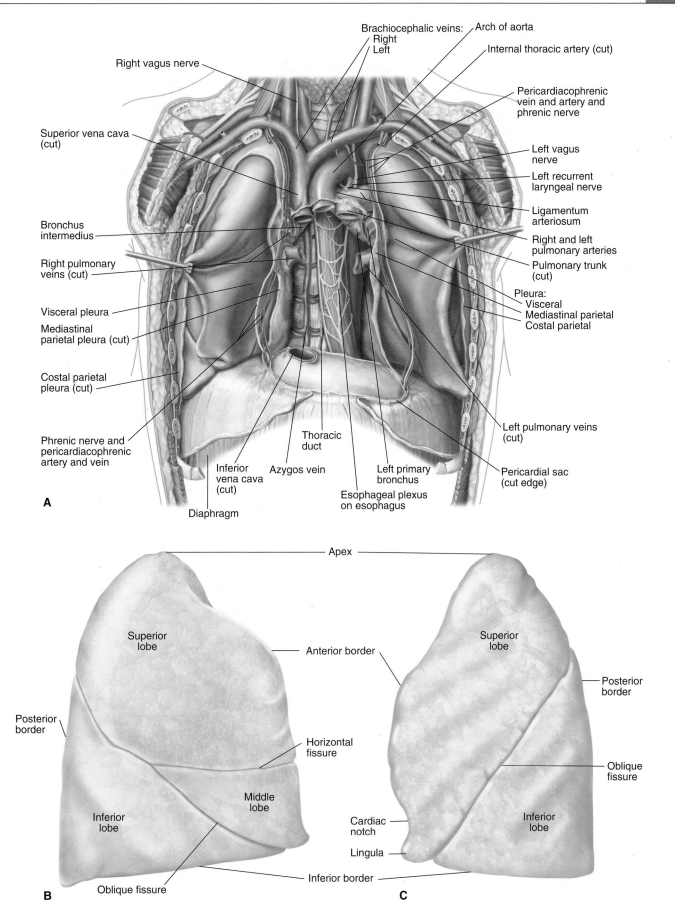

Brachiocephalic veins:
Right
Left

Arch of aorta

Internal thoracic artery (cut)

Right vagus nerve

Pericardiacophrenic
vein and artery and
phrenic nerve

Superior vena cava
(cut)

Left vagus
nerve

Left recurrent
laryngeal nerve

Ligamentum
arteriosum

Bronchus
intermedius

Right and left
pulmonary arteries

Right pulmonary
veins (cut)

Pulmonary trunk
(cut)

Pleura:
Visceral
Mediastinal parietal
Costal parietal

Visceral pleura

Mediastinal
parietal pleura (cut)

Costal parietal
pleura (cut)

Left pulmonary veins
(cut)

Phrenic nerve and
pericardiacophrenic
artery and vein

Thoracic
duct

Pericardial sac
(cut edge)

Inferior
vena cava
(cut)

Azygos vein

Left primary
bronchus

A

Esophageal plexus
on esophagus

Diaphragm

Apex

Superior
lobe

Anterior border

Superior
lobe

Posterior
border

Posterior
border

Horizontal
fissure

Oblique
fissure

Middle
lobe

Inferior
lobe

Cardiac
notch

Inferior
lobe

Lingula

B

Oblique fissure

Inferior border

C

FIG. 1.17A–C. A. Lungs In Situ, Anterior View. **B.** Lung, Right, Lateral View. **C.** Lung, Left, Lateral View.

III. Fissures and Lobes (Fig. 1.17G–O)

A. Left lung: divided into 2 lobes, superior and inferior, by oblique fissure

B. Right lung: divided into 3 lobes; oblique fissure separates inferior from middle and superior lobes, horizontal fissure separates superior and middle lobes

IV. Root of the Lung at the Hilum (Fig. 1.17P,Q)

A. Hilum of lung: the point at which lung root structures enter or exit lung

   1. Like hilum of any organ, this is doorway of lung

   2. Parietal pleura along lung root reflects onto lung at hilum to become visceral pleura

B. Root of lung: collection of structures entering and exiting lung

   1. Right lung

      a. Pulmonary artery lies anterior to superior lobe bronchus

      b. Superior pulmonary vein lies just caudal to artery

      c. Inferior pulmonary vein is inferior to bronchus

   2. Left lung

      a. Pulmonary artery lies most superiorly

      b. Superior pulmonary vein lies anterior to bronchus

      c. Inferior pulmonary vein is inferior to bronchus

V. Clinical Considerations

A. Lung resection (to remove tumors or abscesses)

   1. Pneumonectomy: removal of entire lung

   2. Lobectomy and pulmonary resection: removal of lung lobe in specific cases of bronchiectasis, pulmonary tuberculosis, chronic lung abscesses, and metastatic lesions

   3. Segmentectomy: removal of 1 or more bronchopulmonary segments of lung

B. Pulmonary emboli: obstruction of pulmonary artery by blood clot (embolus)

C. Dyspnea: difficulty in breathing usually seen in patients with asthma, emphysema, or heart failure; tend to use accessory respiratory muscles to help expansion of thoracic cavities

D. Lung percussion: "tapping" on chest wall over lungs with finger to determine if underlying tissues are air-filled (resonant sound), fluid-filled (dull sound), or solid (flat sound)

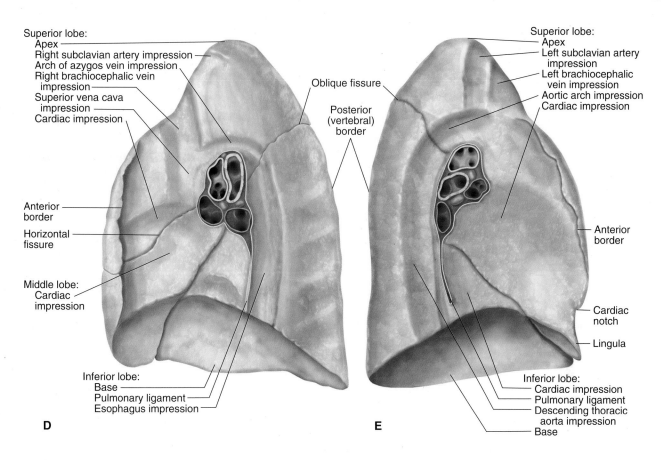

Superior lobe:
  Apex
  Right subclavian artery impression
  Arch of azygos vein impression
  Right brachiocephalic vein impression
  Superior vena cava impression
  Cardiac impression

Oblique fissure

Posterior (vertebral) border

Anterior border

Horizontal fissure

Middle lobe:
  Cardiac impression

Superior lobe:
  Apex
  Left subclavian artery impression
  Left brachiocephalic vein impression
  Aortic arch impression
  Cardiac impression

Anterior border

Cardiac notch

Lingula

Inferior lobe:
  Base
  Pulmonary ligament
  Esophagus impression

Inferior lobe:
  Cardiac impression
  Pulmonary ligament
  Descending thoracic aorta impression
  Base

D

E

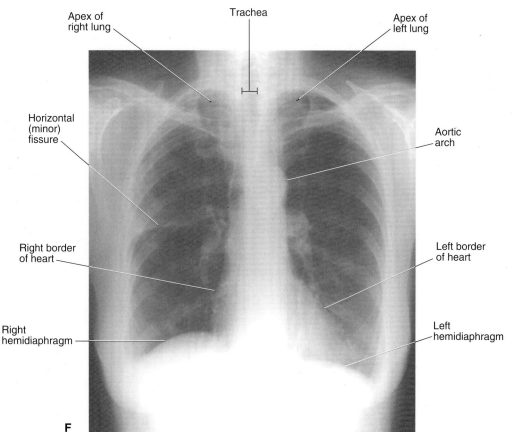

Apex of right lung

Trachea

Apex of left lung

Horizontal (minor) fissure

Aortic arch

Right border of heart

Left border of heart

Right hemidiaphragm

Left hemidiaphragm

F

FIG. 1.17D–F. D. Lung, Right, Medial View. **E.** Lung, Left, Medial View. **F.** Radiograph of the Thorax, PA View.

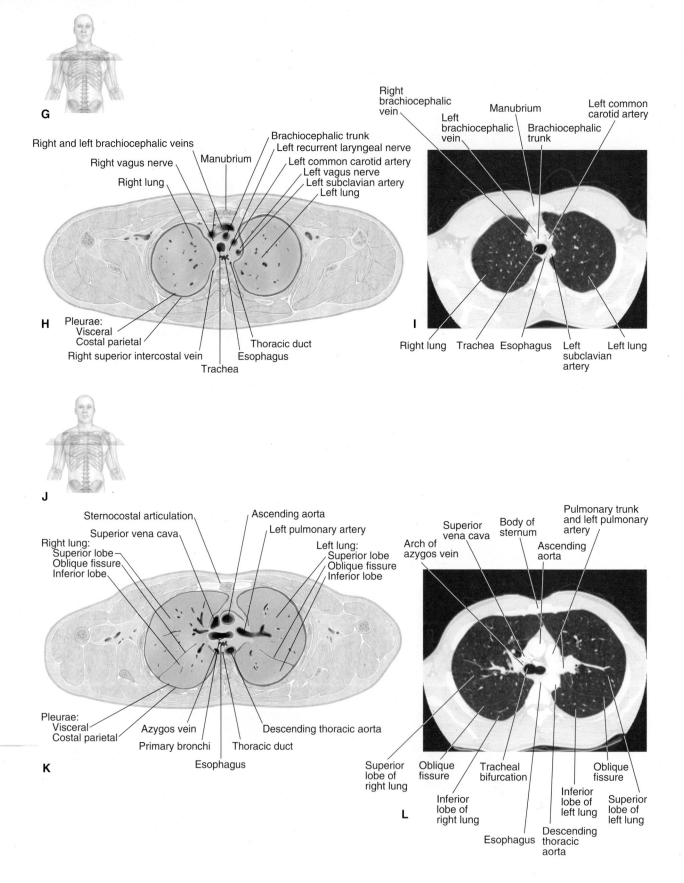

G

Right and left brachiocephalic veins
Right vagus nerve
Right lung
Manubrium
Brachiocephalic trunk
Left recurrent laryngeal nerve
Left common carotid artery
Left vagus nerve
Left subclavian artery
Left lung

H

Pleurae:
Visceral
Costal parietal
Right superior intercostal vein
Trachea
Esophagus
Thoracic duct

Right brachiocephalic vein
Left brachiocephalic vein
Manubrium
Brachiocephalic trunk
Left common carotid artery

I

Right lung   Trachea   Esophagus   Left subclavian artery   Left lung

J

Sternocostal articulation
Superior vena cava
Ascending aorta
Left pulmonary artery
Right lung:
Superior lobe
Oblique fissure
Inferior lobe
Left lung:
Superior lobe
Oblique fissure
Inferior lobe

K

Pleurae:
Visceral
Costal parietal
Azygos vein
Primary bronchi
Esophagus
Thoracic duct
Descending thoracic aorta

Superior vena cava
Arch of azygos vein
Body of sternum
Pulmonary trunk and left pulmonary artery
Ascending aorta

L

Superior lobe of right lung
Oblique fissure
Inferior lobe of right lung
Esophagus
Tracheal bifurcation
Inferior lobe of left lung
Descending thoracic aorta
Oblique fissure
Superior lobe of left lung

FIG. 1.17G–L. **G.** Orientation of Cross Section at T2 Vertebral Level, Anterior View. **H.** Cross Section of Thorax at T2 Vertebral Level. **I.** CT Image with Lung Window at T2 Vertebral Level. **J.** Orientation of Cross Section at T5 Vertebral Level, Anterior View. **K.** Cross Section of Thorax at T5 Vertebral Level. **L.** CT Image with Lung Window at T5 Vertebral Level.

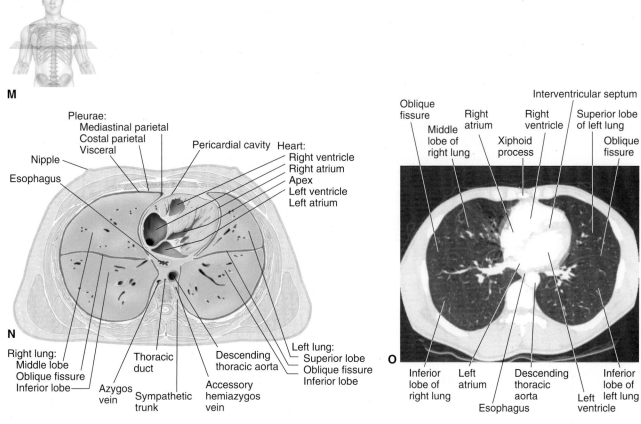

M. Orientation Figure of the Thorax, Anterior View.

Pleurae:
Mediastinal parietal
Costal parietal
Visceral

Nipple

Esophagus

Pericardial cavity

Heart:
Right ventricle
Right atrium
Apex
Left ventricle
Left atrium

Right lung:
Middle lobe
Oblique fissure
Inferior lobe

Azygos vein

Sympathetic trunk

Thoracic duct

Descending thoracic aorta

Accessory hemiazygos vein

Left lung:
Superior lobe
Oblique fissure
Inferior lobe

Oblique fissure

Middle lobe of right lung

Right atrium

Xiphoid process

Interventricular septum

Right ventricle

Superior lobe of left lung

Oblique fissure

Inferior lobe of right lung

Left atrium

Descending thoracic aorta

Esophagus

Left ventricle

Inferior lobe of left lung

FIG. 1.17M–O. M. Orientation Figure of the Thorax, Anterior View. **N.** Cross Section of Thorax at T7 Vertebral Level. **O.** CT Image with Lung Window at T7 Vertebral Level.

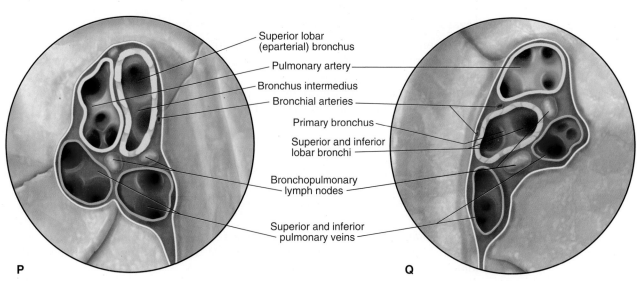

Superior lobar (eparterial) bronchus

Pulmonary artery

Bronchus intermedius

Bronchial arteries

Primary bronchus

Superior and inferior lobar bronchi

Bronchopulmonary lymph nodes

Superior and inferior pulmonary veins

FIG. 1.17P,Q. Lung Hilum. **P.** Right, Medial View. **Q.** Left, Medial View.

Trachea and the Bronchial Tree

I. Trachea (Fig. 1.18A,B)

A. Extent: from C6 to plane of sternal angle (intervertebral disc at T4/T5), where it divides into primary bronchi

B. Dimensions: 9 to 15 cm long, 2.0 to 2.5 cm in diameter, and larger in male than female

C. Shape: nearly cylindrical, flattened posteriorly

D. Structure: U-shaped cartilage, muscle, connective tissue, mucous membrane, and glands

   1. Hyaline cartilage: 16 to 20 "rings" or U-shaped bars, incomplete posteriorly but filled in by smooth muscle (trachealis) and connective tissue where trachea adjoins esophagus

   2. Longitudinal elastic fibers: permit stretch and descent with lungs during inspiration and recoil with lungs during expiration

   3. Carina: ridge on inside of tracheal bifurcation; formed by backward and downward projection of last tracheal cartilage

E. Relations

   1. In neck

      a. Anteriorly (from superior to inferior): isthmus of thyroid, inferior thyroid veins, sternohyoid and sternothyroid muscles, cervical fascia, and jugular venous arch

      b. Laterally: common carotid, lobes of thyroid, inferior thyroid arteries, and recurrent laryngeal nerves (in tracheoesophageal groove)

      c. Posteriorly: esophagus

   2. In thorax

      a. Anteriorly (from superficial to deep): manubrium of sternum, thymus, left brachiocephalic vein, brachiocephalic trunk, arch of aorta, left common carotid artery, and deep cardiac plexus

      b. Laterally

         i. On right: pleura, right vagus, brachiocephalic trunk

         ii. On left: left recurrent laryngeal nerve, arch of aorta, left common carotid and subclavian arteries

F. Surface projections

   1. Bifurcation of trachea at plane of sternal angle

   2. Upper part of primary bronchus in second intercostal space at edge of sternum

   3. Arch of aorta crosses trachea behind manubrium, opposite 1st intercostal space

II. Neurovasculature of the Trachea

A. Supplied mainly by inferior thyroid arteries; in addition, receives branches from bronchial and internal thoracic arteries

B. Drained by inferior thyroid veins

C. Lymphatic vessels drain into adjacent nodes (deep cervical, paratracheal, and tracheobronchial)

D. Innervated by vagus and recurrent laryngeal nerves and sympathetics

III. Primary Bronchi

A. Right: 2.5 cm long

   1. Wider, shorter, and more vertical than left and makes smaller angle with trachea than does left

   2. Azygos vein arches over it; pulmonary artery is at first below, then anterior to it

B. Left: 5.0 cm long

   1. Narrower than right and diverges from trachea at greater angle

   2. Passes behind pulmonary artery, under arch of aorta and anterior to descending thoracic aorta

C. Both are mobile, elastic, and have U-shaped cartilaginous rings, which become plates when bronchi become intrapulmonary at hilum of lungs

D. Blood supply, lymphatic drainage, and nerve supply

   1. Supplied by bronchial arteries and drained by bronchial veins

   2. Lymphatic vessels drain into bronchopulmonary and tracheobronchial nodes

   3. Nerves similar to trachea and arrive via cardiac and pulmonary plexuses

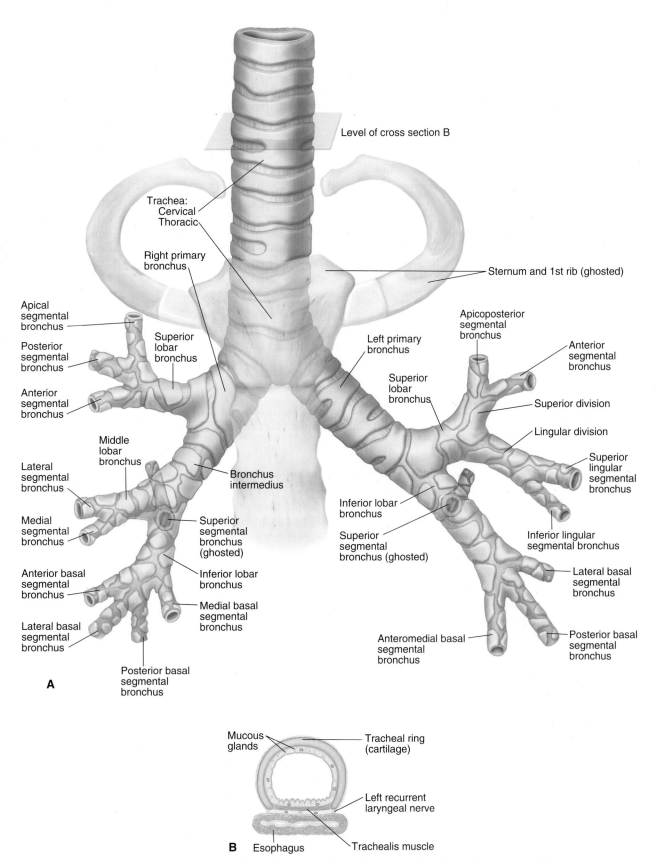

Level of cross section B

Trachea:
Cervical
Thoracic

Right primary
bronchus

Sternum and 1st rib (ghosted)

Apical
segmental
bronchus

Apicoposterior
segmental
bronchus

Posterior
segmental
bronchus

Superior
lobar
bronchus

Left primary
bronchus

Anterior
segmental
bronchus

Anterior
segmental
bronchus

Superior
lobar
bronchus

Superior division

Lingular division

Middle
lobar
bronchus

Bronchus
intermedius

Superior
lingular
segmental
bronchus

Lateral
segmental
bronchus

Medial
segmental
bronchus

Superior
segmental
bronchus
(ghosted)

Inferior lobar
bronchus

Inferior lingular
segmental bronchus

Anterior basal
segmental
bronchus

Superior
segmental
bronchus (ghosted)

Inferior lobar
bronchus

Lateral basal
segmental
bronchus

Lateral basal
segmental
bronchus

Medial basal
segmental
bronchus

Anteromedial basal
segmental
bronchus

Posterior basal
segmental
bronchus

A

Posterior basal
segmental
bronchus

Mucous
glands

Tracheal ring
(cartilage)

Left recurrent
laryngeal nerve

B   Esophagus

Trachealis muscle

FIG. 1.18A,B. A. Trachea and Bronchi, Anterior View. **B.** Trachea and Esophagus, Cross-Sectional View.

IV. Bronchial Branching (Fig. 1.18C,D)

A. Primary (main stem) bronchi give off lobar (secondary) bronchi, which then give off segmental (tertiary) bronchi to bronchopulmonary segments
B. Bronchopulmonary segments are pyramidal in shape with apex toward hilum and base at pleural surface
   1. Each segment has its own segmental bronchus, artery, and vein
   2. Segments are separated by connective tissue septa, which are continuous with visceral pleura

V. Right Primary Bronchus: Gives Rise to 3 Lobar or Secondary Bronchi

A. Superior lobar bronchus
   1. 3 segmental bronchi: apical, posterior, anterior
   2. Lies above pulmonary artery (eparterial); continuation of right bronchus is called **bronchus intermedius**, which divides into middle and inferior lobar bronchi
B. Middle lobar bronchus (2 segmental bronchi): lateral and medial segments
C. Inferior lobar bronchus (5 segmental bronchi): superior, medial basal, anterior basal, lateral basal, posterior basal

VI. Left Primary Bronchus: Gives Rise to 2 Lobar Bronchi

A. Superior lobe bronchus: 2 divisions, superior and lingular
   1. Superior division bronchus (2 segmental bronchi): apicoposterior, anterior
   2. Lingular division bronchus (2 segmental bronchi): superior lingular, inferior lingular
B. Inferior lobe bronchus (4 segmental bronchi): superior, anteromedial basal (sometimes separate), posterior basal, lateral basal

VII. Bronchial Tree

A. Segmental bronchi branch into many smaller divisions known as bronchioles
B. Bronchioles
   1. Terminal (lobular) bronchioles
      a. Last division with typical bronchial structure
      b. Not respiratory in function
      c. Each divides into 2 or more respiratory bronchioles
   2. Respiratory bronchioles: give rise to variable number of alveolar ducts
   3. Alveolar ducts: give off multiple alveolar sacs
   4. Alveolar sacs: gas exchange with pulmonary capillaries occurs through walls of alveolar sacs

VIII. Clinical Considerations

A. Foreign objects more likely to enter right bronchus (larger and more vertical)
B. Emergency tracheotomy
   1. Needed when rima glottidis is closed completely due to spasmodic contraction of laryngeal muscles after severe irritation of mucosa (foreign body, alcohol, etc.)
   2. Opening made in midline, between lower parts of muscular triangles; below 4th tracheal ring, isthmus of thyroid is avoided
C. Tracheostomy
   1. Performed at level of 2nd and 3rd tracheal rings
   2. Isthmus of thyroid is divided; tracheal rings are cut and flapped downward
D. Bronchoscopy: examination of interior of the tracheobronchial tree (using an endoscope) for diagnostic purposes (Fig. 1.18E)
E. Bronchogenic carcinoma: common type of lung cancer arising from bronchial tree epithelium that usually metastasizes widely due to great number of lymphatics in region
F. Carina is very sensitive and associated with cough reflex, being last line of defense before lung is entered

Continued

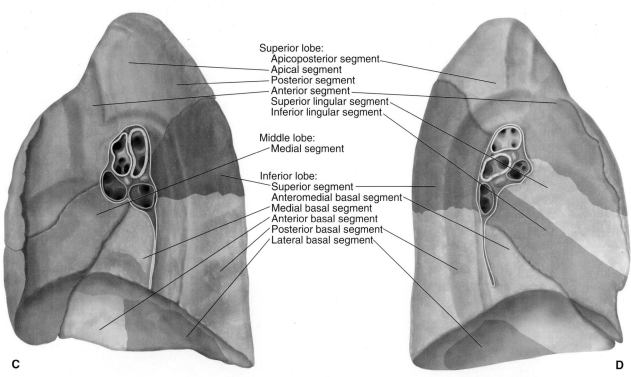

Superior lobe:
  Apicoposterior segment
  Apical segment
  Posterior segment
  Anterior segment
  Superior lingular segment
  Inferior lingular segment

Middle lobe:
  Medial segment

Inferior lobe:
  Superior segment
  Anteromedial basal segment
  Medial basal segment
  Anterior basal segment
  Posterior basal segment
  Lateral basal segment

C   D

FIG. 1.18C,D. Bronchopulmonary Segments, Medial View. **C.** Right Lung. **D.** Left Lung.

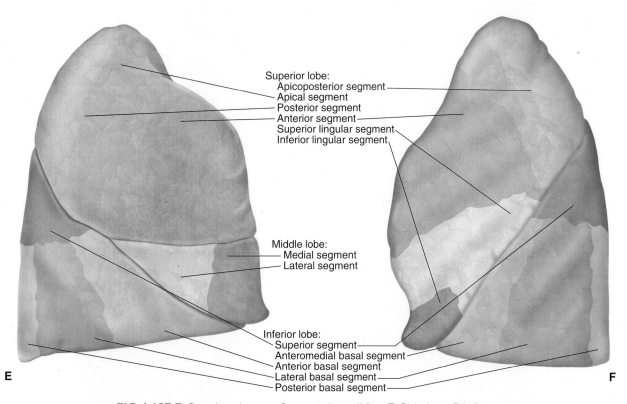

Superior lobe:
  Apicoposterior segment
  Apical segment
  Posterior segment
  Anterior segment
  Superior lingular segment
  Inferior lingular segment

Middle lobe:
  Medial segment
  Lateral segment

Inferior lobe:
  Superior segment
  Anteromedial basal segment
  Anterior basal segment
  Lateral basal segment
  Posterior basal segment

E   F

FIG. 1.18E,F. Bronchopulmonary Segments, Lateral View. **E.** Right Lung. **F.** Left Lung.

G. Lung lobes
   1. Upper lobe related more to anterior chest wall
   2. Middle lobe is anterior part of right lung, not related to posterior chest wall; relates to anterior chest wall between 4th and 6th costal cartilages
   3. Lower lobe primarily associated with posterior chest wall
H. Postural drainage
   1. Gravity used to promote drainage from part of bronchial tree
   2. Patient posture adjusted accordingly
I. Because bronchopulmonary segmental territories are relatively distinct, it is theoretically possible to isolate individual segments without having to remove entire lobe
J. Important to note that although each bronchopulmonary segment is supplied by its own nerve, artery, and vein, during surgical resection of segments, planes between them are crossed by branches of pulmonary veins and sometimes by pulmonary arteries; bronchial arteries also run through interlobular septa to supply visceral pleura

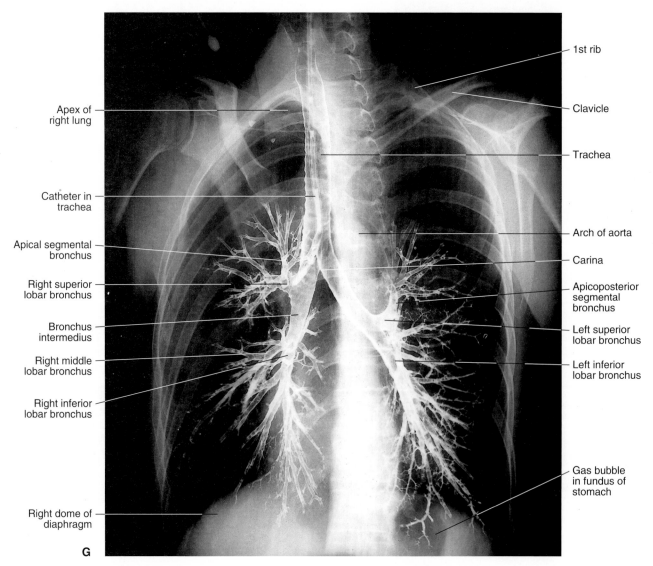

FIG. 1.18G. Bronchogram.

Neurovasculature of the Lungs

I. Blood Supply (Fig. 1.19A,B)

A. Systemic: through bronchial arteries
   1. 2 left bronchial arteries arise from descending thoracic aorta (single right bronchial artery may arise from a left bronchial or right 3rd posterior intercostal artery)
   2. Accompany and supply bronchial tree as far as respiratory bronchioles
B. Pulmonary
   1. Through right and left pulmonary arteries from pulmonary trunk
   2. Forms capillary plexus around alveoli

II. Venous Drainage

A. Systemic: arise from area supplied by bronchial arteries
   1. Vessels converge to form 1 vein at root of each lung
   2. End in azygos on right and in left superior intercostal vein on left
B. Pulmonary: arises in the capillary plexus around the alveoli
   1. Pass through lung substance independent of bronchi and pulmonary arteries
   2. Converge to form 2 veins at hilum of each lung and terminate in left atrium

III. Lymphatics (Fig. 1.19C)

A. Superficial plexus
   1. Lies deep to visceral pleura
   2. Drains tissue along alveolar ducts and pleura
   3. Lymph vessels curve around lung borders to end in bronchopulmonary (hilar) nodes at lung hilum
B. Deep plexus
   1. Located in bronchial submucosa and peribronchial connective tissue
   2. No lymphatics in alveoli
   3. Lymph vessels drain into pulmonary lymph nodes (located along branches of main bronchi)
   4. Lymph follows bronchi and pulmonary vessels to drain into bronchopulmonary nodes at hilum
C. Tracheobronchial nodes
   1. Receives lymph from bronchopulmonary nodes
   2. 2 groups, located above and below tracheal bifurcation: superior and inferior tracheobronchial nodes
D. Paratracheal nodes
   1. Receive lymph from tracheobronchial and mediastinal nodes
   2. Located beside trachea
   3. Channels coalesce to form bronchomediastinal lymph trunks
E. Bronchomediastinal lymph trunks
   1. On right, drains into right lymphatic duct
   2. On left, drains into thoracic duct

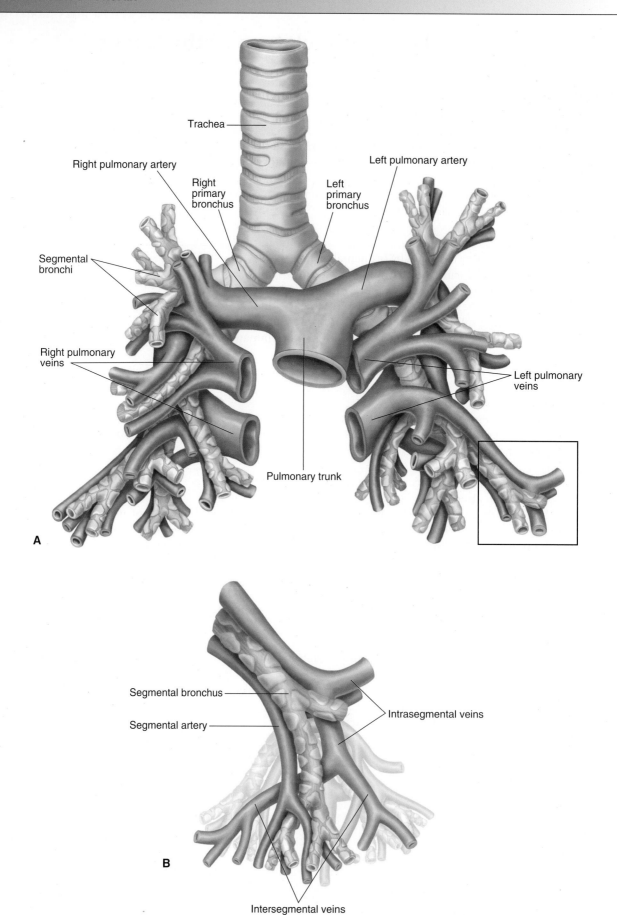

Trachea

Right pulmonary artery

Right primary bronchus

Left primary bronchus

Left pulmonary artery

Segmental bronchi

Right pulmonary veins

Left pulmonary veins

Pulmonary trunk

A

Segmental bronchus

Segmental artery

Intrasegmental veins

Intersegmental veins

B

FIG. 1.19A,B. A. Roots of the Lungs, Anterior View. **B.** Bronchial and Pulmonary Vessels within the Lung.

IV. Nerves

A. Both parasympathetic and sympathetic fibers via anterior and posterior pulmonary plexuses

B. Pulmonary arteries apparently innervated by sympathetic fibers only

C. Smooth muscles and glands of bronchi innervated by parasympathetic fibers

D. Afferent fibers from lung travel with parasympathetic (vagal) fibers

E. Costal and peripheral diaphragmatic pleura supplied by intercostal nerves; central diaphragmatic and mediastinal pleura innervated by phrenic nerve

V. Clinical Considerations

A. Bronchoconstriction: can be alleviated by administering sympathetomimetic drugs to counter bronchial spasm caused by overactivated parasympathetic innervation in lungs

B. Auscultation of lungs: listening to their sounds with stethoscope; assesses airflow through tracheobronchial tree

C. Upper respiratory tract

   1. Conducts air to and from lung and acts as filter and "air conditioner"

   2. Consists of nose, nasopharynx, mouth, oropharynx, larynx, trachea, and bronchi outside lung

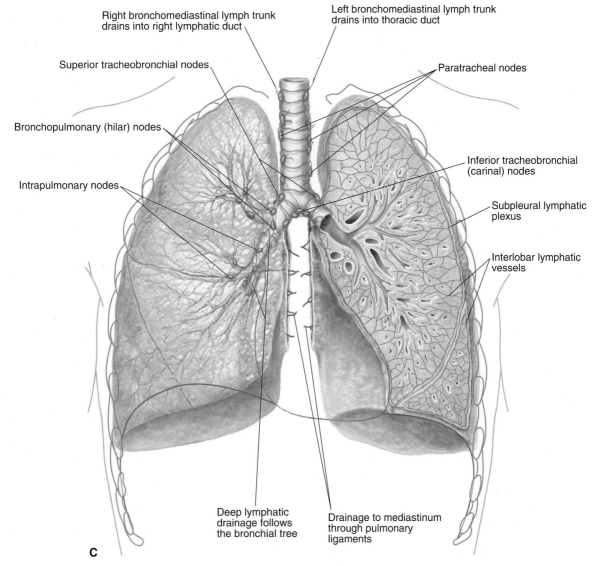

FIG. 1.19C. Lymphatics of the Lung, Anterior View.

Superior Mediastinum

I. Thymus

A. Most anterior structure in superior mediastinum

B. May hang down into anterior mediastinum

II. Brachiocephalic Veins and Superior Vena Cava (Fig. 1.20A,B)

A. Brachiocephalic veins arise as union of internal jugular and subclavian veins

B. Left brachiocephalic vein

    1. Usually receives thoracic duct posteriorly at its beginning

    2. Receives inferior thyroid vein (left or both)

    3. Receives thymic vein

    4. Crosses left to right anterior to aortic arch branches to unite with right brachiocephalic vein

C. Right brachiocephalic vein

    1. Usually receives right lymphatic duct at its beginning

    2. May receive right inferior thyroid vein and right internal thoracic vein

    3. Unites with left brachiocephalic vein to form superior vena cava

D. Superior vena cava

    1. Begins behind right 1st costal cartilage and descends to right 3rd costal cartilage to end in right atrium

    2. Receives azygos arch posteriorly

III. Aortic Arch

A. Continuous with ascending aorta, lying on plane of sternal angle behind manubrium near midline

B. Crosses trachea, coursing toward left and posteriorly, giving off 3 branches

    1. Brachiocephalic trunk

        a. Passes toward right anterior to trachea

        b. Divides behind right sternoclavicular joint into right subclavian and common carotid arteries

    2. Left common carotid artery: passes upward along left side of trachea

    3. Left subclavian artery: arches over apex of lung

IV. Phrenic Nerves (Fig. 1.20C,D)

A. Pass between subclavian vein and artery on both sides

B. Lies along right side of superior vena cava on right and crosses aortic arch laterally on left

C. Pass anterior to lung roots, barely embedded within fibrous pericardial sac, to reach diaphragm

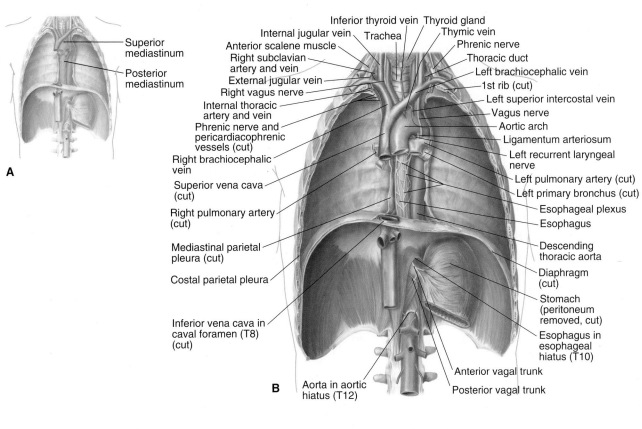

Superior mediastinum

Posterior mediastinum

A

Inferior thyroid vein — Thyroid gland
Internal jugular vein — Trachea — Thyroid gland
Anterior scalene muscle — Thymic vein
Right subclavian artery and vein — Phrenic nerve
External jugular vein — Thoracic duct
Right vagus nerve — Left brachiocephalic vein
Internal thoracic artery and vein — 1st rib (cut)
Phrenic nerve and pericardiacophrenic vessels (cut) — Left superior intercostal vein
Right brachiocephalic vein — Vagus nerve
Superior vena cava (cut) — Aortic arch
Right pulmonary artery (cut) — Ligamentum arteriosum
Mediastinal parietal pleura (cut) — Left recurrent laryngeal nerve
Costal parietal pleura — Left pulmonary artery (cut)
Left primary bronchus (cut)
Esophageal plexus
Esophagus
Descending thoracic aorta
Diaphragm (cut)
Stomach (peritoneum removed, cut)
Esophagus in esophageal hiatus (T10)
Inferior vena cava in caval foramen (T8) (cut)
Aorta in aortic hiatus (T12)
Anterior vagal trunk
Posterior vagal trunk

B

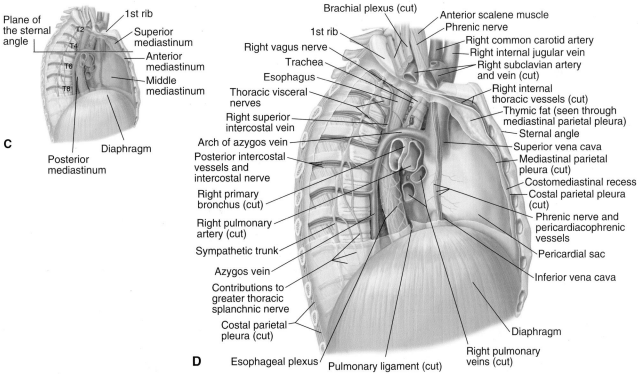

Plane of the sternal angle
1st rib
T2
T4
Superior mediastinum
Anterior mediastinum
T6
Middle mediastinum
T8
Posterior mediastinum
Diaphragm

C

Brachial plexus (cut) — Anterior scalene muscle
1st rib — Phrenic nerve
Right vagus nerve — Right common carotid artery
Trachea — Right internal jugular vein
Esophagus — Right subclavian artery and vein (cut)
Thoracic visceral nerves — Right internal thoracic vessels (cut)
Right superior intercostal vein — Thymic fat (seen through mediastinal parietal pleura)
Arch of azygos vein — Sternal angle
Posterior intercostal vessels and intercostal nerve — Superior vena cava
Right primary bronchus (cut) — Mediastinal parietal pleura (cut)
Right pulmonary artery (cut) — Costomediastinal recess
Sympathetic trunk — Costal parietal pleura (cut)
Azygos vein — Phrenic nerve and pericardiacophrenic vessels
Contributions to greater thoracic splanchnic nerve — Pericardial sac
Costal parietal pleura (cut) — Inferior vena cava
Esophageal plexus — Diaphragm
Pulmonary ligament (cut) — Right pulmonary veins (cut)

D

FIG. 1.20A–D. Superior and Posterior Mediastinum. **A.** Anterior View. **B.** Anterior Structures, Anterior View. **C.** Orientation, Right Lateral View. **D.** Right Lateral View.

V. Vagus nerves (Fig. I.20E,F)

A. Both nerves enter chest lateral to common carotid arteries and posterior to beginning of brachiocephalic veins

B. Right vagus gives off right recurrent laryngeal under right subclavian artery, then lies lateral to trachea and medial to azygos arch

C. Left vagus lies laterally on aortic arch, giving off left recurrent laryngeal, which wraps beneath arch behind ligamentum arteriosum, connecting left pulmonary artery to undersurface of aortic arch

D. Both vagus nerves pass behind roots of lungs

VI. Trachea (Fig. I.20G–I)

A. Lies behind aortic arch, anterior to esophagus, near midline

B. Common carotid arteries ascend to lie laterally

C. Recurrent laryngeal nerves lie within tracheoesophageal groove

D. Ends at sternal angle by branching into primary bronchi

VII. Esophagus

A. Arises in neck as continuation of laryngopharynx

B. Passes through superior mediastinum posterior to trachea

C. Thoracic duct lies along left side in superior mediastinum

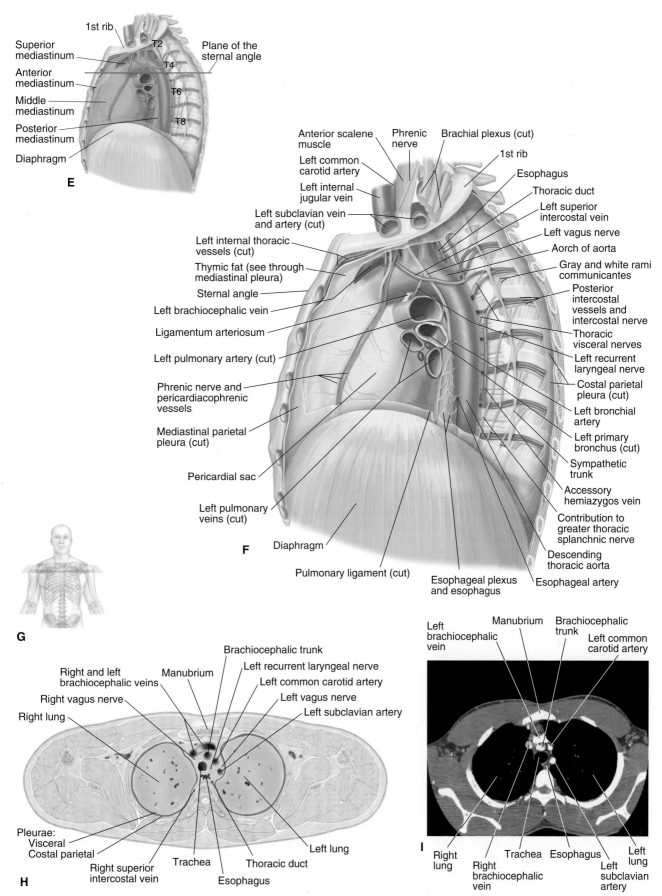

1st rib

Superior mediastinum

Anterior mediastinum

Middle mediastinum

Posterior mediastinum

Diaphragm

T2

T4

T6

T8

Plane of the sternal angle

E

Anterior scalene muscle

Phrenic nerve

Brachial plexus (cut)

Left common carotid artery

1st rib

Esophagus

Left internal jugular vein

Thoracic duct

Left subclavian vein and artery (cut)

Left superior intercostal vein

Left internal thoracic vessels (cut)

Left vagus nerve

Aorch of aorta

Thymic fat (see through mediastinal pleura)

Gray and white rami communicantes

Sternal angle

Posterior intercostal vessels and intercostal nerve

Left brachiocephalic vein

Ligamentum arteriosum

Thoracic visceral nerves

Left pulmonary artery (cut)

Left recurrent laryngeal nerve

Phrenic nerve and pericardiacophrenic vessels

Costal parietal pleura (cut)

Mediastinal parietal pleura (cut)

Left bronchial artery

Left primary bronchus (cut)

Pericardial sac

Sympathetic trunk

Accessory hemiazygos vein

Left pulmonary veins (cut)

Contribution to greater thoracic splanchnic nerve

F

Diaphragm

Descending thoracic aorta

Pulmonary ligament (cut)

Esophageal plexus and esophagus

Esophageal artery

G

Right and left brachiocephalic veins

Manubrium

Brachiocephalic trunk

Left recurrent laryngeal nerve

Right vagus nerve

Left common carotid artery

Right lung

Left vagus nerve

Left subclavian artery

Left brachiocephalic vein

Manubrium

Brachiocephalic trunk

Left common carotid artery

Pleurae:
Visceral
Costal parietal

Right superior intercostal vein

Trachea

Thoracic duct

Left lung

Esophagus

H

I

Right lung

Right brachiocephalic vein

Trachea

Esophagus

Left subclavian artery

Left lung

FIG. I.20E–I. E. Superior and Posterior Mediastinum, Orientation, Left Lateral View. **F.** Left Lateral View. **G.** Orientation of Cross Section at T2 Vertebral Level, Anterior View. **H.** Cross Section of Thorax at T2 Vertebral Level. **I.** CT Image at T2 Vertebral Level.

Posterior Mediastinum

I. Esophagus (Fig. 1.21A–D)

A. Descends along right side of descending thoracic aorta and then crosses in front and to left of aorta

B. Passes through esophageal hiatus of diaphragm at T10

II. Vessels

A. Descending thoracic aorta: on left side of posterior mediastinum (Fig. 1.21E)
   1. Origins of posterior intercostal arteries 3–11 (paired)
   2. Left bronchial arteries (2)
   3. Several esophageal arteries
   4. Inferior phrenic arteries (paired)

B. Azygos vein (Fig. 1.21F)
   1. Originates as union of right subcostal and right ascending lumbar veins
   2. Most posterior structure on right side of posterior mediastinum
   3. Receives terminations of right posterior intercostal veins, right bronchial vein, esophageal veins
   4. Drains to posterior surface of superior vena cava as azygos arch over root of right lung and receives right superior intercostal vein from posterior intercostal veins 2–4 on right

C. Hemiazygos vein
   1. Originates as union of left subcostal and left ascending lumbar vein
   2. Receives posterior intercostal veins 9–11, esophageal veins
   3. Ascends posteriorly on left behind aorta and then crosses midline to join azygos at T9 level, passing behind aorta, thoracic duct, and esophagus

D. Accessory hemiazygos vein
   1. Union of posterior intercostal veins from spaces 5–8; receives left bronchial veins
   2. Crosses midline at T7 or T8 behind aorta and thoracic duct to join azygos vein; may join the hemiazygos as well

E. Other chest wall veins
   1. 1st posterior intercostal veins drain into respective subclavian veins
   2. Superior intercostal veins
      a. Union of posterior intercostal veins 2–4
      b. Drains to azygos arch on right and upward to left brachiocephalic vein on left, lying on aortic arch and left vagus nerve

F. Thoracic duct
   1. Begins at level of L2 beneath right crus of diaphragm, to right of aorta, as occasional dilation called **cisterna chyli** formed by union of right and left lumbar lymph trunks and intestinal trunk
   2. Enters thorax through aortic hiatus (T12 level)
   3. Lies anterior to anterior longitudinal ligament and right posterior intercostal arteries, between azygos vein and descending thoracic aorta
   4. Ascends posterior to esophagus until plane of sternal angle (T4/T5 disc), then deviates to left side of esophagus to continue ascent
   5. Arches forward and to left to drain into union of left internal jugular and subclavian veins
   6. Tributaries: from upper lumbar nodes, lymph nodes in lower posterior intercostal spaces, nodes in posterior intercostal spaces on left side, posterior mediastinal nodes, left jugular, subclavian, and bronchomediastinal lymph trunks near its termination

III. Nerves (Fig. 1.21G)

A. Vagus
   1. Right: enters posterior mediastinum behind root of lung; supplies multiple short branches to posterior pulmonary plexus and then passes onto posterior surface of esophagus to become part of esophageal plexus
   2. Left: passes posterior to root of lung; supplies multiple short branches to posterior pulmonary plexus and then passes onto anterior surface of esophagus to become part of esophageal plexus

B. Thoracic splanchnic nerves: considered with thoracic sympathetic trunk

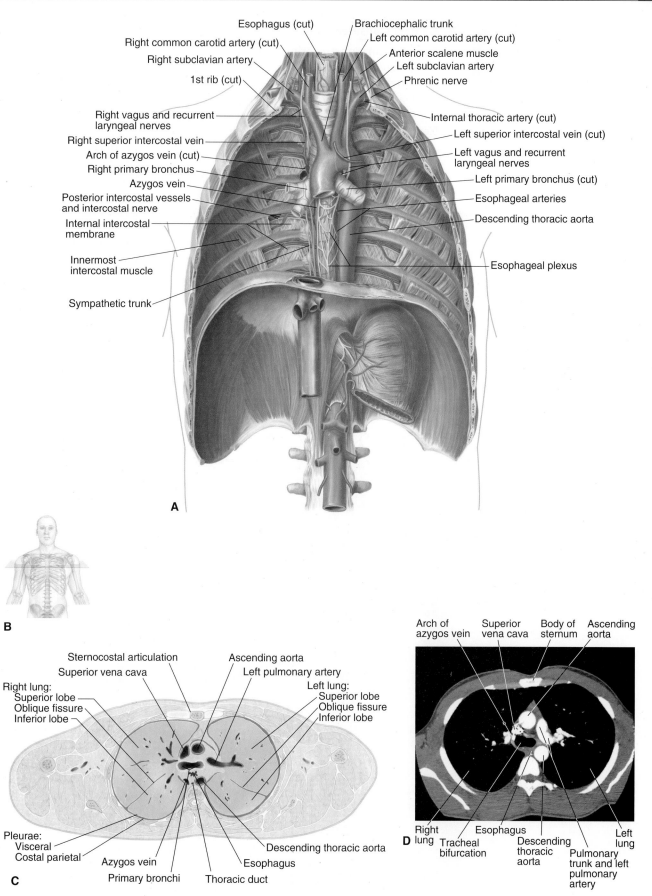

Esophagus (cut)
Brachiocephalic trunk
Right common carotid artery (cut)
Left common carotid artery (cut)
Right subclavian artery
Anterior scalene muscle
Left subclavian artery
1st rib (cut)
Phrenic nerve
Right vagus and recurrent laryngeal nerves
Internal thoracic artery (cut)
Right superior intercostal vein
Left superior intercostal vein (cut)
Arch of azygos vein (cut)
Left vagus and recurrent laryngeal nerves
Right primary bronchus
Left primary bronchus (cut)
Azygos vein
Esophageal arteries
Posterior intercostal vessels and intercostal nerve
Descending thoracic aorta
Internal intercostal membrane
Innermost intercostal muscle
Esophageal plexus
Sympathetic trunk

A

B

Sternocostal articulation
Ascending aorta
Superior vena cava
Left pulmonary artery
Right lung:
 Superior lobe
 Oblique fissure
 Inferior lobe
Left lung:
 Superior lobe
 Oblique fissure
 Inferior lobe
Pleurae:
 Visceral
 Costal parietal
Descending thoracic aorta
Azygos vein
Esophagus
Primary bronchi
Thoracic duct

C

Arch of azygos vein
Superior vena cava
Body of sternum
Ascending aorta
Right lung
Esophagus
Left lung
Tracheal bifurcation
Descending thoracic aorta
Pulmonary trunk and left pulmonary artery

D

FIG. 1.21A–D. A. Superior and Posterior Mediastinum, Anterior View. **B.** Orientation of Cross Section at T5 Vertebral Level, Anterior View. **C.** Cross Section of Thorax at T5 Vertebral Level. **D.** CT Image at T5 Vertebral Level.

IV. Clinical Considerations

A. Aortic aneurysm: ascending aorta or aortic arch may develop an aneurysm, which can be seen on a chest radiograph or MRI angiogram
   1. Patient often has chest pain radiating to back
   2. Dilation may exert pressure on the trachea, esophagus, and left recurrent laryngeal nerve resulting in difficulty in swallowing and breathing

B. Coarctation of aorta
   1. Narrowing of aortic arch or descending aorta that produces obstruction to blood flow to lower part of body
   2. Most commonly seen near ligamentum arteriosum as result of abnormal distribution of smooth muscle associated with ductus arteriosus

C. Chylothorax: leakage of lymph into pleural cavity (chylothorax) at ≈60 to 190 mL/h
   1. Because thoracic duct is very thin walled and carries colorless or white lymph (depending on fat content), it is not as easily seen as blood vessels and may be injured inadvertently during surgery in posterior mediastinum
   2. Also may be ruptured by trauma

D. Azygos system of veins receives esophageal veins, which may become enlarged due to portal hypertension and retrograde passage of blood through left gastric tributaries of esophagus

E. Azygos system of veins is highly variable

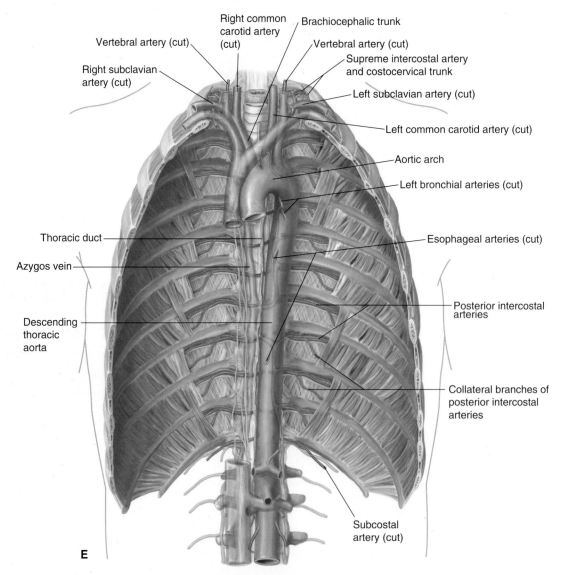

E

FIG. 1.21E. Arteries of the Posterior Thoracic Wall, Anterior View.

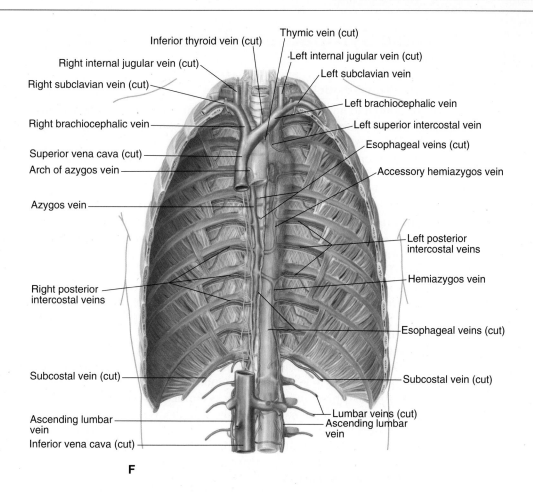

Inferior thyroid vein (cut)
Thymic vein (cut)
Right internal jugular vein (cut)
Left internal jugular vein (cut)
Right subclavian vein (cut)
Left subclavian vein
Right brachiocephalic vein
Left brachiocephalic vein
Left superior intercostal vein
Superior vena cava (cut)
Esophageal veins (cut)
Arch of azygos vein
Accessory hemiazygos vein
Azygos vein
Left posterior intercostal veins
Hemiazygos vein
Right posterior intercostal veins
Esophageal veins (cut)
Subcostal vein (cut)
Subcostal vein (cut)
Lumbar veins (cut)
Ascending lumbar vein
Ascending lumbar vein
Inferior vena cava (cut)

F

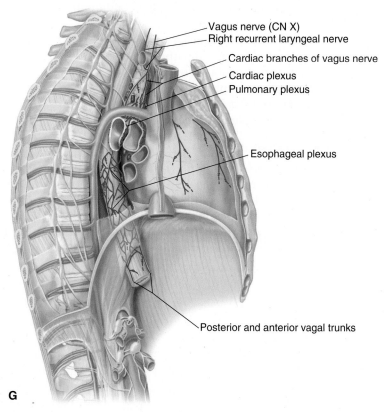

Vagus nerve (CN X)
Right recurrent laryngeal nerve
Cardiac branches of vagus nerve
Cardiac plexus
Pulmonary plexus
Esophageal plexus
Posterior and anterior vagal trunks

G

FIG. 1.21F,G. F. Veins of the Posterior Thoracic Wall, Anterior View. **G.** Vagus Nerve, Right Lateral View.

Thoracic Sympathetic Trunk

I. Thoracic Sympathetic Trunk (Fig. 1.22A,B)

A. Not considered to lie in posterior mediastinum; covered by costal parietal pleura

B. Bilateral chains of ganglia, usually 12 pairs, corresponding to each thoracic nerve; located on or near heads of ribs bilaterally

  1. Interganglionic rami connect adjacent ganglia, crossing posterior intercostal vessels anteriorly

  2. Presynaptic fibers

    a. Arise in intermediolateral cell column of entire thoracic spinal cord and leave cord through anterior roots of spinal nerves

    b. Leave anterior rami of spinal nerves through **white rami communicantes** to join thoracic sympathetic trunk

      i. These may synapse in a ganglion at level of origin

      ii. They may pass superiorly (T1–T4 or 5) to form cervical sympathetic trunk or inferiorly (T9–T12 and L1–L2) to form lumbar and sacral sympathetic trunk

      iii. Some pass through thoracic chain to enter abdomen as **thoracic splanchnic nerves**

  3. Postsynaptic fibers

    a. From thoracic sympathetic ganglia, postsynaptic fibers may return to anterior rami of spinal nerves as **gray rami communicantes**,

    b. Or, they may pass anteroinferiorly as **thoracic visceral nerves** (T1– T4/T5) to enter the cardiac, pulmonary, and esophageal plexuses

C. Thoracic splanchnic nerves

  1. Arise from thoracic sympathetic ganglia, pass anteroinferiorly to lie on vertebral bodies, and enter abdomen by passing through crura of diaphragm

  2. **Greater thoracic splanchnic**

    a. From thoracic sympathetic ganglia T5–T9

    b. Synapses in celiac ganglion, although some fibers synapse directly on cells of suprarenal medulla

  3. **Lesser thoracic splanchnic**

    a. From thoracic sympathetic ganglia T10–T11

    b. Synapses in aorticorenal ganglion

  4. **Least thoracic splanchnic** (inconstant)

    a. From thoracic sympathetic ganglion T12

    b. Synapses in renal plexus

II. Clinical Considerations

A. Because fibers from upper thoracic sympathetic trunk pass upward to create cervical sympathetic trunk, lesions of upper thoracic trunk may lead to **Horner syndrome**, characterized by ptosis (drooping eyelid), miosis (constricted pupil), anhydrosis (lack of sweating), and enophthalmos (sunken eyeball)

B. To treat hyperhydrosis of hand, intentional lesion of upper thoracic sympathetic trunk may be made, which may cause Horner syndrome

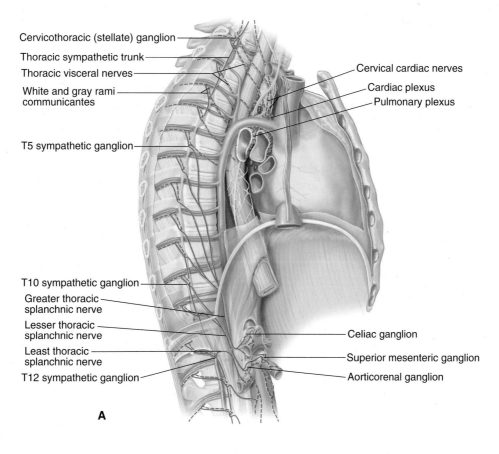

Cervicothoracic (stellate) ganglion

Thoracic sympathetic trunk

Thoracic visceral nerves

White and gray rami communicantes

T5 sympathetic ganglion

T10 sympathetic ganglion

Greater thoracic splanchnic nerve

Lesser thoracic splanchnic nerve

Least thoracic splanchnic nerve

T12 sympathetic ganglion

Cervical cardiac nerves

Cardiac plexus

Pulmonary plexus

Celiac ganglion

Superior mesenteric ganglion

Aorticorenal ganglion

A

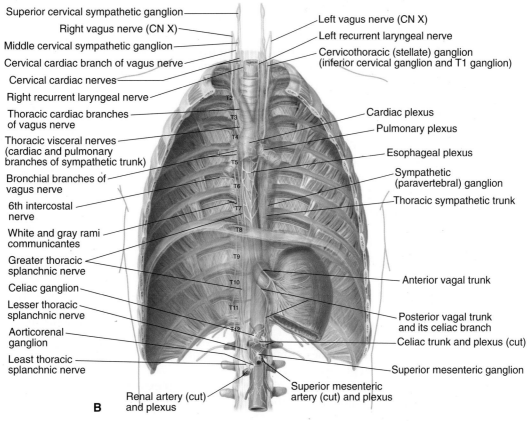

Superior cervical sympathetic ganglion

Right vagus nerve (CN X)

Middle cervical sympathetic ganglion

Cervical cardiac branch of vagus nerve

Cervical cardiac nerves

Right recurrent laryngeal nerve

Thoracic cardiac branches of vagus nerve

Thoracic visceral nerves (cardiac and pulmonary branches of sympathetic trunk)

Bronchial branches of vagus nerve

6th intercostal nerve

White and gray rami communicantes

Greater thoracic splanchnic nerve

Celiac ganglion

Lesser thoracic splanchnic nerve

Aorticorenal ganglion

Least thoracic splanchnic nerve

Left vagus nerve (CN X)

Left recurrent laryngeal nerve

Cervicothoracic (stellate) ganglion (inferior cervical ganglion and T1 ganglion)

Cardiac plexus

Pulmonary plexus

Esophageal plexus

Sympathetic (paravertebral) ganglion

Thoracic sympathetic trunk

Anterior vagal trunk

Posterior vagal trunk and its celiac branch

Celiac trunk and plexus (cut)

Superior mesenteric ganglion

Superior mesenteric artery (cut) and plexus

Renal artery (cut) and plexus

B

FIG. 1.22A,B. A. Sympathetic Nerves In the Thorax, Right Lateral View. **B.** Autonomic Nerves In the Thorax, Anterior View.

Esophagus

I. Extent (Fig. 1.23)

A. Fibromuscular tube from laryngopharynx at level of cricoid cartilage (6th cervical vertebra) to stomach at the level of the 11th thoracic vertebra
B. ≈25 to 30 cm long

II. Course

A. Generally vertically downward but with 2 curvatures
   1. Deviates to left, remains to left through root of neck, gradually reaches midline at T4/T5 intervertebral disc
   2. Shifts toward left as it moves anteriorly toward esophageal hiatus in diaphragm; has posteroanterior flexures corresponding to curves of vertebral column
B. Esophageal hiatus: passes through diaphragm (right crus fibers) at level of T10

III. Relations

A. Cervical portion
   1. Anterior: trachea; recurrent laryngeal nerves ascend in groove between trachea and esophagus
   2. Posterior: vertebral column, prevertebral musculature, sympathetic trunks (posterolaterally)
   3. Lateral: thyroid gland and carotid sheath
B. Thoracic portion
   1. Anterior: trachea, left bronchus, pericardium, left vagus, diaphragm
   2. Posterior: vertebral column, longus colli muscle, right posterior intercostal arteries, thoracic duct, right vagus, descending thoracic aorta (at inferior end)
   3. Left side: aortic arch, left subclavian artery, thoracic duct (posterolateral above T4/T5 disc), pleura, descending aorta
   4. Right side: azygos vein (posterolateral), pleura, right vagus
C. Abdominal portion: short (1 cm); enters stomach at cardia
   1. Right border continuous with lesser curvature of stomach
   2. Left border separated from stomach fundus by cardiac notch
   3. At inferior end, gastroesophageal junction, is **esophageal sphincter**

IV. Blood Supply

A. Arteries
   1. Cervical portion: inferior thyroid artery from thyrocervical trunk
   2. Several small esophageal arteries from descending thoracic aorta
   3. Bronchial arteries
   4. Ascending branch from left gastric artery
   5. Small branches from inferior phrenic arteries
B. Veins
   1. Drain into inferior thyroid, azygos, hemiazygos, accessory hemiazygos, left superior intercostal, left gastric veins
   2. Drainage into gastric veins is site of anastomosis between portal and systemic systems

V. Nerves

A. Recurrent laryngeal nerves supply striated muscle in upper third of organ
B. Parasympathetic
   1. Esophageal branches: from vagi, above root of lung
   2. Esophageal plexus
      a. Below root of lung, vagi form esophageal plexus around esophagus
      b. Postganglionic sympathetic fibers also enter plexus
C. Sympathetic
   1. From upper 4 or 5 thoracic ganglia directly or through branches from cardiac or pulmonary plexuses
   2. From lower thoracic ganglia and thoracic splanchnic nerves

VI. Clinical Considerations

A. Esophageal varices

1. Above diaphragm, esophagus drains to azygos system primarily (systemic or caval system); below diaphragm, tributaries reach left gastric vein (portal system)

2. In portal hypertension, blood may flow retrogradely up left gastric tributaries, greatly dilating these vessels and resulting in varicose veins of lower esophagus

3. One cause of death from portal hypertension is esophageal hemorrhage from rupture of varicose submucosal veins

4. Esophageal constrictions: may be seen in thoracic esophagus

    a. Narrowings of lumen seen in oblique chest radiograms during barium swallow

    b. Esophagus is usually compressed by 4 structures: cricopharyngeus muscle at its beginning, aortic arch, left main bronchus, and diaphragm

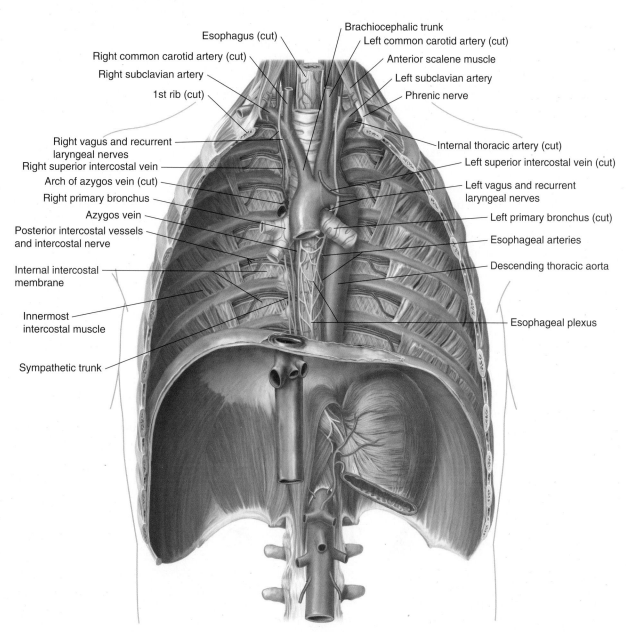

FIG. I.23. Esophagus and Its Relations, Anterior View.

Thoracic Lymphatics

I. Introduction

A. Mediastinal lymph node involvement is common in diseases of chest wall, breast, diaphragm, and intraabdominal or retroperitoneal structures; patterns of nodal enlargement offer clues to origin or nature of disease process

B. Intrathoracic lymph nodes
1. Parietal mediastinal nodes: drain thoracic wall and extrathoracic tissues
2. Visceral mediastinal nodes: concerned with intrathoracic structures
3. Extensive connections exist between parietal and visceral nodal groups as well as within the visceral group itself; 3 mediastinal zones (compartments) described

II. Posterior Mediastinal Zone (Compartment) (Fig. 1.24A)

A. Intercostal (parietal) group: in intercostal spaces and paravertebral areas
1. Afferents: drain intercostal spaces, parietal pleura, and vertebral column
2. Efferents: communicate with posterior mediastinal group and have efferent channels that drain to thoracic duct

B. Posterior mediastinal (visceral) group: along lower esophagus and descending thoracic aorta
1. Afferents
   a. Drain posterior diaphragm, pericardium, esophagus
   b. Communicate with tracheobronchial nodes
2. Efferents: drain predominantly via the thoracic duct

III. Middle Mediastinal Zone (Compartment)

A. Parietal group found mainly around pericardial attachment to diaphragm
1. Afferents: drain diaphragm and parts of liver
2. Efferents: pass anteriorly to parasternal or anterior mediastinal nodes and posteriorly to posterior mediastinal nodes

B. Bronchopulmonary and tracheobronchial nodes
1. Bronchopulmonary nodes: within lung hilum
   a. Afferents: from pulmonary nodes, superficial and deep pulmonary lymphatic plexuses
   b. Efferents: drain to superior and inferior tracheobronchial nodes
2. Inferior tracheobronchial (carinal) nodes: along anterior and inferior aspects of tracheal bifurcation
   a. Afferents: from bronchopulmonary nodes, anterior and posterior mediastinal nodes, heart, pericardium, esophagus
   b. Efferents: drain primarily to right superior tracheobronchial nodes
3. Superior tracheobronchial nodes: located beside tracheal bifurcation, being more numerous on right than left
   a. Azygos node: constant node in right superior tracheobronchial angle near azygos vein
   b. Afferents
      i. From bronchopulmonary nodes, trachea, esophagus
      ii. Communicate with anterior and posterior mediastinal nodes
   c. Efferents: to paratracheal nodes, bronchomediastinal trunks, or right lymphatic or thoracic duct

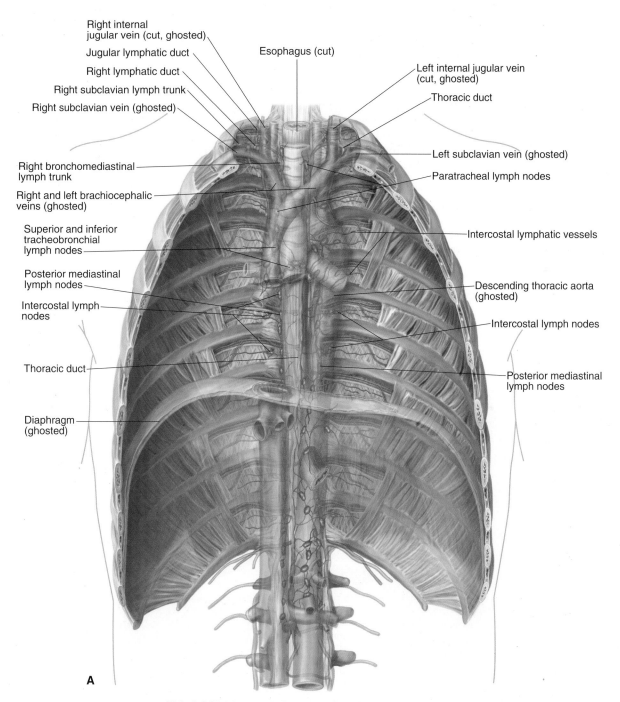

Right internal
jugular vein (cut, ghosted)

Jugular lymphatic duct

Right lymphatic duct

Right subclavian lymph trunk

Right subclavian vein (ghosted)

Esophagus (cut)

Left internal jugular vein
(cut, ghosted)

Thoracic duct

Right bronchomediastinal
lymph trunk

Right and left brachiocephalic
veins (ghosted)

Superior and inferior
tracheobronchial
lymph nodes

Posterior mediastinal
lymph nodes

Intercostal lymph
nodes

Thoracic duct

Diaphragm
(ghosted)

Left subclavian vein (ghosted)

Paratracheal lymph nodes

Intercostal lymphatic vessels

Descending thoracic aorta
(ghosted)

Intercostal lymph nodes

Posterior mediastinal
lymph nodes

A

FIG. 1.24A. Lymphatic Drainage of the Thorax, Anterior View.

IV. Anterior Mediastinal Zone (Compartment) (Fig. 1.24B)

  A. Parasternal group found extrapleurally
    1. Nodes are scattered along internal thoracic arteries and behind anterior intercostal spaces and costal cartilages; a few are directly retrosternal
    2. Afferents
      a. Drain anterior abdominal and thoracic walls, anterior diaphragm, medial parts of breast
      b. Communicate with anterior mediastinal visceral and cervical nodes
    3. Efferents: bronchomediastinal trunks or directly to the right lymphatic on right and thoracic duct on left
  B. Anterior mediastinal group
    1. Most nodes are located along superior vena cava and brachiocephalic veins on right and in front of aorta and carotid artery on left
    2. Afferents: drain mediastinal structures including pericardium, part of heart, thymus, thyroid, diaphragmatic and mediastinal pleura, roots of lungs, bilaterally
    3. Efferents: drain into bronchomediastinal trunk (or right lymphatic or thoracic duct)

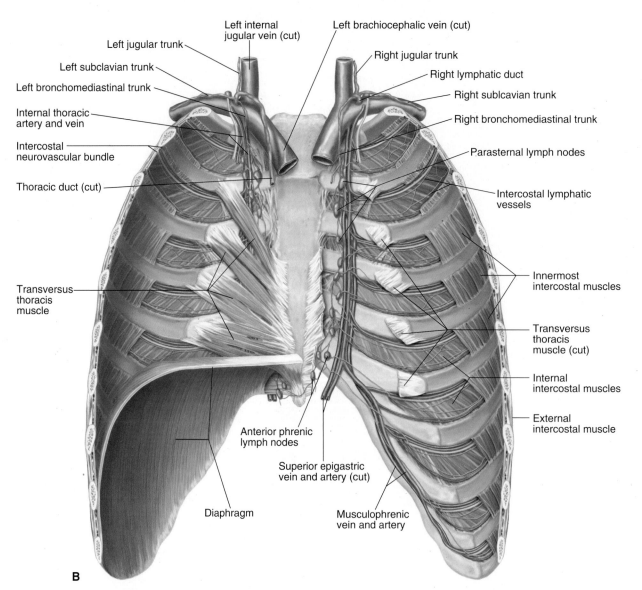

FIG. 1.24B. Lymphatic Drainage of the Thorax, Anterior Chest Wall, Posterior View

Abdomen

Surface Anatomy of the Abdominal Wall

I. Landmark Lines and Planes (Fig. 2.1A)

A. **Midclavicular** or **midinguinal line**: vertical line drawn inferiorly from point halfway between midline and tip of acromion; bisects inguinal ligament vertically

B. **Transumbilical plane**: transverse plane passing through umbilicus

C. **Transpyloric plane**: transverse plane passing halfway between jugular notch and upper border of pubic symphysis; crosses tips of 9th costal cartilages anteriorly and lower 1st lumbar vertebra posteriorly

D. **Subcostal plane**: passes beneath lowest point of costal margin on each side; indicates inferior margin of 10th costal cartilages; lies at level of intervertebral disc between L2 and L3 vertebrae

E. **Intertubercular (transtubercular) plane**: at level of iliac tubercles; crosses body of 5th lumbar vertebra posteriorly

F. **Interspinous plane**: passes through anterior superior iliac spines and sacral promontory

II. Abdominal Quadrants

A. Created by midline and transumbilical plane

B. 4 quadrants
1. Upper right: primarily liver and gallbladder
2. Upper left: primarily stomach and spleen
3. Lower right: primarily cecum, ascending colon, small bowel
4. Lower left: primarily descending and sigmoid colon, small bowel

III. Abdominal Regions (Fig. 2.1C)

A. Created by midclavicular lines and subcostal and intertubercular planes

B. 9 regions
1. **Epigastric region**
   a. Above subcostal plane and between 2 midclavicular lines
   b. Contains pylorus
2. **Right hypochondriac region**
   a. Above subcostal plane and to right of right midclavicular line
   b. Contains liver and hepatic flexure
3. **Left hypochondriac region**
   a. Above subcostal plane and to left of left midclavicular line
   b. Contains spleen and splenic flexure
4. **Umbilical region**
   a. Between subcostal and intertubercular planes and 2 midclavicular lines
   b. Contains jejunum
5. **Right lumbar region**
   a. Between subcostal and intertubercular planes and to right of right midclavicular line
   b. Contains ascending colon
6. **Left lumbar region**
   a. Between subcostal and intertubercular planes and to left of left midclavicular line
   b. Contains descending colon
7. **Hypogastric region**
   a. Below intertubercular plane and between 2 midclavicular lines
   b. Contains rectum and bladder
8. **Right inguinal region**
   a. Below intertubercular plane and to right of right midclavicular line
   b. Contains cecum
9. **Left inguinal region**
   a. Below intertubercular plane and to left of left midclavicular line
   b. Contains sigmoid colon

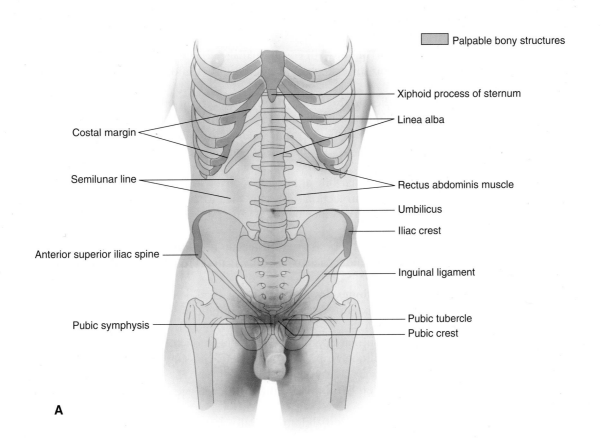

Palpable bony structures

Xiphoid process of sternum

Linea alba

Costal margin

Rectus abdominis muscle

Semilunar line

Umbilicus

Iliac crest

Anterior superior iliac spine

Inguinal ligament

Pubic symphysis

Pubic tubercle

Pubic crest

A

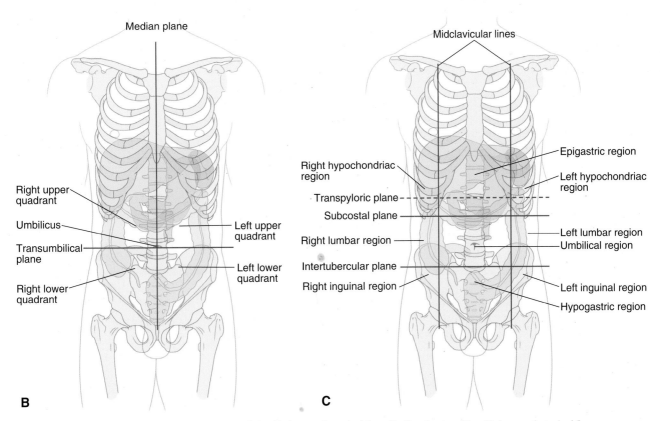

Median plane

Right upper quadrant

Umbilicus

Transumbilical plane

Left upper quadrant

Left lower quadrant

Right lower quadrant

B

Midclavicular lines

Right hypochondriac region

Epigastric region

Left hypochondriac region

Transpyloric plane

Subcostal plane

Right lumbar region

Left lumbar region

Umbilical region

Intertubercular plane

Right inguinal region

Left inguinal region

Hypogastric region

C

FIG. 2.1A–C. **A.** Palpable Features of the Abdomen, Anterior View. **B.** Quadrants of the Abdomen, Anterior View. **C.** Regions of the Abdomen, Anterior View.

IV. Surface Projections of Major Viscera

A. Stomach
 1. Cardiac orifice is behind 7th costal cartilage, 2.5 cm lateral to left border of sternum
 2. Pylorus is on transpyloric plane, 1 cm to right of midline
B. Duodenum
 1. Superior part lies on the transpyloric plane to right of midline
 2. Duodenojejunal flexure lies on transpyloric plane, 2.5 cm to left of midline
C. Ileocecal junction: just below and medial to junction of right midclavicular and intertubercular lines
D. Base of appendix
 1. On right midclavicular line at level of anterior superior iliac spine
 2. **McBurney point**: projection of usual location of base of appendix onto anterior abdominal wall; 1/3 distance between right anterior superior iliac spine and umbilicus
E. Liver
 1. Upper limit of right lobe is at xiphisternal junction; line is continued to right to 5th costal cartilage in midclavicular line, then curves to right and down to 7th rib at side of thorax
 2. Right border continues downward to point 1 cm below costal arch
 3. Upper left limit extends from xiphisternal joint to left 6th costal cartilage 5 cm from midline
 4. Lower limit runs upward parallel to and 1 cm below costal margin to 9th costal cartilage, then extends obliquely upward toward left, crossing midline just above transpyloric plane to 8th costal cartilage
F. Fundus of gallbladder: behind 9th right costal cartilage
G. Umbilicus
 1. Most obvious marking on abdominal wall
 2. Puckered scar representing former site of attachment of umbilical cord in fetus
 3. Position varies, but usually at level of intervertebral disc between L3 and L4

Superficial Veins, Cutaneous Nerves, and Superficial Fascia of the Abdominal Wall

I. Superficial Veins (Fig. 2.2A)

A. **Lateral thoracic vein**
   1. Drains from upper anterolateral abdominal and thoracic wall, including venous plexus of mammary gland
   2. Drains to axillary vein

B. **Superficial epigastric vein**
   1. Drains from anterior abdominal wall below umbilicus
   2. Drains to proximal end of great saphenous vein at saphenous hiatus

C. **Superficial circumflex iliac vein**
   1. Drains from lower lateral abdominal wall and upper thigh
   2. Drains to proximal end of great saphenous vein at saphenous hiatus

D. **Superficial external pudendal vein**
   1. Drains from superficial tissues of penis/clitoris and pubic region
   2. Drains to proximal end of great saphenous vein at saphenous hiatus

E. **Thoracoepigastric vein**
   1. Frequent connection between lateral thoracic and tributaries to superficial epigastric and superficial circumflex iliac veins
   2. Terminates in both axillary and great saphenous veins

II. Cutaneous Nerves

A. **Thoracoabdominal nerves**
   1. Lower intercostal nerves (T7–T11) and subcostal nerve (T12)
   2. Pass deep to costal margin to descend obliquely between internal abdominal oblique and transversus abdominis muscles
   3. Give lateral and anterior cutaneous branches
      a. Lateral cutaneous branch of T12 supplies skin over hip
      b. Anterior cutaneous branch of T10 supplies skin around umbilicus
      c. Anterior cutaneous branches penetrate rectus abdominis muscle and anterior lamina of rectus sheath to reach skin

B. **Iliohypogastric** and **ilioinguinal nerves**
   1. Branch from L1 from lumbar plexus usually as common trunk that divides variably on inner aspect of posterior abdominal wall
   2. Lateral cutaneous branches supply skin of upper lateral buttock
   3. Anterior cutaneous branches
      a. Iliohypogastric distributes over pubis
      b. Anterior cutaneous branch of ilioinguinal becomes anterior labial or anterior scrotal branch for skin of this region

C. Dermatomes of the abdominal wall (Fig. 2.2B,C)
   1. Follow oblique linear distributions of thoracoabdominal nerves
   2. Key dermatome landmarks
      a. T7 located over xiphoid process
      b. T10 located around umbilicus
      c. T12 located suprapubically

III. Superficial Fascia

A. 2 layers that become more distinct in lower anterior abdominal wall
   1. Outer fatty layer (Camper fascia)
      a. Varies greatly in thickness
      b. Generally thickens inferiorly, pronounced over iliac crests laterally
   2. Inner membranous layer (Scarpa fascia)
      a. Covers investing fascia of external abdominal oblique muscle
      b. Attaches inferior to inguinal ligament to fascia lata of upper thigh

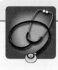

IV. Clinical Considerations

A. Enlargement of thoracoepigastric vein
  1. May result from blockage of either superior or inferior vena cava
  2. To determine which vena cava is obstructed
      a. Compress segment of dilated vein between 2 fingers
      b. When fingers alternately lift, the direction from which vein refills most rapidly indicates direction of blood flow

B. **Portal hypertension**
  1. Restriction of portal blood flow through liver
      a. Due to cirrhosis or cancer
      b. May enlarge small **paraumbilical veins** that lie within falciform ligament of liver
  2. Enlarged paraumbilical veins carry blood to veins of anterior abdominal wall, causing their enlargement or varicosity
  3. Varicose anterior abdominal wall veins present as **caput medusae** due to tortuous veins radiating from umbilicus

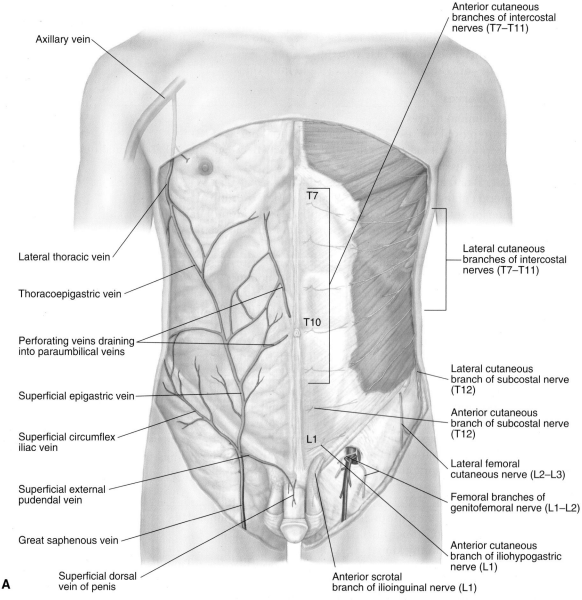

FIG. 2.2A. Superficial Veins and Cutaneous Nerves of the Abdomen, Anterior View.

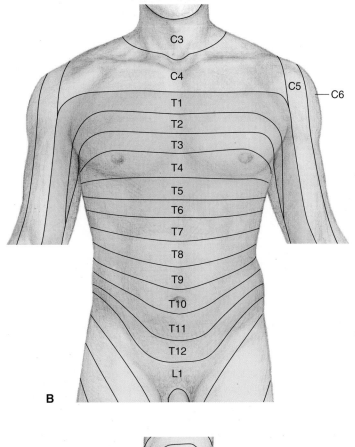

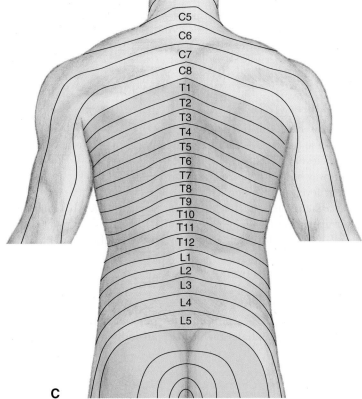

FIG. 2.2B,C. Dermatomes of the Thorax and Abdomen. **B.** Anterior View.
C. Posterior View.

Muscles of the Abdominal Wall

I. Muscles of the Abdominal Wall (Fig. 2.3A–D)

Muscle	Origin	Insertion	Action	Nerve
External abdominal oblique	Lower 8 ribs	Linea alba, pubic crest and tubercle, anterior superior iliac spine and anterior half of iliac crest	Flexes and laterally bends the trunk; compresses abdomen	Intercostal (T7–T11), subcostal (T12), iliohypogastric and ilioinguinal nerves (L1)
Internal abdominal oblique	Thoracolumbar fascia, anterior 2/3 of iliac crest, lateral 2/3 of inguinal ligament	Lower 3 or 4 ribs, linea alba, pubic crest, and pecten	Same as above	Same as above
Transversus abdominis	Lower 6 ribs, thoracolumbar fascia, anterior 3/4 of the iliac crest, lateral 1/3 of inguinal ligament	Linea alba, pubic crest, and pecten	Same as above	Same as above
Rectus abdominis	Pubic crest and symphysis	Xiphoid process of sternum and costal cartilages 5–7	Flexes trunk; compresses abdomen	Intercostal (T 7–T11) and subcostal nerves (T12)
Pyramidalis	Pubic crest, anterior to rectus abdominis	Linea alba	Draws linea alba inferiorly	Subcostal nerve (T12)
Quadratus lumborum	Posterior part of iliac crest and iliolumbar ligament	Transverse processes of L1–L4 and 12th rib	Laterally bends trunk, fixes 12th rib	Subcostal nerve (T12) and branches of anterior rami of spinal nerves L1–L4
Psoas major	Bodies and transverse processes of lumbar vertebrae	Lesser trochanter of femur (with iliacus) via iliopsoas tendon	Flexes thigh; flexes and laterally bends lumbar vertebral column	Branches of anterior rami of spinal nerves L2–L4
Iliacus	Iliac fossa and iliac crest; ala of sacrum	Lesser trochanter of femur (with psoas major)	Flexes thigh; if thigh is fixed, it flexes pelvis on thigh	Femoral nerve (L2–L4)
Cremaster	Inguinal ligament	Forms thin network of muscle fascicles around spermatic cord and testis (or round ligament of uterus within inguinal canal)	Elevates testis (not well developed in females)	Genital branch of genitofemoral nerve (L1–L2)

II. Special Features

A. **Tendinous intersections** or bands
   1. 3 transverse tendinous bands usually interrupt rectus abdominis muscle
      a. Near level of xiphoid
      b. Halfway between xiphoid and umbilicus
      c. Near level of umbilicus
   2. Firmly attached to anterior lamina of the rectus sheath, causing surface markings called **linea transversae** (marking "6-pack abs")
B. Compression of abdominal wall increases intraabdominal pressure, useful for bodily functions
   1. Forced exhalation (blowing)
   2. Defecation
   3. Parturition (childbearing)
   4. Heimlich maneuver: grasping choking person from behind and compressing abdominal wall causes forced exhalation and may dislodge foreign body from airway

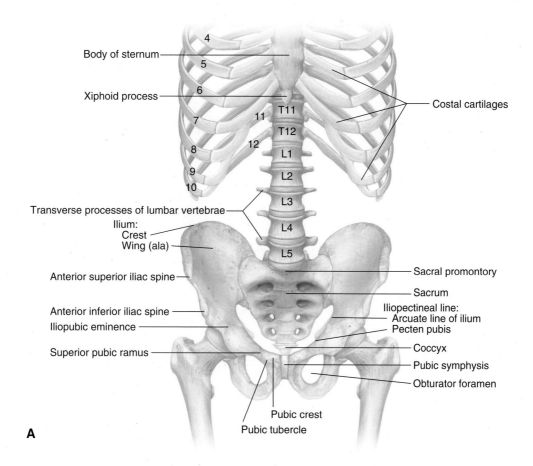

4
Body of sternum
5
Xiphoid process
6
T11
7   11
T12
8   12
L1
9
L2
10
L3
Transverse processes of lumbar vertebrae
L4
Ilium:
  Crest
  Wing (ala)
L5
Anterior superior iliac spine
Anterior inferior iliac spine
Iliopubic eminence
Superior pubic ramus

Costal cartilages
Sacral promontory
Sacrum
Iliopectineal line:
  Arcuate line of ilium
  Pecten pubis
Coccyx
Pubic symphysis
Obturator foramen

Pubic crest
Pubic tubercle

A

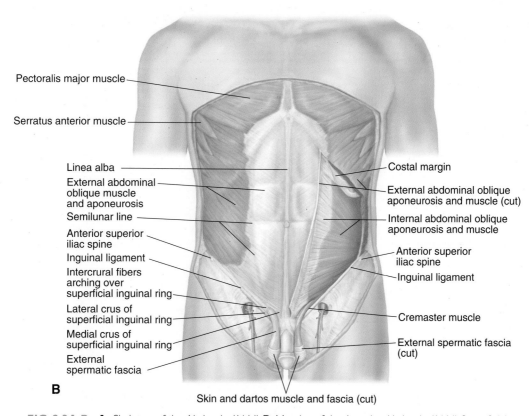

Pectoralis major muscle
Serratus anterior muscle

Linea alba
External abdominal oblique muscle and aponeurosis
Semilunar line
Anterior superior iliac spine
Inguinal ligament
Intercrural fibers arching over superficial inguinal ring
Lateral crus of superficial inguinal ring
Medial crus of superficial inguinal ring
External spermatic fascia

Costal margin
External abdominal oblique aponeurosis and muscle (cut)
Internal abdominal oblique aponeurosis and muscle
Anterior superior iliac spine
Inguinal ligament
Cremaster muscle
External spermatic fascia (cut)

B

Skin and dartos muscle and fascia (cut)

FIG. 2.3A,B.   A. Skeleton of the Abdominal Wall. **B.** Muscles of the Anterior Abdominal Wall, Superficial Dissection.

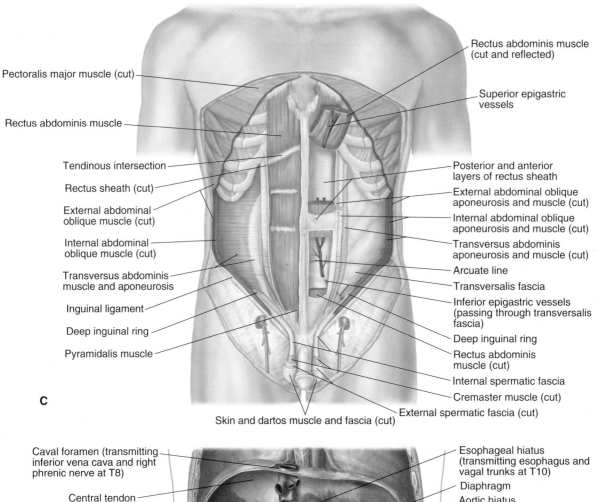

Pectoralis major muscle (cut)

Rectus abdominis muscle

Tendinous intersection

Rectus sheath (cut)

External abdominal oblique muscle (cut)

Internal abdominal oblique muscle (cut)

Transversus abdominis muscle and aponeurosis

Inguinal ligament

Deep inguinal ring

Pyramidalis muscle

Rectus abdominis muscle (cut and reflected)

Superior epigastric vessels

Posterior and anterior layers of rectus sheath

External abdominal oblique aponeurosis and muscle (cut)

Internal abdominal oblique aponeurosis and muscle (cut)

Transversus abdominis aponeurosis and muscle (cut)

Arcuate line

Transversalis fascia

Inferior epigastric vessels (passing through transversalis fascia)

Deep inguinal ring

Rectus abdominis muscle (cut)

Internal spermatic fascia

Cremaster muscle (cut)

External spermatic fascia (cut)

Skin and dartos muscle and fascia (cut)

C

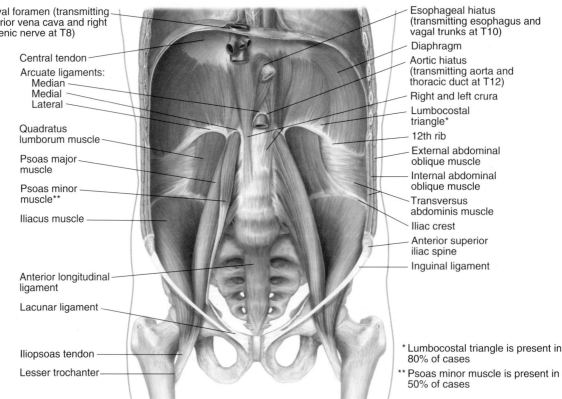

Caval foramen (transmitting inferior vena cava and right phrenic nerve at T8)

Central tendon

Arcuate ligaments:
    Median
    Medial
    Lateral

Quadratus lumborum muscle

Psoas major muscle

Psoas minor muscle**

Iliacus muscle

Anterior longitudinal ligament

Lacunar ligament

Iliopsoas tendon

Lesser trochanter

Esophageal hiatus (transmitting esophagus and vagal trunks at T10)

Diaphragm

Aortic hiatus (transmitting aorta and thoracic duct at T12)

Right and left crura

Lumbocostal triangle*

12th rib

External abdominal oblique muscle

Internal abdominal oblique muscle

Transversus abdominis muscle

Iliac crest

Anterior superior iliac spine

Inguinal ligament

* Lumbocostal triangle is present in 80% of cases

** Psoas minor muscle is present in 50% of cases

D

FIG. 2.3C,D. **C.** Muscles of the Anterior Abdominal Wall, Deeper Dissection. **D.** Muscles of the Posterior Abdominal Wall, Superficial Dissection.

Abdominal Aponeuroses, Rectus Sheath, and Neurovasculature of the Abdominal Wall

I. General Organization of the Abdominal Wall (Fig. 2.4A–C)

A. Skin, subcutaneous connective tissue (superficial fascia), muscles and their investing fasciae and aponeuroses, deep (transversalis) fascia, extraperitoneal fat, and parietal peritoneum

B. Fascial layers (superficial to deep)

   1. Subcutaneous connective tissue (superficial fascia): consists of 2 layers below umbilicus

      a. Superficial fatty layer (Camper fascia)

      b. Deep membranous layer (Scarpa fascia), attached inferiorly to fascia lata of upper thigh

   2. Investing fascia (epimysium): surrounds each of the 3 muscle layers

   3. Endo-abdominal (transversalis) fascia: very thin layer lining entire internal surface of abdominal wall

   4. Parietal peritoneum: lines abdominal cavity and located deep to transversalis fascia (which it is separated from by variable amount of extraperitoneal fat)

II. Aponeurosis of External Abdominal Oblique Muscle

A. Covers anterior abdominal wall and forms important features of abdominal wall

B. **Linea alba**

   1. Midline fibrous band extending from xiphoid process to pubic symphysis

   2. Intermingling of fibers from external and internal abdominal oblique and transversus abdominis

C. **Inguinal ligament**

   1. Extends from anterior superior iliac spine to pubic tubercle

   2. Lowest fibers curve inward

D. **Lacunar ligament**

   1. Fibers from medial end of inguinal ligament that curve inward

   2. Attaches to pectineal ligament along pubic pecten

E. **Reflected inguinal ligament**

   1. Fibers passing upward and medially from bony attachment of lacunar ligament to reach linea alba

F. **Superficial inguinal ring**

   1. Triangular gap in aponeurosis, superolateral to pubis, for passage of spermatic cord or round ligament of uterus

   2. Framed by lateral and medial crura united by intercrural fibers

G. Anterior layer of anterior lamina of rectus sheath

III. Rectus Sheath

A. Basic formation
  1. Composed of aponeuroses of external and internal abdominal oblique and transversus abdominis muscles
  2. Posterior and anterior layers pass on either surface of rectus abdominis muscle
B. **Arcuate line** (semicircular line of Douglas)
  1. Line on posterior wall of rectus sheath below which only transversalis fascia makes up posterior layer of rectus sheath
  2. Usually midway between umbilicus and pubic crest
C. Rectus sheath above arcuate line
  1. Anterior lamina
      a. External abdominal oblique aponeurosis
      b. Anterior layer of internal abdominal oblique aponeurosis (internal abdominal oblique splits to surround rectus abdominis)
  2. Posterior lamina
      a. Posterior layer of internal abdominal oblique aponeurosis
      b. Transversus abdominis aponeurosis
D. Rectus sheath below arcuate line
  1. Anterior lamina
      a. Aponeurosis of external abdominal oblique
      b. Aponeurosis of internal abdominal oblique
      c. Aponeurosis of transversus abdominis
  2. Posterior lamina is deficient: only transversalis fascia
E. Structures within rectus sheath
  1. Rectus abdominis and pyramidalis muscles
  2. Superior and inferior epigastric vessels behind and within rectus abdominis
      a. Superior epigastric artery descends from internal thoracic artery, passes deep to costal cartilage, and enters rectus sheath
          i. In sheath, it is at first behind and then enters muscle
          ii. Anastomoses with inferior epigastric artery
      b. Inferior epigastric artery arises from external iliac artery above inguinal ligament
          i. It courses upward and medially, pierces transversalis fascia, and passes anterior to arcuate line to enter rectus sheath
          ii. At origin, it lies medial to deep inguinal ring
  3. Anterior ends of lower 5 intercostal and subcostal vessels and nerves
      a. Enter rectus sheath laterally
      b. Pass through rectus abdominis, innervating it, then penetrate anterior rectus sheath to reach skin as anterior cutaneous branches
F. **Linea semilunaris:** slight surface depression that indicates lateral border of rectus abdominis muscle
G. **Linea transversae:** transverse grooves overlying tendinous intersections of rectus abdominis muscles

IV. Conjoined Tendon (Falx Inguinalis)

A. Formed by aponeuroses of internal abdominal oblique and transversus abdominis uniting to insert onto pubic crest and medial portion of pectineal ligament
B. Many diverse opinions exist on exact anatomy and on preferred names of structures in region of insertion of internal abdominal oblique and transversus abdominis muscles, particularly on whether a conjoined tendon or falx inguinalis (i.e., the 2 muscles combined) is ever formed lateral to lateral border of rectus muscle
  1. Current majority opinion equates conjoined (conjoint) tendon and falx inguinalis
  2. Minority opinion
      a. Conjoint tendon represents common aponeurotic fibers of insertion
      b. Falx inguinalis represents crescentic muscular fibers arching over inguinal canal, which function to close off and prevent herniation into the canal when abdominal wall contracts and intraabdominal pressure increases

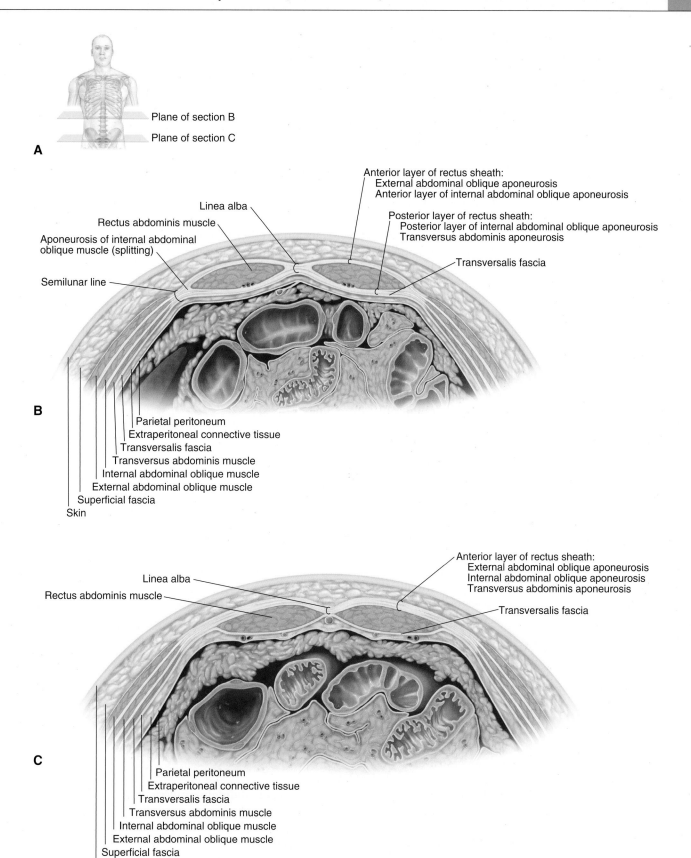

Plane of section B

Plane of section C

A

Anterior layer of rectus sheath:
External abdominal oblique aponeurosis
Anterior layer of internal abdominal oblique aponeurosis

Linea alba

Rectus abdominis muscle

Aponeurosis of internal abdominal oblique muscle (splitting)

Posterior layer of rectus sheath:
Posterior layer of internal abdominal oblique aponeurosis
Transversus abdominis aponeurosis

Semilunar line

Transversalis fascia

B

Parietal peritoneum
Extraperitoneal connective tissue
Transversalis fascia
Transversus abdominis muscle
Internal abdominal oblique muscle
External abdominal oblique muscle
Superficial fascia
Skin

Anterior layer of rectus sheath:
External abdominal oblique aponeurosis
Internal abdominal oblique aponeurosis
Transversus abdominis aponeurosis

Linea alba

Rectus abdominis muscle

Transversalis fascia

C

Parietal peritoneum
Extraperitoneal connective tissue
Transversalis fascia
Transversus abdominis muscle
Internal abdominal oblique muscle
External abdominal oblique muscle
Superficial fascia
Skin

FIG. 2.4A–C. **A.** Planes of Section. **B.** Rectus Sheath, Cross Section Superior to Arcuate Line. **C.** Rectus Sheath, Cross Section Inferior to Arcuate Line.

V. Nerves (Fig. 2.4D)

A. Innervation of muscles of anterolateral abdominal wall
  1. Thoracoabdominal (lower intercostal, T7–T11) nerves
  2. Subcostal (T12) nerve
  3. Iliohypogastric (L1) nerve
  4. Ilioinguinal (L1) nerve

B. Thoracoabdominal nerves
  1. T7–T11 intercostal nerves supply thoracic as well as abdominal wall
  2. T7–T9 pass between costal margin and chondral attachments of diaphragm
  3. T7–T12
      a. Pass anteriorly around trunk between internal abdominal oblique and transversus abdominis muscles
      b. Penetrate lateral edge of rectus sheath to enter it behind rectus abdominis muscle
      c. Pierce rectus abdominis, innervating it, to pass through anterior lamina of rectus sheath and become anterior cutaneous branches
      d. Common nerve supply explains contraction of abdominal muscles when cold hands are applied to abdomen

C. Subcostal nerve (T12)
  1. Enters abdomen behind lateral arcuate ligament, courses downward and laterally behind kidney on anterior surface of quadratus lumborum, pierces transversus abdominis, and passes between it and internal abdominal oblique
  2. Supplies muscles and skin of lower abdominal wall and skin suprapubically

D. Iliohypogastric and ilioinguinal nerves
  1. From anterior ramus of L1 from lumbar plexus
  2. Common branch lies on posterior abdominal wall on anterior surface of quadratus lumborum
  3. Splits into superior branch (iliohypogastric) and inferior branch (ilioinguinal)
  4. Both nerves pass through transversus abdominis to lie between it and internal abdominal oblique initially
  5. Above anterior superior iliac spine, both nerves pass through internal abdominal oblique to lie between it and external abdominal oblique muscle and aponeurosis
      a. Iliohypogastric lies parallel to and superior to inguinal canal
      b. Ilioinguinal travels medially within inguinal canal
  6. Both nerves innervate muscles and skin of lower abdominal wall
      a. Iliohypogastric supplies skin over pubis
      b. Ilioinguinal passes through superficial inguinal ring to become anterior labial/scrotal and supply skin of this region

VI. Arteries (Fig. 2.4E)

A. Posterior intercostal arteries
  1. Travel with thoracoabdominal nerves
  2. Supply lateral abdominal wall primarily

B. Superficial epigastric artery
  1. Usually small branch of femoral artery
  2. Passes upward with vein to supply superficial fascia of lower abdominal wall

C. Superior epigastric artery
  1. Terminal branch of internal thoracic artery
  2. Becomes embedded in upper portion of rectus abdominis muscle

D. Inferior epigastric artery
  1. From distal end of external iliac artery
  2. Passes into rectus sheath deep to rectus abdominis
  3. Primary supply to lower anterior abdominal wall

E. Superficial circumflex iliac artery
  1. Usually small branch of femoral artery
  2. Passes superolaterally with vein to supply superficial fascia of lower lateral abdominal wall

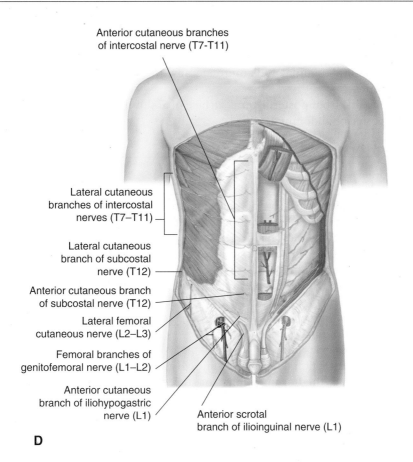

Anterior cutaneous branches
of intercostal nerve (T7-T11)

Lateral cutaneous
branches of intercostal
nerves (T7–T11)

Lateral cutaneous
branch of subcostal
nerve (T12)

Anterior cutaneous branch
of subcostal nerve (T12)

Lateral femoral
cutaneous nerve (L2–L3)

Femoral branches of
genitofemoral nerve (L1–L2)

Anterior cutaneous
branch of iliohypogastric
nerve (L1)

Anterior scrotal
branch of ilioinguinal nerve (L1)

D

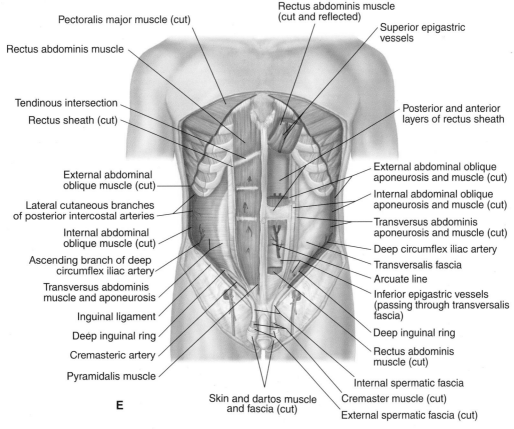

Pectoralis major muscle (cut)

Rectus abdominis muscle

Rectus abdominis muscle
(cut and reflected)

Superior epigastric
vessels

Tendinous intersection

Rectus sheath (cut)

Posterior and anterior
layers of rectus sheath

External abdominal
oblique muscle (cut)

Lateral cutaneous branches
of posterior intercostal arteries

Internal abdominal
oblique muscle (cut)

Ascending branch of deep
circumflex iliac artery

Transversus abdominis
muscle and aponeurosis

Inguinal ligament

Deep inguinal ring

Cremasteric artery

Pyramidalis muscle

External abdominal oblique
aponeurosis and muscle (cut)

Internal abdominal oblique
aponeurosis and muscle (cut)

Transversus abdominis
aponeurosis and muscle (cut)

Deep circumflex iliac artery

Transversalis fascia

Arcuate line

Inferior epigastric vessels
(passing through transversalis
fascia)

Deep inguinal ring

Rectus abdominis
muscle (cut)

Internal spermatic fascia

Skin and dartos muscle
and fascia (cut)

Cremaster muscle (cut)

External spermatic fascia (cut)

E

FIG. 2.4D,E. **D.** Nerves of the Anterior Abdominal Wall. **E.** Arteries of the Anterior Abdominal Wall.

F. **Deep circumflex iliac artery**
  1. From distal end of external iliac artery
  2. Travels deep and parallel to inguinal ligament
  3. Supplies lower abdominal wall anterolaterally
G. **Lumbar arteries**
  1. Usually 4 pairs, from posterolateral surface of abdominal aorta
  2. Supply posterior abdominal wall

VII. Veins: Follow Arteries

VIII. Clinical Considerations

A. Vertical incision along linea semilunaris denervates part of rectus abdominis muscle; vertical incision through rectus only denervates medial part
B. Superficial abdominal reflex
  1. Elicited with patient supine if quickly stroked horizontally lateral to medial toward umbilicus
  2. Contraction of abdominal muscles is usually felt (may not be seen in obese patients)
  3. Any injury to abdominal skin results in a fast, reflex contraction of abdominal muscles
C. **Cremasteric reflex**
  1. Contraction of cremaster muscle elicited by stroking skin on medial side of upper thigh using applicator stick or tongue depressor
  2. Results in elevation of testis on same side
  3. Active in children, but a hyperactive reflex may mimic an undescended testis

Inguinal Canal, Spermatic Cord, and Hernia

I. Special Features of the Lower Abdominal Wall (Fig. 2.5A–D)

A. **Conjoined tendon (falx inguinalis)**
1. Union of fibers of internal abdominal oblique and transversus abdominis muscles
2. Arises from lateral end of inguinal ligament and arches over spermatic cord/round ligament of uterus
3. Inserts aponeurotically onto pubic crest and medial portion of pectineal ligament (Fig. 2.5E–H)

B. **Cremaster muscle**
1. Arises from inguinal ligament as lowermost fibers of internal abdominal oblique muscle and sends long loops along spermatic cord and testis
2. Inserts on pubis

C. **Transversalis fascia**
1. Deep fascia that lines entire abdomen deep to transversus abdominis muscle
2. Forms posterior lamina of rectus sheath below arcuate line

D. **Interfoveolar ligament**
1. Thickening of transversalis fascia forming medial boundary of deep inguinal ring
2. Roughly parallels inferior epigastric vessels

E. **Medial and lateral inguinal fossae**
1. Lie superior to inguinal ligament, separated by inferior epigastric vessels
2. Medial inguinal fossa contains **inguinal triangle** (Hesselbach), bounded medially by lateral edge of rectus abdominis, laterally by inferior epigastric vessels, and below by inguinal ligament

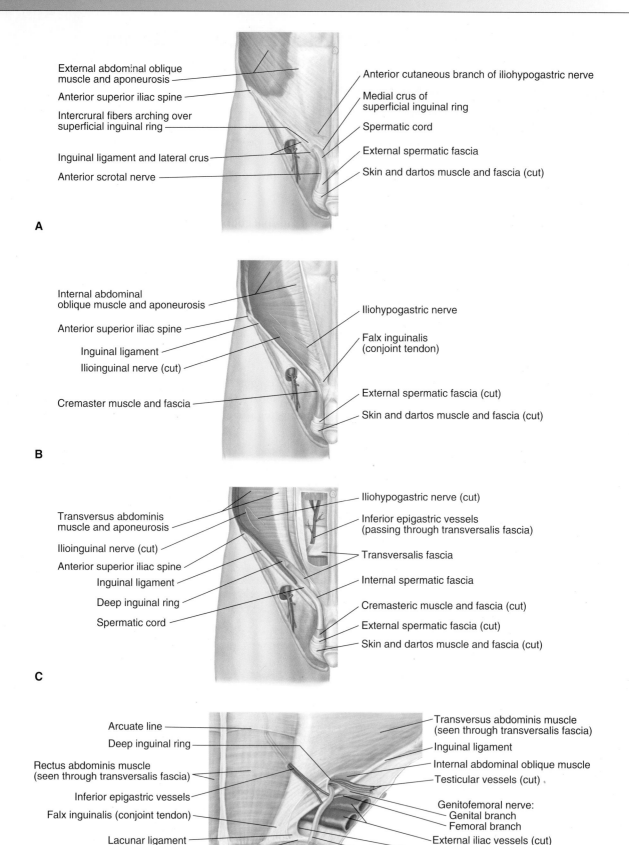

External abdominal oblique muscle and aponeurosis

Anterior superior iliac spine

Intercrural fibers arching over superficial inguinal ring

Inguinal ligament and lateral crus

Anterior scrotal nerve

Anterior cutaneous branch of iliohypogastric nerve

Medial crus of superficial inguinal ring

Spermatic cord

External spermatic fascia

Skin and dartos muscle and fascia (cut)

A

Internal abdominal oblique muscle and aponeurosis

Anterior superior iliac spine

Inguinal ligament

Ilioinguinal nerve (cut)

Cremaster muscle and fascia

Iliohypogastric nerve

Falx inguinalis (conjoint tendon)

External spermatic fascia (cut)

Skin and dartos muscle and fascia (cut)

B

Transversus abdominis muscle and aponeurosis

Ilioinguinal nerve (cut)

Anterior superior iliac spine

Inguinal ligament

Deep inguinal ring

Spermatic cord

Iliohypogastric nerve (cut)

Inferior epigastric vessels (passing through transversalis fascia)

Transversalis fascia

Internal spermatic fascia

Cremasteric muscle and fascia (cut)

External spermatic fascia (cut)

Skin and dartos muscle and fascia (cut)

C

Arcuate line

Deep inguinal ring

Rectus abdominis muscle (seen through transversalis fascia)

Inferior epigastric vessels

Falx inguinalis (conjoint tendon)

Lacunar ligament

Pectineal ligament

Transversus abdominis muscle (seen through transversalis fascia)

Inguinal ligament

Internal abdominal oblique muscle

Testicular vessels (cut)

Genitofemoral nerve:
Genital branch
Femoral branch

External iliac vessels (cut)

Femoral ring

Ductus deferens (cut)

Obturator artery and nerve entering obturator canal

D

FIG. 2.5A–D. A, B, and **C.** Spermatic Cord and Inguinal Canal. **D.** Formation of the Spermatic Cord and Deep Inguinal Ring.

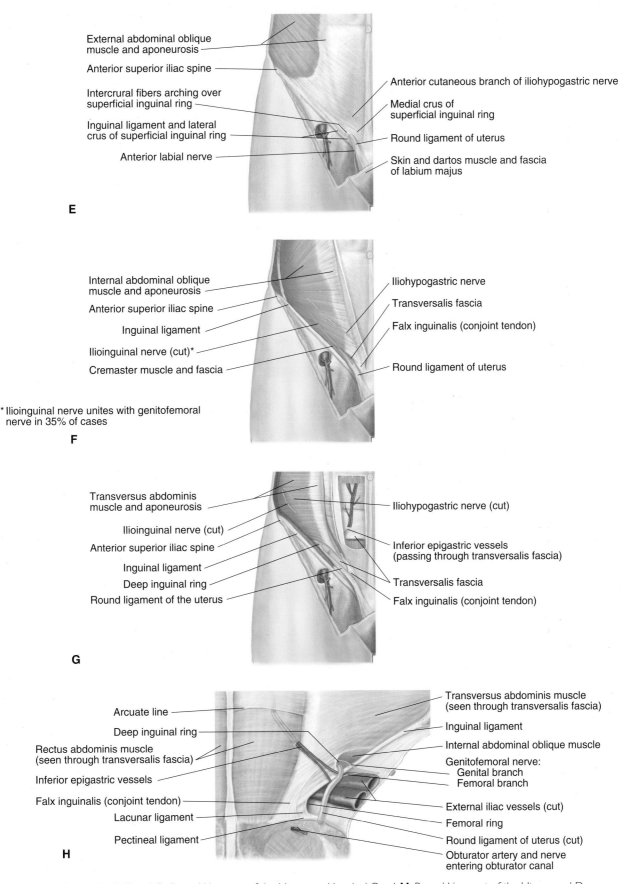

External abdominal oblique muscle and aponeurosis

Anterior superior iliac spine

Intercrural fibers arching over superficial inguinal ring

Inguinal ligament and lateral crus of superficial inguinal ring

Anterior labial nerve

Anterior cutaneous branch of iliohypogastric nerve

Medial crus of superficial inguinal ring

Round ligament of uterus

Skin and dartos muscle and fascia of labium majus

E

Internal abdominal oblique muscle and aponeurosis

Anterior superior iliac spine

Inguinal ligament

Ilioinguinal nerve (cut)*

Cremaster muscle and fascia

Iliohypogastric nerve

Transversalis fascia

Falx inguinalis (conjoint tendon)

Round ligament of uterus

* Ilioinguinal nerve unites with genitofemoral nerve in 35% of cases

F

Transversus abdominis muscle and aponeurosis

Ilioinguinal nerve (cut)

Anterior superior iliac spine

Inguinal ligament

Deep inguinal ring

Round ligament of the uterus

Iliohypogastric nerve (cut)

Inferior epigastric vessels (passing through transversalis fascia)

Transversalis fascia

Falx inguinalis (conjoint tendon)

G

Arcuate line

Deep inguinal ring

Rectus abdominis muscle (seen through transversalis fascia)

Inferior epigastric vessels

Falx inguinalis (conjoint tendon)

Lacunar ligament

Pectineal ligament

Transversus abdominis muscle (seen through transversalis fascia)

Inguinal ligament

Internal abdominal oblique muscle

Genitofemoral nerve:
Genital branch
Femoral branch

External iliac vessels (cut)

Femoral ring

Round ligament of uterus (cut)

Obturator artery and nerve entering obturator canal

H

FIG. 2.5E–H. E, F, and **G.** Round Ligament of the Uterus and Inguinal Canal. **H.** Round Ligament of the Uterus and Deep Inguinal Ring.

II. Inguinal Canal (Fig. 2.5I,J)

A. Extent: 4 cm, from deep inguinal ring to superficial inguinal ring

B. Course: oblique, running parallel to and just above inguinal ligament

C. Boundaries

    1. Anterior wall: external abdominal oblique aponeurosis along entire length; internal abdominal oblique muscle on lateral 1/3

    2. Posterior wall: from medial to lateral, reflected inguinal ligament and conjoined tendon on medial 1/3, and transversalis fascia (over entire length)

    3. Roof: arching fibers of internal abdominal oblique and transversus abdominis muscles

    4. Floor: inguinal ligament and lacunar ligament (medially)

D. Contents

    1. Male, **spermatic cord**: ductus deferens, deferential vessels, testicular artery, pampiniform plexus of veins, genital branch of genitofemoral nerve, lymphatics, and autonomic nerves (Fig. 2.5K)

    2. Female, **round ligament of uterus** and genital branch of genitofemoral nerve

    3. Both sexes

        a. Ilioinguinal nerve

        b. Cremasteric muscle and artery (both small in female)

III. Coverings of Spermatic Cord

A. **External spermatic fascia**: prolongation of deep fascia of external abdominal oblique muscle at superficial inguinal ring

B. **Cremasteric muscle and fascia**: derived from internal abdominal oblique muscle and fascia

C. **Internal spermatic fascia**: from transversalis fascia at deep inguinal ring

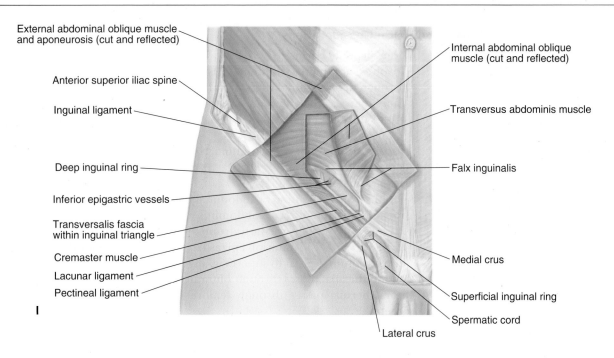

External abdominal oblique muscle and aponeurosis (cut and reflected)

Anterior superior iliac spine

Inguinal ligament

Deep inguinal ring

Inferior epigastric vessels

Transversalis fascia within inguinal triangle

Cremaster muscle

Lacunar ligament

Pectineal ligament

I

Internal abdominal oblique muscle (cut and reflected)

Transversus abdominis muscle

Falx inguinalis

Medial crus

Superficial inguinal ring

Spermatic cord

Lateral crus

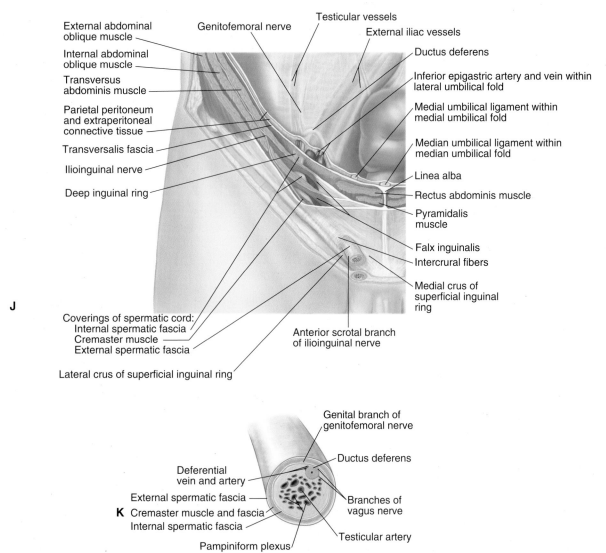

External abdominal oblique muscle

Internal abdominal oblique muscle

Transversus abdominis muscle

Parietal peritoneum and extraperitoneal connective tissue

Transversalis fascia

Ilioinguinal nerve

Deep inguinal ring

J

Coverings of spermatic cord:
Internal spermatic fascia
Cremaster muscle
External spermatic fascia

Lateral crus of superficial inguinal ring

Genitofemoral nerve

Testicular vessels

External iliac vessels

Ductus deferens

Inferior epigastric artery and vein within lateral umbilical fold

Medial umbilical ligament within medial umbilical fold

Median umbilical ligament within median umbilical fold

Linea alba

Rectus abdominis muscle

Pyramidalis muscle

Falx inguinalis

Intercrural fibers

Medial crus of superficial inguinal ring

Anterior scrotal branch of ilioinguinal nerve

Genital branch of genitofemoral nerve

Ductus deferens

Deferential vein and artery

External spermatic fascia

K Cremaster muscle and fascia

Internal spermatic fascia

Pampiniform plexus

Branches of vagus nerve

Testicular artery

FIG. 2.5I–K. **I.** Inguinal Canal in the Male. **J.** Inguinal Region in the Male, Exploded View. **K.** Spermatic Cord.

IV. Clinical Considerations

A. **Indirect inguinal hernia** (Fig. 2.5L,M)

  1. Involves abdominal contents (usually small or large bowel) pushing through deep inguinal ring, lateral to inferior epigastric vessels; represents more than 2/3rds of inguinal hernias

  2. Passes through inguinal canal alongside spermatic cord or round ligament within coverings of cord

  3. Passes through superficial inguinal ring, commonly passing into scrotum or labium majus

B. **Direct inguinal hernia** (Fig. 2.5N)

  1. Results from weakening of abdominal wall just lateral to superficial inguinal ring and margin of rectus abdominis muscle

  2. Hernia sac pushes forward from abdomen in inguinal (Hesselbach) triangle, medial to inferior epigastric vessels, and passes through medial end of inguinal canal to superficial inguinal ring

C. **Obturator hernia**: passes through obturator canal

D. **Femoral hernia**: passes through femoral ring and canal lateral to lacunar ligament

E. **Umbilical hernia**: passes through umbilical ring, usually in newborns, but may occur due to aging, obesity, and surgical or traumatic wounds

F. **Epigastric hernia**: in epigastric area through linea alba between xiphoid process and umbilicus

  1. Seen in people over age 40 years and associated with obesity

  2. Sac consists of peritoneum covered by fatty subcutaneous tissue and skin

G. **Spigelian hernia**: occurs along semilunar line

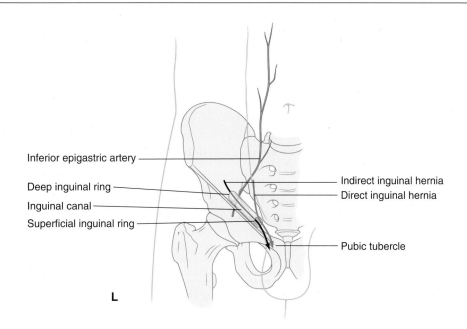

Inferior epigastric artery

Deep inguinal ring

Inguinal canal

Superficial inguinal ring

Indirect inguinal hernia

Direct inguinal hernia

Pubic tubercle

L

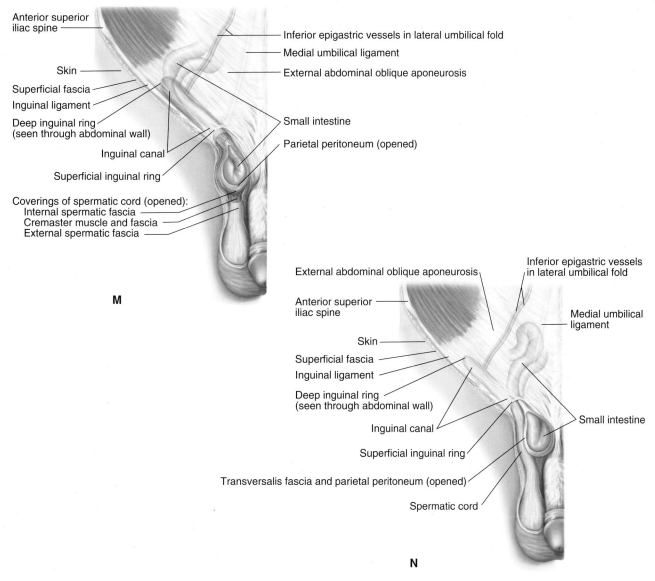

Anterior superior iliac spine

Inferior epigastric vessels in lateral umbilical fold

Medial umbilical ligament

External abdominal oblique aponeurosis

Skin

Superficial fascia

Inguinal ligament

Deep inguinal ring
(seen through abdominal wall)

Small intestine

Parietal peritoneum (opened)

Inguinal canal

Superficial inguinal ring

Coverings of spermatic cord (opened):
Internal spermatic fascia
Cremaster muscle and fascia
External spermatic fascia

M

External abdominal oblique aponeurosis

Inferior epigastric vessels in lateral umbilical fold

Anterior superior iliac spine

Medial umbilical ligament

Skin

Superficial fascia

Inguinal ligament

Deep inguinal ring
(seen through abdominal wall)

Small intestine

Inguinal canal

Superficial inguinal ring

Transversalis fascia and parietal peritoneum (opened)

Spermatic cord

N

FIG. 2.5L-N. L. Types of Inguinal Hernias. **M.** Indirect Inguinal Hernia. **N.** Direct Inguinal Hernia.

Peritoneum

I. Fundamentals (Fig. 2.6A–C)

A. Serous layer of abdomen

B. Has parietal and visceral layers

C. Forms peritoneal ligaments

1. Double layers of peritoneum that connect viscera to each other and to body wall

2. Often transmit blood vessels

D. Forms **fusion fascia**

1. 4 gut structures become secondarily retroperitoneal during development

a. Duodenum (except 1st and 4th parts)

b. Pancreas (except tail)

c. Ascending colon

d. Descending colon

2. Relatively avascular plane lying behind these organs

3. Organs may be mobilized by cutting through fusion fascia

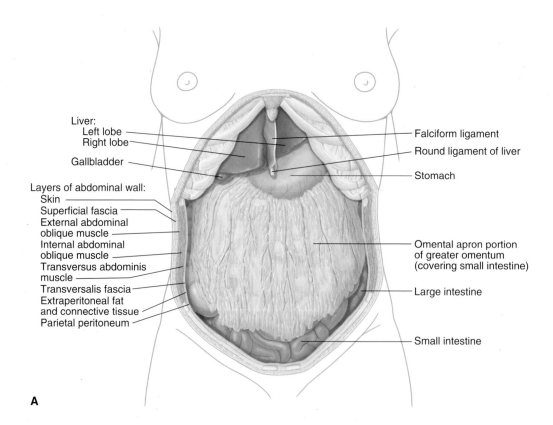

Liver:
Left lobe
Right lobe
Gallbladder

Layers of abdominal wall:
Skin
Superficial fascia
External abdominal oblique muscle
Internal abdominal oblique muscle
Transversus abdominis muscle
Transversalis fascia
Extraperitoneal fat and connective tissue
Parietal peritoneum

Falciform ligament
Round ligament of liver
Stomach

Omental apron portion of greater omentum (covering small intestine)
Large intestine
Small intestine

A

FIG. 2.6A. Peritoneum, Omental Apron.

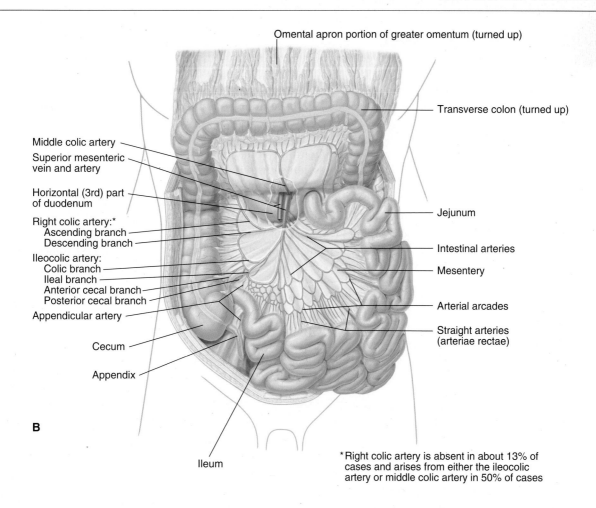

Omental apron portion of greater omentum (turned up)

Transverse colon (turned up)

Middle colic artery

Superior mesenteric
vein and artery

Horizontal (3rd) part
of duodenum

Right colic artery:*
Ascending branch
Descending branch

Ileocolic artery:
Colic branch
Ileal branch
Anterior cecal branch
Posterior cecal branch

Appendicular artery

Cecum

Appendix

Jejunum

Intestinal arteries

Mesentery

Arterial arcades

Straight arteries
(arteriae rectae)

Ileum

B

*Right colic artery is absent in about 13% of
cases and arises from either the ileocolic
artery or middle colic artery in 50% of cases

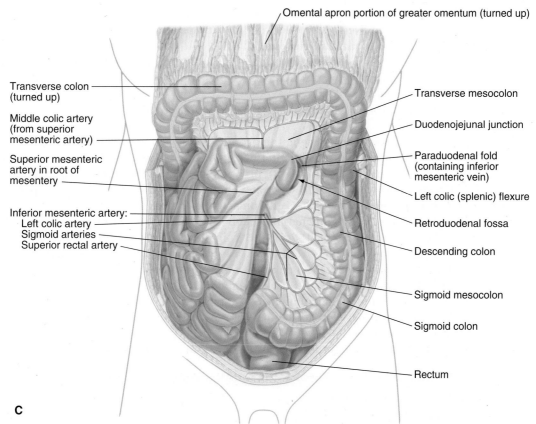

Omental apron portion of greater omentum (turned up)

Transverse colon
(turned up)

Middle colic artery
(from superior
mesenteric artery)

Superior mesenteric
artery in root of
mesentery

Inferior mesenteric artery:
Left colic artery
Sigmoid arteries
Superior rectal artery

Transverse mesocolon

Duodenojejunal junction

Paraduodenal fold
(containing inferior
mesenteric vein)

Left colic (splenic) flexure

Retroduodenal fossa

Descending colon

Sigmoid mesocolon

Sigmoid colon

Rectum

C

FIG. 2.6B,C. Peritoneum. **B.** Transverse Mesocolon and the Mesentery. **C.** Transverse and Sigmoid Mesocolon.

II. Peritoneal Cavity

A. Potential space between layers of peritoneum

B. 2 subdivisions

   1. Main peritoneal cavity (greater sac): surrounds but does not contain most GI tract organs

   2. **Omental bursa** (lesser sac): diverticulum from main peritoneal cavity, behind stomach primarily (Fig. 2.6D,E)

     a. Boundaries

       i. Anteriorly: lesser omentum, stomach, gastrocolic ligament

       ii. Posteriorly: pancreas, left suprarenal gland and left kidney

       iii. Inferiorly: transverse mesocolon

       iv. Left: hilum of spleen, gastrosplenic and splenorenal ligament

       v. Right: opens to greater peritoneal sac at omental foramen

     b. **Omental (epiploic) foramen** (of Winslow)

       i. Opening between main peritoneal cavity (greater sac) and lesser sac (omental bursa)

       ii. Boundaries

         a) Anteriorly: hepatoduodenal ligament

         b) Posteriorly: inferior vena cava

         c) Superiorly: caudate lobe of liver

         d) Inferiorly: duodenum

     c. Subdivisions

       i. Superior recess: between caudate lobe of liver and diaphragm

       ii. Inferior recess: includes all of remaining lower part

III. Ligaments and Folds of Peritoneum

A. **Falciform ligament** (Fig. 2.6F)

   1. Sickle-shaped peritoneal fold attaching liver to anterior abdominal wall from umbilicus superiorly

   2. Contains round ligament of liver and paraumbilical veins

B. **Coronary ligaments of liver**

   1. Anterior layer formed by splitting of falciform ligament to right and left sides

   2. Posterior layer is lower, from back of right lobe to right suprarenal and kidney

   3. Bare area of liver lies between anterior and posterior layers of coronary ligament

C. **Left and right triangular ligaments**

   1. Formed by fusion of anterior and posterior layers of coronary ligaments laterally

   2. Left triangular more distinct, connecting left lobe to diaphragm

D. **Lesser omentum**

   1. Extends from lesser curvature of stomach to liver

   2. 2 parts

     a. **Hepatogastric ligament**: thin, connects stomach to undersurface of liver

     b. **Hepatoduodenal ligament**: thick, connects 1st part of duodenum to porta hepatis, contains bile duct (to right), proper hepatic artery (to left), and portal vein (behind)

E. **Greater omentum**: hangs from greater curvature of stomach; has multiple parts

   1. **Gastrocolic ligament**: between stomach and transverse colon

   2. **Gastrosplenic (gastrolienal) ligament**: from stomach to spleen

   3. **Splenorenal (lienorenal) ligament**: from left kidney to spleen

   4. **Omental apron**: hangs from transverse colon; filled with variable amount of fat

F. **Transverse mesocolon**: from pancreas on posterior abdominal wall to transverse colon

G. **Phrenicocolic ligament**: fold of peritoneum from left colic flexure to diaphragm, helps support spleen (sustentaculum lienis)

H. **Mesentery** (proper): broad, fanlike fold of peritoneum suspending jejunum and ileum from posterior body wall (Fig. 2.6G)

I. **Sigmoid mesocolon**: from posterior body wall to sigmoid colon

IV. Peritoneal Folds and Fossa of the Anterior Abdominal Wall (Fig. 2.6H,I)

A. **Median umbilical fold**

   1. In midline

   2. Peritoneum covering median umbilical ligament (urachus), which extends from apex of bladder to umbilicus

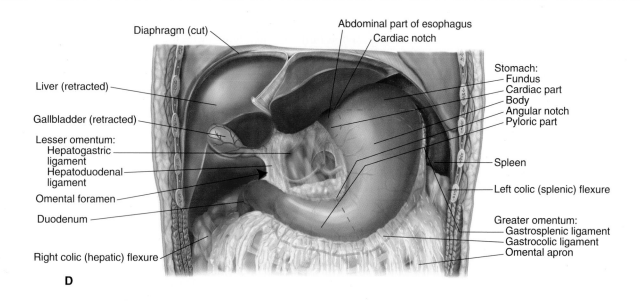

D.

- Diaphragm (cut)
- Abdominal part of esophagus
- Cardiac notch
- Liver (retracted)
- Gallbladder (retracted)
- Lesser omentum:
  - Hepatogastric ligament
  - Hepatoduodenal ligament
- Omental foramen
- Duodenum
- Right colic (hepatic) flexure
- Stomach:
  - Fundus
  - Cardiac part
  - Body
  - Angular notch
  - Pyloric part
- Spleen
- Left colic (splenic) flexure
- Greater omentum:
  - Gastrosplenic ligament
  - Gastrocolic ligament
  - Omental apron

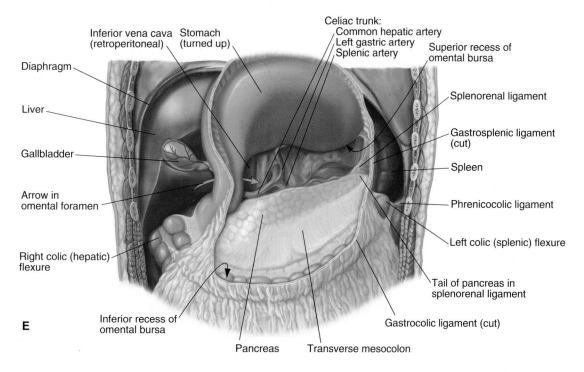

E.

- Inferior vena cava (retroperitoneal)
- Stomach (turned up)
- Diaphragm
- Liver
- Gallbladder
- Arrow in omental foramen
- Right colic (hepatic) flexure
- Inferior recess of omental bursa
- Pancreas
- Transverse mesocolon
- Celiac trunk:
  - Common hepatic artery
  - Left gastric artery
  - Splenic artery
- Superior recess of omental bursa
- Splenorenal ligament
- Gastrosplenic ligament (cut)
- Spleen
- Phrenicocolic ligament
- Left colic (splenic) flexure
- Tail of pancreas in splenorenal ligament
- Gastrocolic ligament (cut)

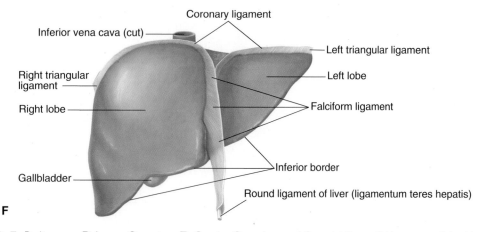

F.

- Inferior vena cava (cut)
- Coronary ligament
- Right triangular ligament
- Right lobe
- Gallbladder
- Left triangular ligament
- Left lobe
- Falciform ligament
- Inferior border
- Round ligament of liver (ligamentum teres hepatis)

FIG. 2.6D–F. Peritoneum. **D.** Lesser Omentum. **E.** Greater Omentum and Omental Bursa. **F.** Ligaments of the Liver.

B. **Medial umbilical folds** (paired)
  1. Peritoneum covering medial umbilical ligaments, which are ligamentous remnants of distal ends of umbilical arteries
C. **Lateral umbilical folds**: peritoneum covering inferior epigastric vessels
D. **Lateral and medial inguinal fossae**: depressions in peritoneum on either side of lateral umbilical folds
E. **Supravesical fossae**: between median and medial umbilical folds, above bladder

V. Clinical Considerations

A. Major functions of peritoneum are to minimize friction and resist infection; it exudes a small amount of peritoneal fluid, and in response to injury (or infection) it tends to wall it off or localize it
B. **Ascites**
  1. Accumulation of serous fluid in peritoneal cavity
  2. Often due to liver damage such as cirrhosis
C. **Peritonitis**
  1. Inflammation of peritoneum due to infection
  2. Adhesions may result that can lead to chronic pain or visceral obstruction due to **volvulus** (intestine twists around an adhesion)
  3. General peritonitis can be life threatening
D. Irritation of parietal peritoneum produces reflex spasm of body wall muscles; wall becomes "boardlike" (rigid), and breathing is rapid and shallow
E. **Paracentesis**: surgical puncture of peritoneal cavity for aspiration or drainage of fluid
F. **Peritoneal dialysis**
  1. Soluble substances and excess water are removed by transfer across peritoneum using dilute sterile solution introduced into peritoneal cavity on one side and drained from the other
  2. Temporary procedure; long term requires renal dialysis

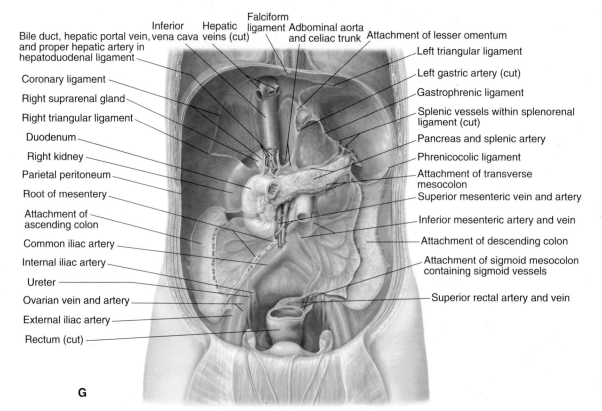

FIG. 2.6G. Peritoneal Attachments on the Posterior Abdominal Wall.

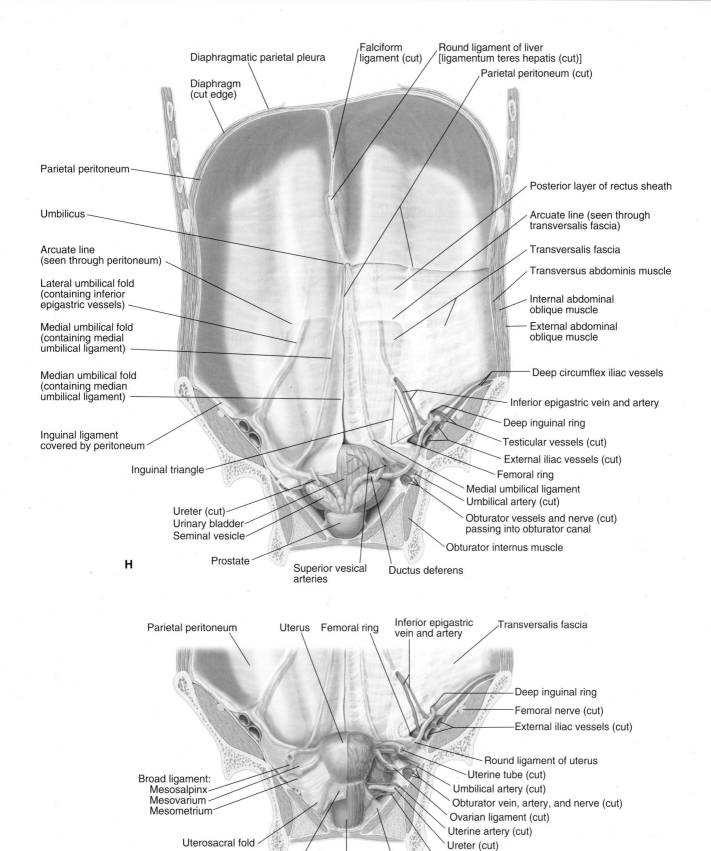

Diaphragmatic parietal pleura

Falciform ligament (cut)

Round ligament of liver [ligamentum teres hepatis (cut)]

Diaphragm (cut edge)

Parietal peritoneum (cut)

Parietal peritoneum

Umbilicus

Arcuate line (seen through peritoneum)

Lateral umbilical fold (containing inferior epigastric vessels)

Medial umbilical fold (containing medial umbilical ligament)

Median umbilical fold (containing median umbilical ligament)

Inguinal ligament covered by peritoneum

Inguinal triangle

Ureter (cut)

Urinary bladder

Seminal vesicle

Prostate

Superior vesical arteries

Ductus deferens

Posterior layer of rectus sheath

Arcuate line (seen through transversalis fascia)

Transversalis fascia

Transversus abdominis muscle

Internal abdominal oblique muscle

External abdominal oblique muscle

Deep circumflex iliac vessels

Inferior epigastric vein and artery

Deep inguinal ring

Testicular vessels (cut)

External iliac vessels (cut)

Femoral ring

Medial umbilical ligament

Umbilical artery (cut)

Obturator vessels and nerve (cut) passing into obturator canal

Obturator internus muscle

H

Parietal peritoneum

Uterus

Femoral ring

Inferior epigastric vein and artery

Transversalis fascia

Broad ligament:
Mesosalpinx
Mesovarium
Mesometrium

Uterosacral fold

Rectouterine pouch

Vagina

Deep inguinal ring

Femoral nerve (cut)

External iliac vessels (cut)

Round ligament of uterus

Uterine tube (cut)

Umbilical artery (cut)

Obturator vein, artery, and nerve (cut)

Ovarian ligament (cut)

Uterine artery (cut)

Ureter (cut)

Vaginal artery (cut)

Uterosacral ligament (cut)

I

FIG. 2.6H,I. Peritoneal Folds and Fossae on the Inner Anterior Abdominal Wall. **H.** Male. **I.** Female.

Small Intestine: Parts and Relations

I. Fundamentals of the Small Intestine (Small Bowel)

A. 3 parts
1. Duodenum (discussed in Section 2.13)
2. Jejunum
3. Ileum

B. Jejunum and ileum are suspended from posterior abdominal wall by mesentery (proper) (Fig. 2.7A,B)

II. Duodenojejunal Junction (Flexure)

A. Point where ascending part of duodenum turns sharply anteroinferiorly to become jejunum

B. Located at upper border of L2 vertebra on left side

C. **Suspensory muscle of duodenum** (ligament of Treitz)
1. Musculofibrous band, from right crus of diaphragm to ascending duodenum
2. Acts as physiological sphincter

D. Duodenal folds and fossae
1. **Paraduodenal fold**: peritoneal fold to left of ascending duodenum; contains inferior mesenteric vein and ascending branch of left colic artery
2. **Paraduodenal fossa**: small pocket medial to paraduodenal fold
3. **Retroduodenal fossa**: lies behind ascending part of duodenum, anterior to aorta

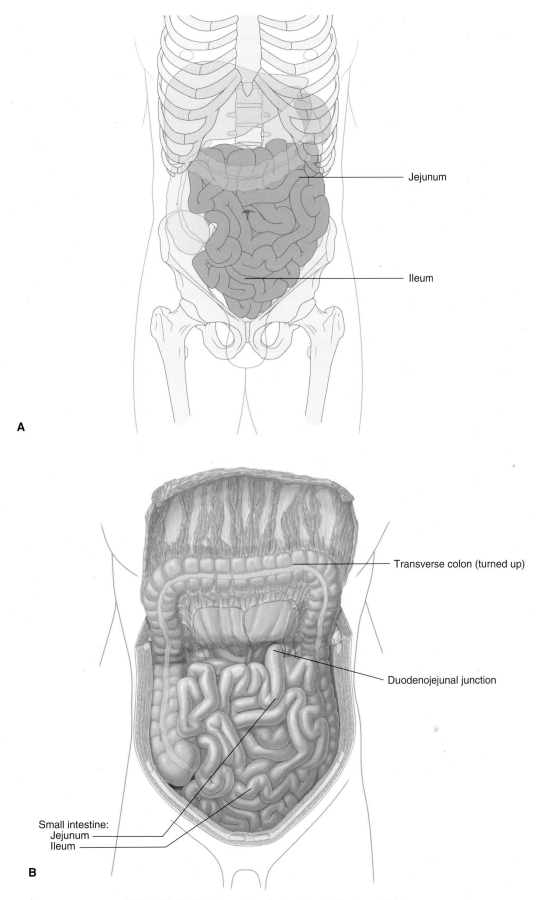

Jejunum

Ileum

A

Transverse colon (turned up)

Duodenojejunal junction

Small intestine:
Jejunum
Ileum

B

FIG. 2.7A,B. Small Intestine. **A.** Location. **B.** Parts and Relations.

III. Jejunum (Fig. 2.7C)

A. Upper 2/5 of small bowel (8 ft or 2.4m)
B. Primarily located in umbilical region
C. Thicker walled than ileum; lined with prominent circular folds (plicae circulares) of mucous membrane
D. Mesenteric fat typically scant, although variable
E. Vascular arcades between adjacent intestinal branches are relatively simple
F. **Vasa recta** (arteria recta) are relatively long, when compared to ileum

IV. Ileum (Fig. 2.7D)

A. Lower 3/5 of small bowel (12 ft, or 3.6 m)
B. Located primarily in hypogastric region and pelvis (especially lower ileum)
C. Thinner walled than jejunum
   1. Circular folds are small in upper ileum and absent in terminal ileum
   2. Aggregated lymph nodules (Peyer patches) seen in antimesenteric border
D. Abundant fat in mesentery
E. Multiple (3–4 arches) vascular arcades between adjacent intestinal branches
F. Vasa recta (arteria recta) are relatively short, when compared to jejunum
G. Ends at ileocecal junction

V. Clinical Considerations (Fig. 2.7E)

A. **Meckel diverticulum**: present in 2% of population
   1. Location: usually about 2 ft proximal from ileocecal valve on antimesenteric border of ileum
   2. Usually about 2 in long
     a. May contain gastric and/or pancreatic tissue
     b. End may be free or attached to abdominal wall
   3. Caused by failure of fetal vitelline duct to completely degenerate
   4. May become inflamed and produce appendicitis-like pain
B. **Enterostomy**
   1. Surgical procedure to create artificial fistulous opening between lumen of small bowel and body surface
   2. May be either jejunostomy or ileostomy
   3. May be temporary or permanent

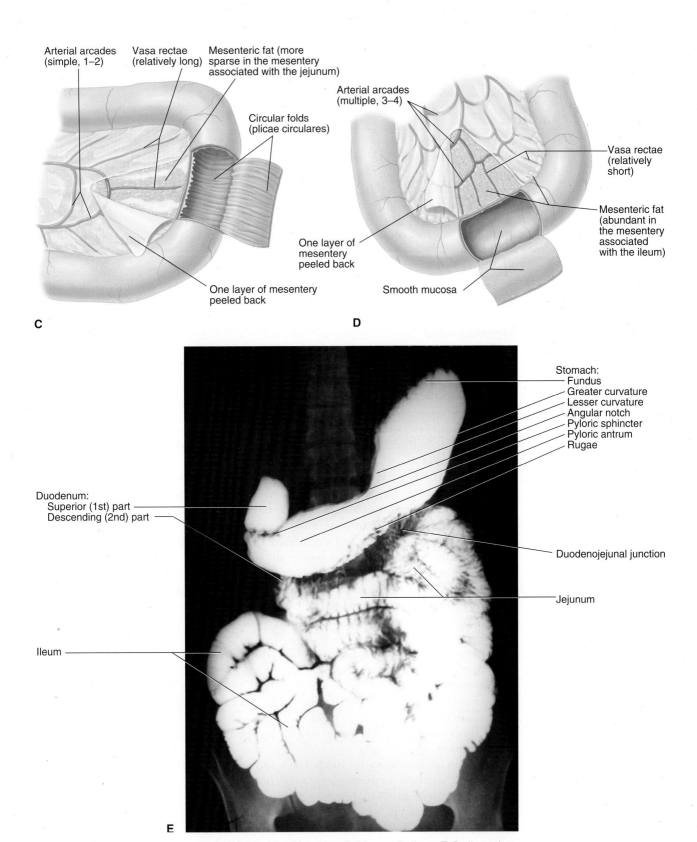

Arterial arcades
(simple, 1–2)

Vasa rectae
(relatively long)

Mesenteric fat (more
sparse in the mesentery
associated with the jejunum)

Circular folds
(plicae circulares)

One layer of mesentery
peeled back

One layer of
mesentery
peeled back

C

Arterial arcades
(multiple, 3–4)

Vasa rectae
(relatively
short)

Mesenteric fat
(abundant in
the mesentery
associated
with the ileum)

Smooth mucosa

D

Stomach:
Fundus
Greater curvature
Lesser curvature
Angular notch
Pyloric sphincter
Pyloric antrum
Rugae

Duodenum:
Superior (1st) part
Descending (2nd) part

Duodenojejunal junction

Jejunum

Ileum

E

FIG. 2.7C–E. Small Intestine. **C.** Jejunum. **D.** Ileum. **E.** Radiograph.

Large Intestine: Parts and Relations

I. Extent

A. From terminal ileum to anus (Fig. 2.8A)
B. Approximately 5 ft, or 1.5 m long

II. Parts

A. **Cecum** (Fig. 2.8B)
  1. Blind pouch that extends caudally below ileocecal valve
    a. Located in right iliac fossa above inguinal ligament
    b. Shape varies; covered by peritoneum
  2. **Ileocecal valve**
    a. Papilla-like with 2 lips that project into lumen of cecum
    b. Lips merge on either side of opening, forming membranous ridges (the frenula of the valve)
  3. **Appendix**
    a. Long, narrow tube (8.2 cm), which begins at inferior end of cecum; position varies
    b. Suspended by mesoappendix containing appendicular artery
B. Colon
  1. **Ascending colon**
    a. Begins at ileocecal valve and ascends through right lumbar and hypochondriac regions to visceral surface of liver to right of gallbladder, then bends sharply to left as right colic (hepatic) flexure to continue as transverse colon
    b. Approximately 5–8 in long
    c. Anterior surface and sides covered by peritoneum; paracolic gutter lies to right
    d. Secondarily retroperitoneal; posteriorly, fused to body wall over iliacus, quadratus lumborum, and transversus abdominis muscles and lateral part of right kidney
  2. **Transverse colon**
    a. Longest (18–20 in) and most movable portion of large bowel
    b. From right colic (hepatic) flexure in right hypochondriac region, arches across umbilical region and then upward into left hypochondriac region, where it bends caudally at left colic flexure (splenic) below spleen
    c. Invested in peritoneum and suspended from body wall by transverse mesocolon (which attaches along inferior border of pancreas)
  3. **Descending colon** (Fig. 2.8C)
    a. Extends caudally from left colic (splenic) flexure through left hypochondriac and lateral (lumbar) regions along lateral border of left kidney; at caudal end of kidney bends medially and descends in groove between psoas and quadratus lumborum muscles to crest of ilium
    b. Covered anteriorly and on sides with peritoneum; paracolic gutter lies to left
    c. Secondarily retroperitoneal
    d. **Phrenicocolic ligament**
      i. Fold of peritoneum connecting splenic flexure to diaphragm opposite 10th or 11th rib
      ii. Bloodless and may be cut in mobilizing splenic flexure or during splenectomy
  4. **Sigmoid colon**
    a. Begins in left iliac fossa, crosses pelvic brim, and then curves to midline at 3rd sacral segment, where it turns inferiorly to become rectum
    b. Average length 10–15 in, but may vary from 5–35 in
    c. Usually completely invested with peritoneum and suspended from posterior abdominal wall by sigmoid mesocolon
    d. Crossed anteriorly by coils of small intestine
C. **Rectum and anal canal** (see Sections 3.10 and 3.11)

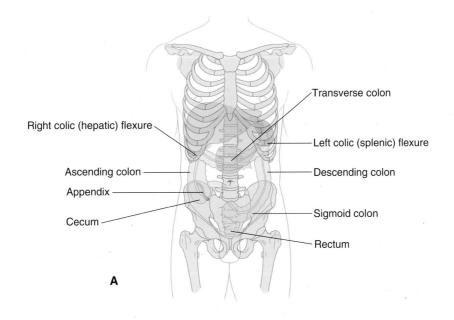

A

Transverse colon

Right colic (hepatic) flexure

Left colic (splenic) flexure

Ascending colon

Descending colon

Appendix

Cecum

Sigmoid colon

Rectum

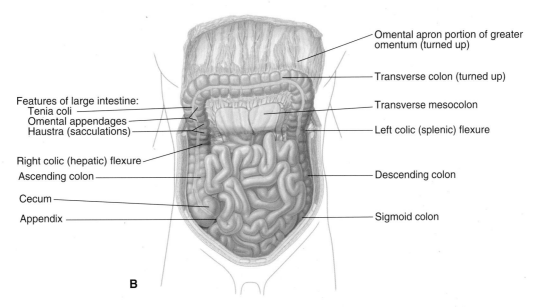

B

Omental apron portion of greater omentum (turned up)

Features of large intestine:
Tenia coli
Omental appendages
Haustra (sacculations)

Transverse colon (turned up)

Transverse mesocolon

Left colic (splenic) flexure

Right colic (hepatic) flexure

Ascending colon

Descending colon

Cecum

Appendix

Sigmoid colon

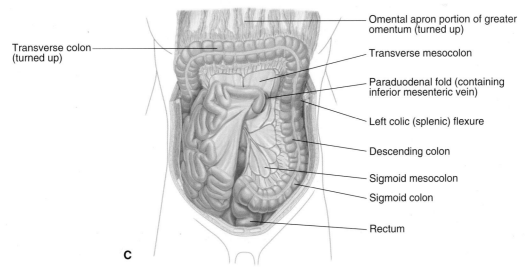

C

Omental apron portion of greater omentum (turned up)

Transverse colon (turned up)

Transverse mesocolon

Paraduodenal fold (containing inferior mesenteric vein)

Left colic (splenic) flexure

Descending colon

Sigmoid mesocolon

Sigmoid colon

Rectum

FIG. 2.8A–C. Large Intestine. **A.** Location. **B, C.** Parts and Relations.

III. Special Characteristics of Cecum and Colon (Fig. 2.8D)

A. Teniae coli
  1. Longitudinal smooth muscle is aggregated into 3 narrow bands called teniae
  2. All 3 teniae come together at root of appendix
B. Sacculations (haustra): outpocketing of wall of bowel
C. Semilunar folds: crescent-shaped folds of mucosal lining between haustra
D. Omental (epiploic) appendages: small fat-filled tabs of peritoneum attached along teniae

IV. Peritoneal Folds and Fossae

A. Anterior cecal fold: fold of peritoneum over anterior cecal branch of ileocolic artery (Fig. 2.8E,F)
B. Ileocecal fold (bloodless fold of Treves): below ileocecal junction
C. Mesoappendix: peritoneal fold suspending appendix from mesentery, passing posterior to terminal ileum
D. Retrocecal (cecal) fossa: behind cecum

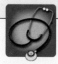 V. Clinical Considerations

A. McBurney point
  1. Point 3–4 cm along line from right anterior superior iliac spine to umbilicus
  2. Used to locate root of appendix (Fig. 2.8G)
B. Colostomy: artificial opening between colon and skin, often performed after partial colectomy
C. Diverticulitis: inflammation of abnormal outpocketings chiefly in sigmoid colon
D. Most tumors of large intestine occur in sigmoid colon and rectum and frequently are seen near rectosigmoid junction
  1. Other common sites of colon carcinoma are ascending and descending colon
  2. Tumors in ascending colon are relatively symptom free compared to those in descending colon
E. Diverticulosis
  1. Multiple external evaginations (outpocketings) of mucosa of sigmoid colon
  2. Primarily affects middle-aged and older people
F. Colonoscopy
  1. Viewing of interior of colon using long, fiberoptic endoscope (colonoscope) inserted into colon through anus and rectum
  2. Used to perform minor surgery (i.e., take biopsies, remove polyps, and check for colon cancer)
G. Colitis: chronic inflammation of colon
  1. **Ulcerative colitis** (Crohn disease): severe inflammation with ulceration of colon and rectum
  2. **Colectomy** may be necessary, in which terminal ileum and colon, as well as rectum and anal canal, are removed
H. Volvulus of sigmoid colon
  1. Twisting and rotation of mobile loop of sigmoid colon and mesocolon that can lead to obstruction of lumen
  2. Can result in constipation, ischemia of looped segment, and eventually colonic fecal impaction and even necrosis of bowel loop

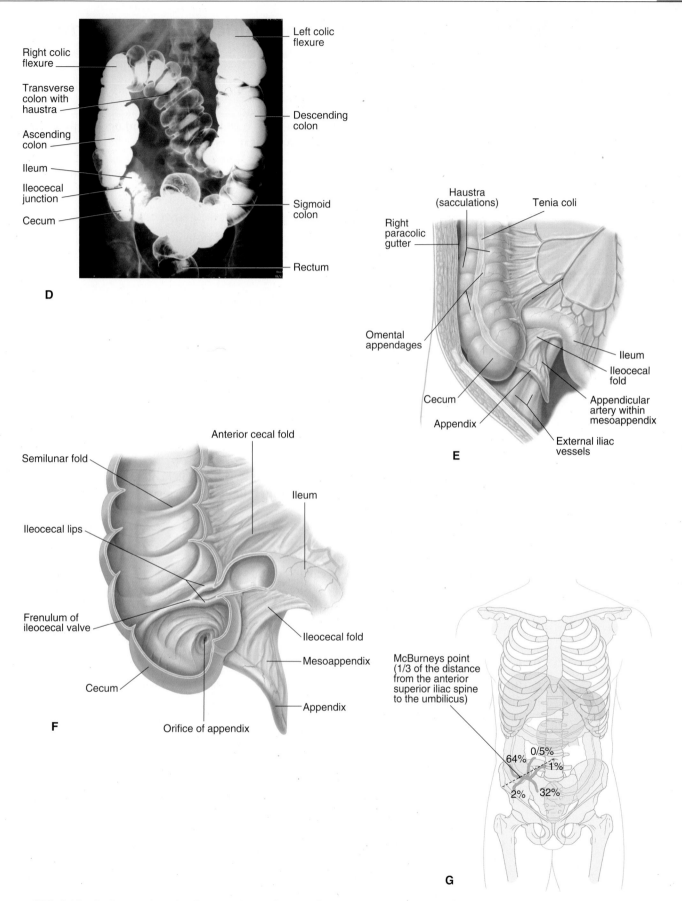

FIG. 2.8D–G. D. Large Intestine: Radiograph with Contrast. **E.** Ileocecal Junction, Exterior. **F.** Ileocecal Junction, Interior. **G.** Vermiform Appendix Variations.

Small and Large Intestine: Blood Supply, Lymph Drainage, and Innervation

I. Superior Mesenteric Artery (Fig. 2.9A)

A. Branches anteriorly from abdominal aorta at L1 vertebral level, behind neck of pancreas

B. Crosses 3rd part of duodenum to left of superior mesenteric vein

C. Branches

    1. **Inferior pancreaticoduodenal artery**: to pancreas and duodenum (see Section 2.15)

    2. **Middle colic artery**

       a. Passes anteroinferiorly in transverse mesocolon

       b. Branches near border of transverse colon

          i. Right: anastomoses with ascending branch of right colic artery

          ii. Left: anastomoses with ascending branch of left colic artery

    3. **Intestinal arteries**: usually 12–15

       a. Supply jejunum and ileum

       b. Pass within mesentery, running roughly parallel with each other

       c. Each divides into 2 branches, which unite with branches from adjoining arteries, forming arches (arterial arcades) with convexities toward intestine

          i. In jejunum, usually only 1 arcade prior to branching of straight arteries (vasa or arteria recta) that pass to gut wall

          ii. In ileum, arcades become more numerous, up to 5 generations of arches prior to branching of vasa recta, which are much shorter than in jejunum

    4. **Right colic artery**

       a. Passes to right, behind peritoneum, crossing anterior to ovarian/testicular vessels, right ureter, and psoas major muscle

       b. Branches

          i. Descending: anastomoses with superior branch of ileocolic artery

          ii. Ascending: courses superiorly to join middle colic artery

    5. **Ileocolic artery** (Fig. 2.9B)

       a. Passes inferiorly and to right into right iliac fossa

       b. Branches

          i. Ascending (colic): to ascending colon

          ii. Anterior and posterior cecal: to cecum

          iii. Appendicular: descends posterior to terminal ileum within mesoappendix; usually from ileal or posterior cecal branch

          iv. Ileal: passes to left on ileum to anastomose with last intestinal branch of superior mesenteric artery

II. Inferior Mesenteric Artery (Fig. 2.9C)

A. Branches from anterior surface of abdominal aorta at level of L3 vertebra

B. Passes inferiorly toward left

C. Branches

    1. **Left colic artery**

       a. Passes toward left, behind peritoneum, in front of left psoas major muscle, and crosses left ureter and gonadal vessels

       b. Branches

          i. Ascending: ascends in front of left kidney to enter transverse mesocolon, and anastomoses with left branch of middle colic artery

          ii. Descending: descends to join highest sigmoid artery

    2. **Sigmoid arteries**: 2 or 3

       a. Pass inferolaterally behind peritoneum, but anterior to psoas major muscle, ureter, and gonadal vessels; enters sigmoid mesocolon

       b. Superiormost sigmoid artery anastomoses with left colic artery

       c. Inferiormost sigmoid artery anastomoses with superior rectal artery

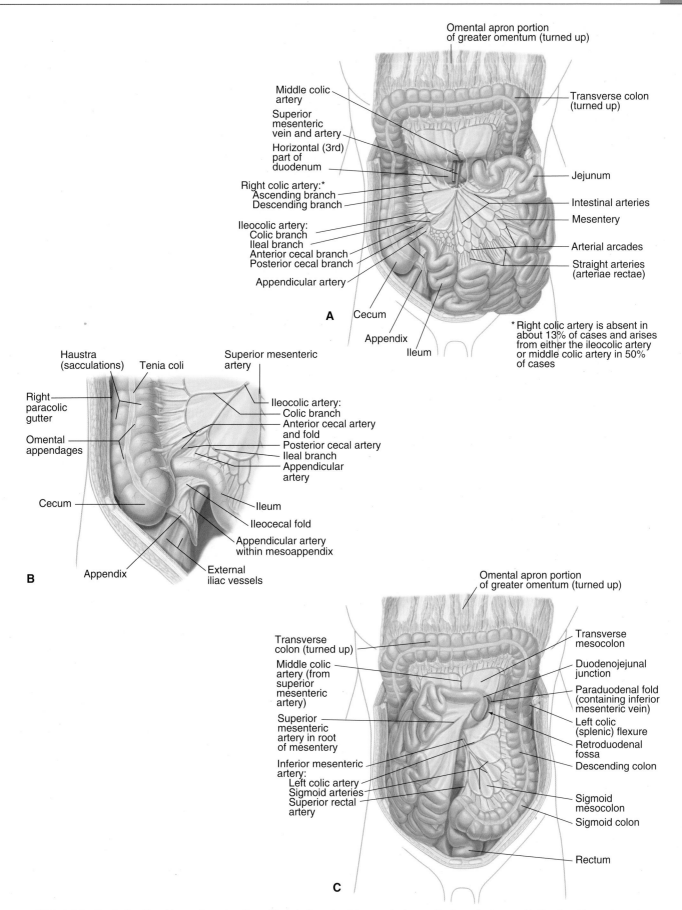

Omental apron portion of greater omentum (turned up)

Middle colic artery

Superior mesenteric vein and artery

Horizontal (3rd) part of duodenum

Right colic artery:*
Ascending branch
Descending branch

Ileocolic artery:
Colic branch
Ileal branch
Anterior cecal branch
Posterior cecal branch

Appendicular artery

Transverse colon (turned up)

Jejunum

Intestinal arteries

Mesentery

Arterial arcades

Straight arteries (arteriae rectae)

Cecum

Appendix

Ileum

A

* Right colic artery is absent in about 13% of cases and arises from either the ileocolic artery or middle colic artery in 50% of cases

Haustra (sacculations)

Tenia coli

Superior mesenteric artery

Right paracolic gutter

Omental appendages

Cecum

Ileocolic artery:
Colic branch
Anterior cecal artery and fold
Posterior cecal artery
Ileal branch
Appendicular artery

Ileum

Ileocecal fold

Appendicular artery within mesoappendix

Appendix

External iliac vessels

B

Transverse colon (turned up)

Middle colic artery (from superior mesenteric artery)

Superior mesenteric artery in root of mesentery

Inferior mesenteric artery:
Left colic artery
Sigmoid arteries
Superior rectal artery

Omental apron portion of greater omentum (turned up)

Transverse mesocolon

Duodenojejunal junction

Paraduodenal fold (containing inferior mesenteric vein)

Left colic (splenic) flexure

Retroduodenal fossa

Descending colon

Sigmoid mesocolon

Sigmoid colon

Rectum

C

FIG. 2.9A–C. **A.** Small and Large Intestine: Blood Supply, Superior Mesenteric Artery. **B.** Ileocolic Artery. **C.** Small and Large Intestine: Blood Supply, Inferior Mesenteric Artery.

3. **Superior rectal artery**
   a. Passes into pelvis by crossing left common iliac vessels
   b. Branches: divides at third sacral segment giving 1 branch to either side of rectum

III. Portal Vein

A. Formed behind neck of pancreas by union of splenic and superior mesenteric veins
B. Lies within hepatoduodenal ligament posterior to bile duct and proper hepatic artery
C. Tributaries
   1. **Inferior mesenteric vein**: begins in rectum as superior rectal vein and drains sigmoid and descending colon; usually joins splenic vein behind pancreas, but may join superior mesenteric vein
   2. **Splenic vein**: receives inferior mesenteric and veins from pancreas and stomach
   3. **Superior mesenteric vein**
      a. Receives veins from stomach, pancreas, duodenum, jejunum, ileum, cecum, appendix, and ascending and transverse colon
      b. Lies to right of superior mesenteric artery as they cross 3rd part of duodenum anteriorly
D. Branches into right and left branches within hilum of liver (porta hepatis)

IV. Lymphatics (Fig. 2.9D,E)

A. Small intestine: from lacteals in villi; lymph vessels in wall of jejunum and ileum pass in mesentery to numerous small superior mesenteric nodes
B. Large intestine
   1. Vessels and nodes follow arterial supply
   2. Ileocolic, right colic, and middle colic nodes drain to superior mesenteric nodes near origin of superior mesenteric artery
   3. Small nodes near descending colon, sigmoid colon, and upper rectum drain to inferior mesenteric nodes near origin of inferior mesenteric artery

V. Nerves

A. Small intestine and large intestine to splenic flexure: derived from vagus (parasympathetic) and thoracic splanchnic nerves (sympathetic) via celiac and superior mesenteric ganglia and superior mesenteric plexus
B. Large intestine from splenic flexure to anus: pelvic splanchnic nerves (parasympathetic) and lumbar splanchnic nerves (sympathetic)

VI. Clinical Considerations

A. **Marginal artery** (Fig. 2.9F)
   1. Anastomosis of branches of colic arteries, forming continuous channel along mesenteric border of large bowel
   2. Enables ligation of inferior mesenteric artery at origin
B. Referred pain in small bowel
   1. Experienced in areas of 9th, 10th and 11th thoracic nerves
   2. Usually in umbilical region and may spread to lumbar region and back

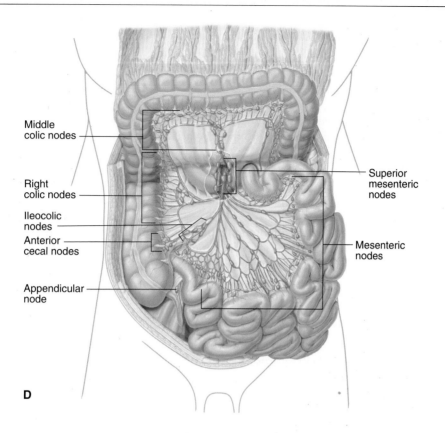

Middle colic nodes

Right colic nodes

Ileocolic nodes

Anterior cecal nodes

Appendicular node

Superior mesenteric nodes

Mesenteric nodes

D

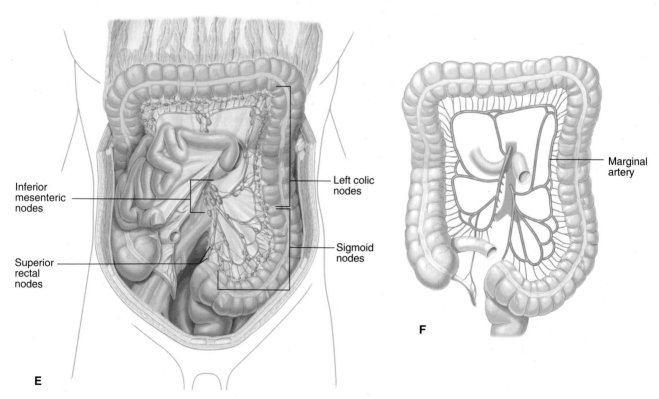

Inferior mesenteric nodes

Superior rectal nodes

Left colic nodes

Sigmoid nodes

Marginal artery

E

F

FIG. 2.9D–F. **D,E.** Lymphatics of the Large Intestine. **F.** Marginal Artery.

Stomach: Parts and Relations

I. Surface Projection (Fig. 2.10A)

A. Gastroesophageal junction: located at level of xiphoid process and T11 vertebra

B. Pylorus: located at L1 vertebral level

C. Size and shape of body of stomach is variable and changes with stages of digestion

II. Parts of Stomach (Fig. 2.10B)

A. **Cardia**

1. **Gastroesophageal junction:** junction of abdominal end of esophagus (1– 2 cm) with stomach

2. Esophagus enters abdomen by passing through diaphragm at T10 vertebral level, then opens toward left into stomach at cardiac orifice

3. Right side of esophagus is continuous with lesser curvature

B. **Fundus**

1. Domed portion superior to horizontal line through cardiac opening

2. Often filled with air in upright posture

C. **Body**

1. Lies to left of midline, below fundus

2. Marked by 2 curvatures

   a. **Greater curvature**

      i. Left or convex border; faces left and inferiorly

      ii. Greater omentum attaches along it

   b. **Lesser curvature**

      i. Right or concave border; faces right and superiorly

      ii. Continuous with right side of esophagus

      iii. Lesser omentum (hepatogastric ligament portion) attaches along it

      iv. Marked by angular incisure (and often an angular vein) that separates body from pyloric region

D. **Pylorus**

1. **Pyloric antrum:** continuous with body, marked by angular notch, or incisure

2. **Pyloric canal:** constricted passage through **pyloric sphincter** made of circular muscle fibers

3. Pyloric canal opens into 1st part of duodenum toward right

III. Relations of the Stomach

A. Anterior surface

1. Entire surface is covered with peritoneum

2. Left half is in contact with diaphragm; right half is in contact with left and quadrate lobes of liver and abdominal wall

B. Posterior surface (Fig. 2.10C)

1. Entire surface is covered with peritoneum except near cardiac opening, where gastrophrenic ligament is attached

2. Contacts peritoneum covering diaphragm, spleen, left suprarenal gland, upper part of left kidney, pancreas, left colic flexure, and upper surface of transverse mesocolon

IV. Special Features (Fig. 2.10D)

A. Muscular coat made up of 3 layers of smooth muscle (rather than 2 typical of gut structures)

1. Outer longitudinal coat

2. Intermediate circular coat

3. Inner oblique, chiefly at cardia and spreading to anterior and posterior surfaces

B. Muscularis externis of lower esophagus

1. Although not very thick, often referred to as esophageal, or cardiac, sphincter

2. Functions are physiologic and not truly anatomic, but it prevents reflux into esophagus

C. Pyloric sphincter: greatly thickened circular muscular layer of pylorus that controls rate of discharge of stomach contents into duodenum

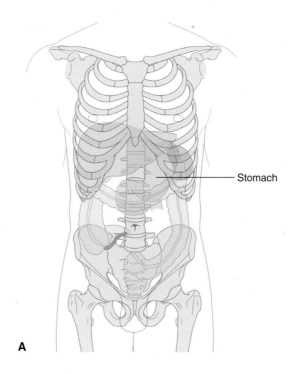

A

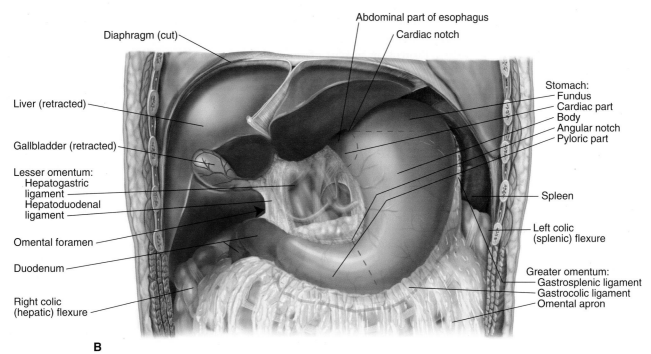

B

FIG. 2.10A,B. Stomach. **A.** Location. **B.** Parts and Relations, Anterior View.

V. Clinical Considerations

A. Stomach ulcer

1. Due to an excess of acid secretion associated with vagal nerve involvement

2. Bleeding peptic ulcer is usually located posteriorly, whereas perforating type is located anteriorly

3. Gastric ulcers are open mucosal lesions of stomach, whereas pyloric ulcers usually involve pyloric canal or, more frequently, the duodenum

4. If ulcer erodes into gastric or splenic arteries, excessive bleeding into peritoneal cavity can result

5. Recurrent peptic ulcer treated by vagotomy may have persistent pain because pain impulses from stomach are carried by visceral afferents that accompany sympathetic nerves

B. Stomach carcinoma

1. Mass may be felt if located in stomach or pyloric area

2. Biopsies of gastric lesions of mucosa are taken and seen with a gastroscope

3. Very difficult to remove all lymph nodes because of extensive lymphatic drainage

C. Partial **gastrectomy** (stomach removal)

1. Most common operation performed on stomach in cases of duodenal ulcer, gastric ulcer, or malignancy (total gastrectomy is rare)

2. Because arterial anastomoses provide good collateral circulation, 1 or more arteries can be ligated without serious consequences

3. Partial gastrectomy to remove a carcinoma requires removing all regional lymph nodes involved

D. **Gastrojejunosotomy**

1. Establishes a direct connection between stomach and jejunum

2. Indicated by pyloric obstruction and low gastric acidity

3. May be palliative measure for relief of pyloric obstruction due to inoperable carcinoma

E. **Hiatal hernia**

1. Protrusion of part of stomach into posterior mediastinum via esophageal hiatus of diaphragm

2. Seen most often after middle age due to weakening of muscular part of diaphragm

3. Major types

   a. Paraesophageal: less common

      i. Cardia remains in normal position, but a pouch of peritoneum, often with part of fundus extends through hiatus anterior to esophagus

      ii. No regurgitation of gastric content

   b. Sliding

      i. Abdominal esophagus, cardia, and parts of fundus slide up through hiatus into thorax (usually on bending over or lying down)

      ii. Some regurgitation of stomach contents into esophagus

F. Pyloric spasm

1. Spasmodic contraction of pyloric sphincter may occur in 2–12-week-old infants, preventing food from passing easily into duodenum

2. Stomach fills up, causing discomfort and vomiting

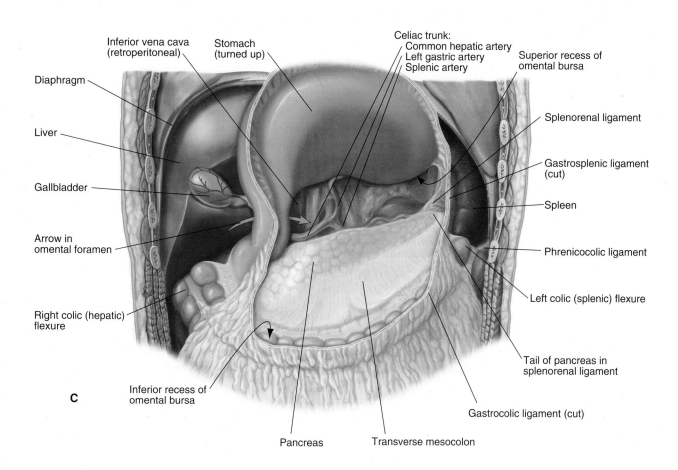

Inferior vena cava (retroperitoneal)

Diaphragm

Liver

Gallbladder

Arrow in omental foramen

Right colic (hepatic) flexure

C

Stomach (turned up)

Celiac trunk:
Common hepatic artery
Left gastric artery
Splenic artery

Superior recess of omental bursa

Splenorenal ligament

Gastrosplenic ligament (cut)

Spleen

Phrenicocolic ligament

Left colic (splenic) flexure

Tail of pancreas in splenorenal ligament

Gastrocolic ligament (cut)

Inferior recess of omental bursa

Pancreas

Transverse mesocolon

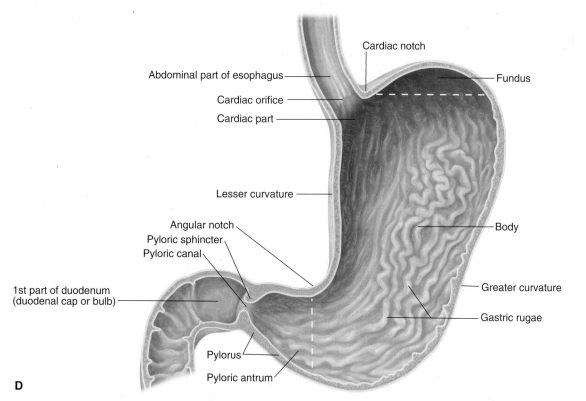

Cardiac notch

Abdominal part of esophagus

Cardiac orifice

Cardiac part

Fundus

Lesser curvature

Body

Angular notch
Pyloric sphincter
Pyloric canal

1st part of duodenum (duodenal cap or bulb)

Greater curvature

Gastric rugae

Pylorus

Pyloric antrum

D

FIG. 2.10C,D. **C.** Stomach Elevated: Parts and Relations, Anterior View. **D.** Stomach Interior.

Stomach: Blood Supply, Lymph Drainage, and Innervation

I. Blood Supply (Fig. 2.11A)

A. Arteries: all derived directly or indirectly from celiac trunk

1. **Left gastric artery**: directly from celiac, runs upward and to left across posterior wall of omental bursa to reach superior end of lesser curvature, which it follows
2. **Right gastric artery**: branches from proper hepatic artery, runs to left along lesser curvature to anastomose with left gastric
3. **Right gastro-omental** (gastroepiploic) **artery**: one of terminal branches of gastroduodenal artery from common hepatic artery, runs toward left along greater curvature within gastrocolic ligament
4. **Left gastro-omental** (gastroepiploic) **artery**: from splenic artery, through gastrosplenic (gastrolienal) ligament; runs from left to right along greater curvature within gastrocolic ligament to meet right gastro-omental
5. **Short gastric arteries**: 5 to 7 small branches from splenic artery to fundus and greater curvature above left gastro-omental (gastroepiploic) artery

B. Veins: venous drainage directly or indirectly into portal vein

1. **Short gastric veins**: from greater curvature and fundus to splenic vein
2. **Left gastro-omental** (gastroepiploic) **vein**: along greater curvature to splenic vein
3. **Right gastro-omental** (gastroepiploic) **vein**: from right end of greater curvature to superior mesenteric vein
4. **Left gastric (coronary) vein**: runs right to left along lesser curvature to reach posterior abdominal wall and drain to portal vein; accompanies left gastric artery
5. **Right gastric vein**: small; receives prepyloric vein (of Mayo; useful in identifying pylorus); accompanies right gastric artery; drains to portal vein

II. Lymphatic Drainage (Fig. 2.11B)

A. Visceral nodes

1. Gastric nodes
   a. Superior (left gastric) along left gastric artery
   b. Inferior along right half of greater curvature
2. Hepatic nodes: Subdivided into groups
   a. Along hepatic artery
   b. Near neck of gallbladder
   c. In angle between superior and descending duodenum
3. Pancreaticosplenic nodes: along splenic artery

B. Lymph vessels

1. Along lesser curvature follow left gastric artery to superior gastric nodes
2. From fundus and body (to left of esophagus) along left gastro-omental artery to pancreaticosplenic nodes
3. From right part of greater curvature to inferior gastric and hepatic nodes
4. From pyloric region into hepatic and superior gastric nodes
5. Drainage is eventually to paraaortic nodes around celiac trunk

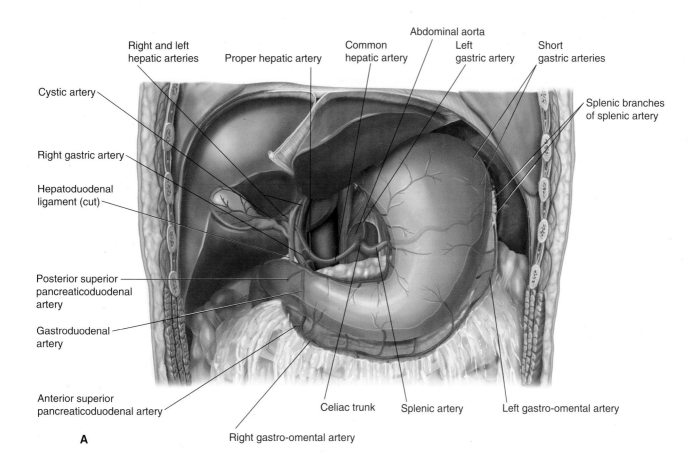

Right and left hepatic arteries

Cystic artery

Proper hepatic artery

Common hepatic artery

Abdominal aorta

Left gastric artery

Short gastric arteries

Splenic branches of splenic artery

Right gastric artery

Hepatoduodenal ligament (cut)

Posterior superior pancreaticoduodenal artery

Gastroduodenal artery

Anterior superior pancreaticoduodenal artery

Celiac trunk

Splenic artery

Left gastro-omental artery

Right gastro-omental artery

A

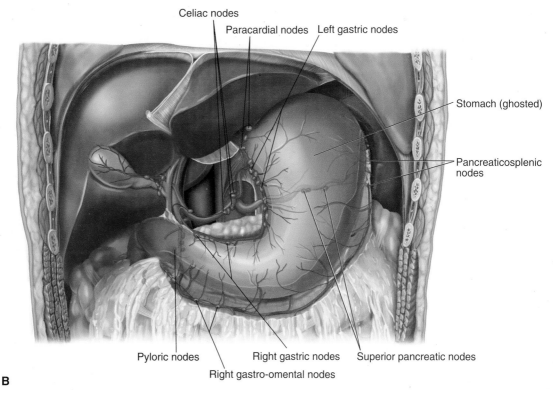

Celiac nodes

Paracardial nodes

Left gastric nodes

Stomach (ghosted)

Pancreaticosplenic nodes

Pyloric nodes

Right gastric nodes

Right gastro-omental nodes

Superior pancreatic nodes

B

FIG. 2.11A,B. Stomach. **A.** Blood Supply. **B.** Lymph Drainage.

III. Nerve Supply (Fig. 2.11 C,D)

A. Parasympathetic
1. Presynaptic fibers from posterior vagal trunk posteriorly and anterior vagal trunk anteriorly
2. Synapse within walls of stomach

B. Sympathetic
1. Presynaptic fibers mainly in greater thoracic splanchnic nerves (from T5– T9 segments of spinal cord)
2. Synapse in celiac ganglia beside celiac trunk
3. Postsynaptic fibers form perivascular celiac plexus to distribute along vessels

IV. Clinical Considerations

A. **Vagotomy**: section of vagal trunks as they enter abdomen
1. Because vagal trunks largely control secretion of acid by parietal cells of stomach and excess acid secretion is associated with peptic ulcers (either in stomach or duodenum), procedure may reduce acid production (often in conjunction with resection of ulcerated area)
2. Procedure largely replaced recently by more effective drug therapies

B. Stomach cancer produces metastases in liver because venous drainage is via portal vein

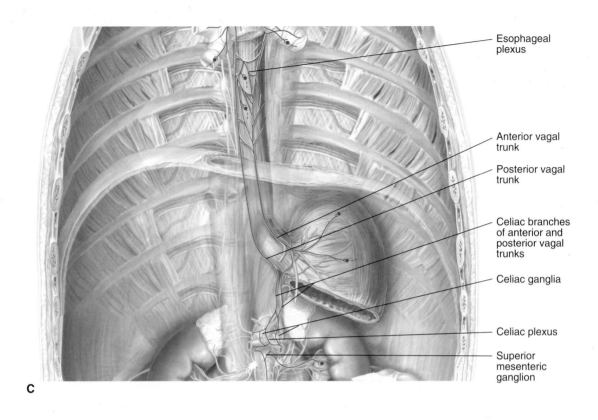

Esophageal plexus

Anterior vagal trunk

Posterior vagal trunk

Celiac branches of anterior and posterior vagal trunks

Celiac ganglia

Celiac plexus

Superior mesenteric ganglion

C

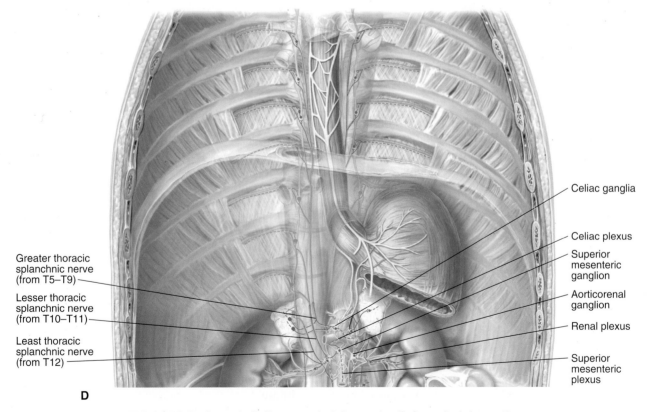

Celiac ganglia

Celiac plexus

Superior mesenteric ganglion

Aorticorenal ganglion

Renal plexus

Superior mesenteric plexus

Greater thoracic splanchnic nerve (from T5–T9)

Lesser thoracic splanchnic nerve (from T10–T11)

Least thoracic splanchnic nerve (from T12)

D

FIG. 2.11C,D. Stomach. **C.** Parasympathetic Innervation. **D.** Sympathetic Innervation.

Spleen: Parts and Relations

I. Fundamentals of the Spleen

A. Lymphatic organ interposed in bloodstream
B. Develops within dorsal mesogastrium, the dorsal mesentery of stomach

II. Surface Projection (Fig. 2.12A)

A. Long axis in line with left 10th rib
B. Extent
   1. Medially to 4 cm from posterior midline
   2. Laterally to left 9th intercostal space in midaxillary line
   3. Superiorly to left 9th rib
   4. Inferiorly to left 11th rib

III. Relations (Fig. 2.12B)

A. Diaphragmatic surface
   1. Related to diaphragm, which separates it from 9th, 10th, and 11th ribs and left lung and pleura
   2. Convex, smooth; faces upward, backward, and to left
B. Visceral relations (Fig. 2.12C,D)
   1. Gastric
      a. Contacts posterior left side of stomach and tail of pancreas
      b. Concave; faces anteriorly, superiorly, and medially
   2. Renal
      a. Related to upper anterior surface of left kidney
      b. Flattened; faces medially and inferiorly
   3. Colic
      a. Related to left colic flexure
      b. Small and slightly concave, at anterior extremity
C. Posterosuperior extremity: directed toward vertebral column
D. Anteroinferior extremity: rests on left colic flexure and phrenicocolic ligament

IV. Support

A. Splenorenal (lienorenal) ligament
   1. Reflection of peritoneum running from diaphragm and anterior aspect of left kidney to hilum of spleen
   2. Contains splenic vessels and tail of pancreas
B. Gastrosplenic (gastrolienal) ligament
   1. Part of greater omentum between spleen and stomach
   2. Contains short gastric and left gastro-omental (gastroepiploic) vessels
C. Phrenicocolic ligament
   1. Suspends left colic flexure from diaphragm
   2. Supports inferior surface of spleen

V. Blood Supply

A. Splenic artery
   1. From celiac artery
   2. Large, tortuous course across posterior wall of omental bursa along upper border of pancreas
   3. Runs through splenorenal ligament to hilum of spleen
   4. Divides into 6 or more branches in hilum
B. Splenic vein
   1. Arises from union of 6 or more veins that emerge from hilum
   2. Runs on posterior surface of pancreas, below artery, and ends behind neck of pancreas by joining superior mesenteric vein to form portal vein
   3. Usually receives inferior mesenteric vein behind body of pancreas

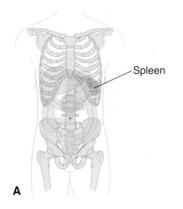

A

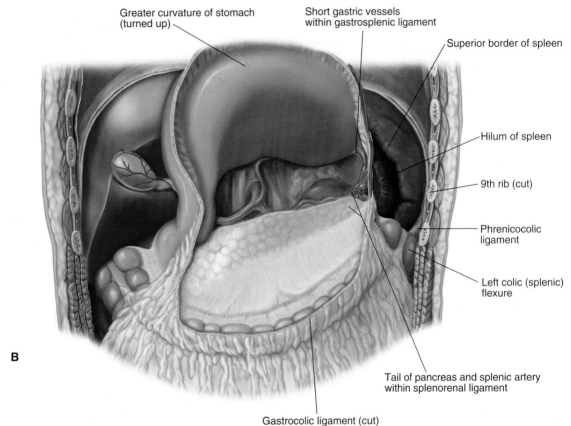

Greater curvature of stomach (turned up)

Short gastric vessels within gastrosplenic ligament

Superior border of spleen

Hilum of spleen

9th rib (cut)

Phrenicocolic ligament

Left colic (splenic) flexure

Tail of pancreas and splenic artery within splenorenal ligament

Gastrocolic ligament (cut)

B

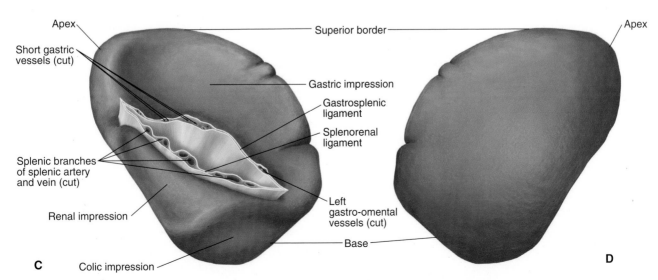

Apex

Short gastric vessels (cut)

Superior border

Apex

Gastric impression

Gastrosplenic ligament

Splenorenal ligament

Splenic branches of splenic artery and vein (cut)

Renal impression

Left gastro-omental vessels (cut)

Base

Colic impression

C

D

FIG. 2.12A–D. Spleen. **A.** Location. **B.** Relations, Anterior View. **C.** Visceral Surface. **D.** Diaphragmatic Surface.

VI. Lymphatic Drainage: Into Pancreaticosplenic Nodes

VII. Nerves

A. Chiefly postsynaptic sympathetic fibers
B. From celiac plexus to blood vessels, capsule, and trabeculae of organ

VIII. Functions

A. Storage of red blood cells, which can be forced back into circulation during respiratory crisis by contraction of smooth muscle in capsule and trabeculae
B. Destruction of worn-out red blood cells
C. Removal of foreign material from bloodstream
D. Production of mononuclear leukocytes

IX. Clinical Considerations

A. **Splenomegaly** (abnormal enlargement of spleen): hypertrophic spleen due to overactivity of macrophage system can be removed without any apparent ill effects
B. **Splenic rupture**: although protected under costal margin, spleen is more prone to rupture than any other abdominal organ due to its thin capsule and soft and pulpy parenchyma, causing severe bleeding into peritoneal cavity, eventually leading to shock
   1. Repair is difficult and entire spleen is usually removed (splenectomy)
   2. Total splenectomy does not usually create serious side effects (in adults) because other organs (liver and bone marrow) take over its function
C. **Accessory spleens**
   1. Very common, but tend to be small and resemble lymph nodes
   2. Should be removed if spleen is removed
   3. May develop prenatally near splenic hilum or be embedded in pancreatic tail between layers of gastrosplenic ligament, in infracolic compartment, in mesentery, or near ovary or testis
D. Splenic needle biopsy or injection: for diagnostic purposes or for injecting radiopaque material into spleen for visualization of the hepatic portal vein

Duodenum: Parts and Relations

I. Fundamentals of the Duodenum

A. First and shortest part of small intestine

B. Extends from pylorus to duodenojejunal junction, 25 cm long

II. Parts and Relations (Fig. 2.13A,B)

A. **Superior (1st) part**
   1. Extends from pylorus to right, under quadrate lobe of liver to neck of gallbladder, where it bends sharply inferiorly
   2. Nearly completely covered by peritoneum except at neck of gallbladder
   3. Hepatoduodenal ligament attached to upper border
   4. Related above and anteriorly to liver and gallbladder; posteriorly to gastroduodenal artery, bile duct, and portal vein; below and posteriorly to pancreas

B. **Descending (2nd) part**
   1. Extends from level of neck of gallbladder at first lumbar vertebra, along right side of vertebral column to upper body of L3
   2. Covered anteriorly by peritoneum, except where crossed by transverse mesocolon
   3. Related posteriorly to medial surface of right kidney and structures at its hilum, inferior vena cava, and psoas major muscle; anteriorly to liver, transverse colon, coils of jejunum; medially to head of pancreas and bile duct; and laterally to right colic flexure
   4. Bile duct and main pancreatic duct pierce wall about 7 cm below pylorus; accessory pancreatic duct is 2 cm superior to this

C. **Horizontal (inferior or 3rd) part**
   1. Passes from right to left at level of L3 vertebral body
   2. Covered anteriorly by peritoneum, except near midline, where crossed by superior mesenteric vessels
   3. Related anteriorly to superior mesenteric vessels, which cross it; posteriorly to right crus of diaphragm, inferior vena cava, and aorta; and superiorly to pancreas

D. **Ascending (4th) part**
   1. Rises superiorly to left of aorta to upper border of L2, where it turns sharply to join jejunum
   2. Covered anteriorly by peritoneum
   3. Related posteriorly to left psoas major muscle and left renal vessels; and on right to uncinate process of pancreas
   4. Connected to right crus of diaphragm by suspensory muscle of duodenum

III. Structural Characteristics (Fig. 2.13C,D)

A. Retroperitoneal (secondarily, due to fusion to posterior body wall during development) except for 1st part

B. Plicae circulares (circular folds of submucosa): numerous and well developed in duodenum, beginning in descending part

C. Duodenal glands (of Brunner): compound tubuloalveolar glands of mucous type found in submucosa

D. Numerous large villi

E. **Major duodenal papilla** with sphincter of ampulla (of Oddi) around bile duct and main pancreatic duct (**hepatopancreatic ampulla**) within wall of duodenum

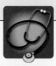

IV. Clinical Considerations

A. **Duodenal ulcers**

1. Most (65%) occur within 4 cm of pylorus and more frequently on anterior wall of superior part of duodenum

2. Tend to recur, and several cycles of ulceration and scar tissue healing can permanently narrow 1st part of duodenum and deform duodenal cap, or bulb (superior part of duodenum as seen on barium meal)

3. If ulcer penetrates duodenal wall, duodenal contents may enter peritoneal cavity and lead to peritonitis

4. Because superior duodenum is related to liver, gallbladder, and pancreas, any of these may adhere to inflamed site and become eroded and ulcerated

5. Erosion of gastroduodenal artery (a posterior relation of superior part of duodenum) leads to severe hemorrhage into peritoneal cavity and peritonitis

B. **Duodenal bulb or cap**: barium passing through pylorus forms a mushroom-shaped cap in 1st part of duodenum, which empties in a few seconds

C. **Kocher maneuver**: because duodenum is secondarily retroperitoneal, both it and attached head of pancreas can be reflected from posterior body wall viscera (right kidney) without endangering blood vessels

D. Because superior (1st) part of duodenum is not supplied from the arcades but by small branches from gastroduodenal artery, it has poorest blood supply

E. Anomalies relatively uncommon and include atresia (discontinuity of lumen) and stenosis (complete or incomplete)

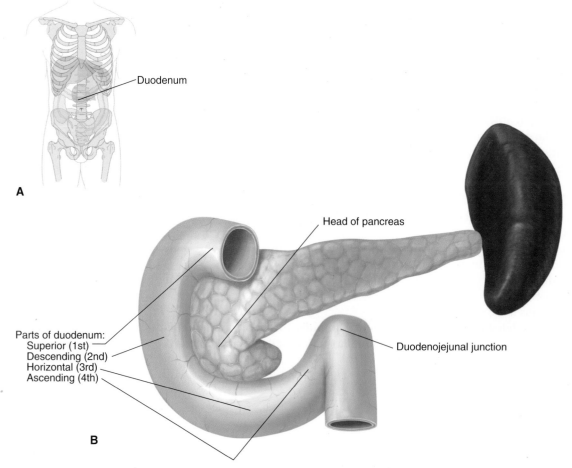

Duodenum

A

Head of pancreas

Duodenojejunal junction

Parts of duodenum:
Superior (1st)
Descending (2nd)
Horizontal (3rd)
Ascending (4th)

B

FIG. 2.13A,B. Duodenum. **A.** Location. **B.** Parts, Anterior View.

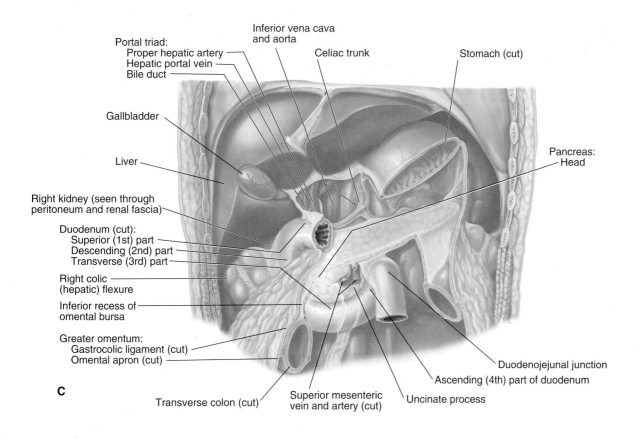

Portal triad:
Proper hepatic artery
Hepatic portal vein
Bile duct

Inferior vena cava
and aorta

Celiac trunk

Stomach (cut)

Gallbladder

Liver

Pancreas:
Head

Right kidney (seen through
peritoneum and renal fascia)

Duodenum (cut):
Superior (1st) part
Descending (2nd) part
Transverse (3rd) part

Right colic
(hepatic) flexure

Inferior recess of
omental bursa

Greater omentum:
Gastrocolic ligament (cut)
Omental apron (cut)

Duodenojejunal junction

Ascending (4th) part of duodenum

Uncinate process

C

Transverse colon (cut)

Superior mesenteric
vein and artery (cut)

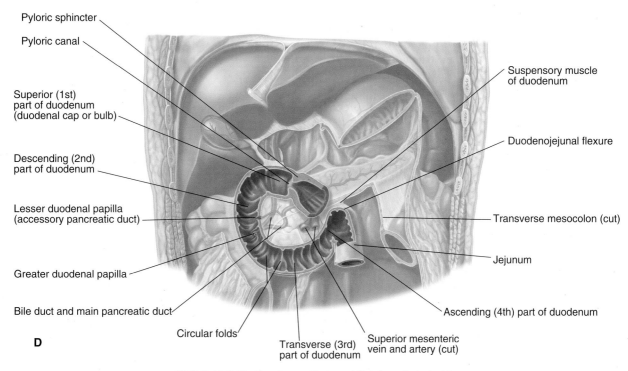

Pyloric sphincter

Pyloric canal

Superior (1st)
part of duodenum
(duodenal cap or bulb)

Descending (2nd)
part of duodenum

Lesser duodenal papilla
(accessory pancreatic duct)

Greater duodenal papilla

Bile duct and main pancreatic duct

Suspensory muscle
of duodenum

Duodenojejunal flexure

Transverse mesocolon (cut)

Jejunum

Ascending (4th) part of duodenum

D

Circular folds

Transverse (3rd)
part of duodenum

Superior mesenteric
vein and artery (cut)

FIG. 2.13C,D. Duodenum. Parts and Relations, Anterior View.

Pancreas: Parts and Relations

I. Fundamentals of the Pancreas (Fig. 2.14A)

A. Soft, fleshy gland with little connective tissue
B. Possesses both endocrine and exocrine gland components
  1. Endocrine: islets of Langerhans
  2. Exocrine: compound tubuloalveolar, serous secretion

II. Parts and Relations (Fig. 2.14B,C)

A. **Head**
  1. Broad, right extremity; lies within curve of duodenum
  2. **Uncinate process**
    a. Prolongation of inferior border of head to left
    b. Crossed by superior mesenteric vessels with superior mesenteric vein on right
  3. Anterior surface: most of right side is separated from transverse colon by areolar tissue (no peritoneum); lower part of anterior surface below transverse colon is covered by peritoneum; in contact with coils of small intestine
  4. Posterior surface: lacks peritoneum; in contact with inferior vena cava, bile duct, renal veins, right crus of diaphragm, and aorta
B. **Neck**
  1. Constricted portion to left of head
  2. Above, it adjoins pylorus
  3. Behind, it is related to origin of portal vein
C. **Body**
  1. Anterior surface: separated from stomach by omental bursa
  2. Posterior surface: lacks peritoneum; related to aorta, splenic vein, left kidney and vessels, left suprarenal, origin of superior mesenteric artery, and crura of diaphragm
  3. Inferior surface: peritoneal; related to duodenojejunal junction, coils of jejunum, and left colic flexure
  4. Anteroinferior border: attachment of transverse mesocolon
  5. Superior border: related to celiac trunk, with common hepatic artery to right and splenic artery to left
D. **Tail**
  1. Left extremity
  2. Extends to hilum of spleen, in splenorenal ligament

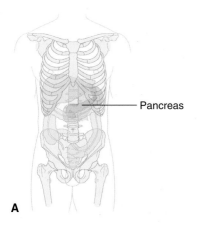

A

Pancreas

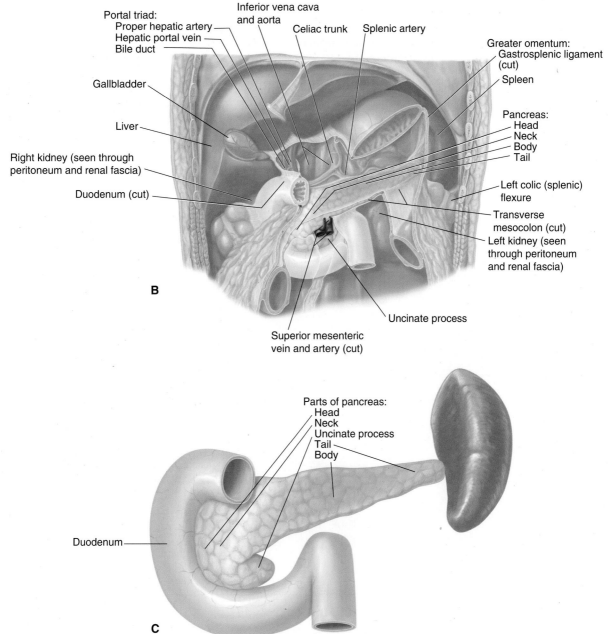

Portal triad:
Proper hepatic artery
Hepatic portal vein
Bile duct

Inferior vena cava
and aorta
Celiac trunk

Splenic artery

Greater omentum:
Gastrosplenic ligament
(cut)
Spleen

Gallbladder

Liver

Pancreas:
Head
Neck
Body
Tail

Right kidney (seen through
peritoneum and renal fascia)

Left colic (splenic)
flexure

Duodenum (cut)

Transverse
mesocolon (cut)
Left kidney (seen
through peritoneum
and renal fascia)

B

Uncinate process

Superior mesenteric
vein and artery (cut)

Parts of pancreas:
Head
Neck
Uncinate process
Tail
Body

Duodenum

C

FIG. 2.14A–C. Pancreas. **A.** Location. **B.** Parts and Relations, Anterior View. **C.** Ducts, Anterior View.

III. Ducts (Fig. 2.14D)

A. **Main pancreatic duct** (of Wirsung)

   1. Extends toward right, reaches neck of pancreas, where it turns caudally and dorsally and unites with bile duct to form hepatopancreatic ampulla (of Vater)

   2. **Hepatopancreatic ampulla** passes obliquely through wall of descending duodenum and opens through common orifice into its lumen at major duodenal papilla

B. **Accessory pancreatic duct** (minor of Santorini) drains upper part of head, enters duodenum at minor duodenal papilla above major papilla

IV. Clinical Considerations

A. Hypertrophy of head may cause portal or bile duct obstruction

B. Degeneration of islets of Langerhans leads to diabetes mellitus

C. **Pancreatitis**: serious inflammatory condition of exocrine pancreas

   1. May develop due to "stone" obstruction of hepatopancreatic ampulla, which blocks pancreatic duct so that pancreatic juice cannot be released

   2. Bile may also "back up," causing pain

D. Pancreatic carcinoma

   1. Pancreatic head involvement accounts for most cases of extrahepatic obstruction of biliary ducts

   2. Difficult to diagnose unless in head and compresses bile duct, causing obstructive jaundice; because metastasizes to liver very early via hepatic portal vein, surgical resection almost futile

   3. Most people with pancreatic cancer develop ductular adenocarcinoma with frequent back pain

E. Accessory pancreatic tissue can develop in the stomach, duodenum, ileum or ileal (Meckel) diverticulum

   1. Stomach most common location

   2. May have insulin- and glucagon-producing islet cells

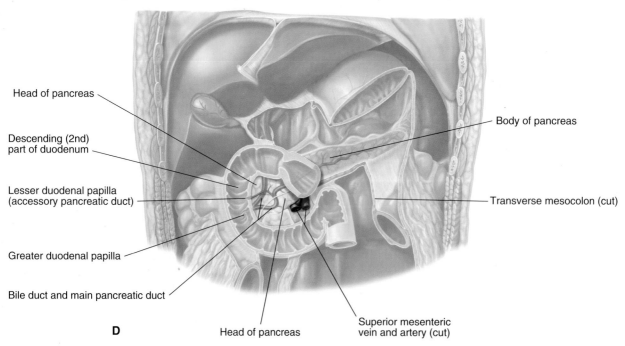

FIG. 2.14D. Pancreas: Ducts.

Duodenum, Pancreas, and Spleen: Blood Supply, Lymph Drainage, and Innervation

I. Arterial Supply (Fig. 2.15A,B)

A. Duodenum and head of pancreas
  1. Proximal half of duodenum and upper head: supplied by **anterior** and **posterior superior pancreaticoduodenal arteries**
  2. Distal half of duodenum and lower head: supplied by **inferior pancreaticoduodenal artery**, which has anterior and posterior branches
  3. Pancreaticoduodenal arteries anastomose to form anterior and posterior arterial arcades, which occupy angle between duodenum and pancreas
  4. Superior part, in addition to above, is also supplied by supraduodenal, right gastric, right gastro-omental, and retroduodenal arteries
  5. Because arteries approach duodenum through its concavity, incision along right edge of descending part of duodenum will mobilize organ and head of pancreas without endangering their blood supplies

B. Spleen and body and tail of pancreas supplied by branches of **splenic artery**
  1. **Dorsal pancreatic artery**: supplies region near neck of pancreas
  2. **Great pancreatic artery**: supplies middle of body
  3. **Pancreatic branches**: multiple small
  4. **Caudal pancreatic branches**: to tail
  5. **Splenic branches**: splenic artery splits into 6 or more branches that enter hilum of spleen

II. Venous Drainage

A. Veins generally follow arteries but are more variable and drain into portal venous system
B. Spleen and body and tail of pancreas drain into **splenic vein**
C. Head of pancreas drains into superior mesenteric vein primarily
D. A few tributaries enter portal vein directly

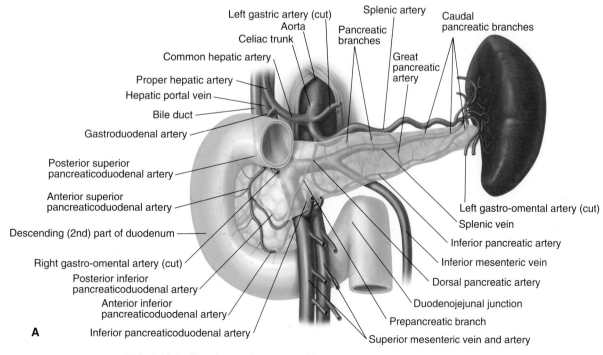

FIG. 2.15A. Duodenum, Pancreas, and Spleen. **A.** Blood Supply, Anterior View.

III. Lymphatic Drainage (Fig. 2.15C)

A. Lymph vessels on anterior and posterior surfaces of duodenum drain into anterior and posterior collecting vessels and nodes that lie in front of and behind pancreas, anastomose freely with each other, and ultimately drain into thoracic duct

B. Anterior efferent vessels follow arteries and drain upward via **pancreaticoduodenal nodes** to gastroduodenal nodes and finally into celiac nodes

C. Posterior efferent vessels pass behind head of pancreas and drain downward into superior mesenteric nodes (found around origin of superior mesenteric artery)

IV. Nerve Supply

A. Sympathetic supply
  1. Presynaptic fibers from greater thoracic splanchnic nerves synapse in celiac ganglion
  2. Postsynaptic fibers pass to organs on respective arteries (within celiac and superior mesenteric plexuses)
  3. Sympathetics decrease motility and secretion and cause vasoconstriction

B. Parasympathetic supply
  1. Derived entirely from vagus nerves, which become vagal trunks within abdomen
     a. **Anterior vagal trunk**
        i. Continues from anterior surface of esophagus onto lesser curvature and anterior surface of stomach as anterior gastric nerve
        ii. Enters free edge of lesser omentum and gives fibers to liver, gallbladder, and a few to duodenum
     b. **Posterior vagal trunk**
        i. From right posterolateral surface of esophagus, sends branches to posterior surface of stomach (posterior gastric nerve), but also a large celiac branch to join celiac ganglia (which does not synapse there)
        ii. Fibers continue through and reach organs to be innervated
        iii. Synapse occurs in intrinsic ganglia in walls of organs innervated
  2. Parasympathetics increase peristalsis and gastric secretion and relate to vasodilation

C. Sensory fibers
  1. Found in greater thoracic splanchnic nerves
  2. Pain associated with distention or violent contraction

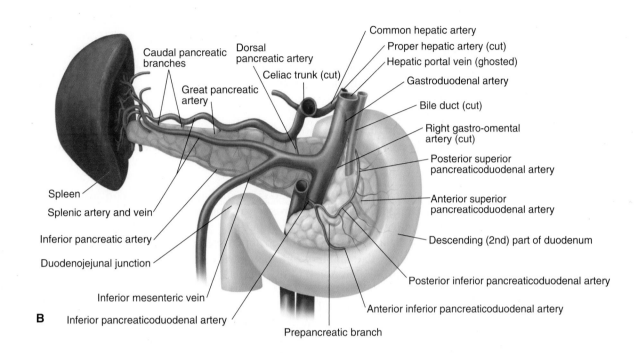

Caudal pancreatic branches

Dorsal pancreatic artery

Common hepatic artery

Proper hepatic artery (cut)

Hepatic portal vein (ghosted)

Great pancreatic artery

Celiac trunk (cut)

Gastroduodenal artery

Bile duct (cut)

Right gastro-omental artery (cut)

Posterior superior pancreaticoduodenal artery

Anterior superior pancreaticoduodenal artery

Spleen

Splenic artery and vein

Inferior pancreatic artery

Duodenojejunal junction

Descending (2nd) part of duodenum

Posterior inferior pancreaticoduodenal artery

Inferior mesenteric vein

Anterior inferior pancreaticoduodenal artery

B Inferior pancreaticoduodenal artery

Prepancreatic branch

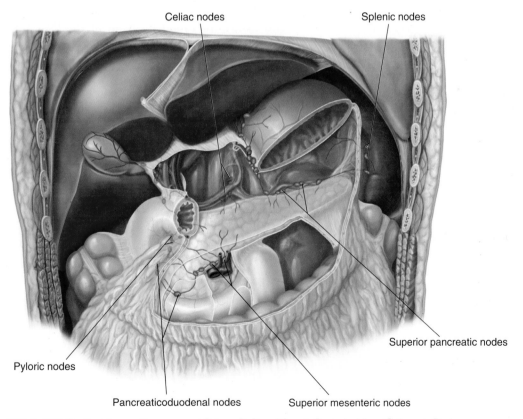

Celiac nodes

Splenic nodes

Superior pancreatic nodes

Pyloric nodes

C

Pancreaticoduodenal nodes

Superior mesenteric nodes

FIG. 2.15B,C. Duodenum, Pancreas, and Spleen. **B.** Blood Supply, Posterior View. **C.** Lymph Drainage.

Liver: Parts and Relations

I. Surfaces (Fig. 2.16A,B)

A. Diaphragmatic
1. Anterior
   a. Faces diaphragm, which separates liver from 6th to 10th ribs and cartilages on right and from 7th and 8th cartilages on left
   b. Covered by peritoneum except along attachment of falciform ligament
2. Superior (Fig. 2.16C)
   a. Under dome of diaphragm, which separates it from lungs on right and heart on left
   b. Covered by peritoneum except posteriorly, at edge of bare area, posterior to anterior lamina of coronary ligament
3. Posterior
   a. Fitted against vertebral column and crura of diaphragm with concavity
   b. **Bare area**: large area between coronary ligaments not covered by peritoneum
   c. Sulcus for inferior vena cava to right of this
   d. **Fissure for ligamentum venosum** to left of vena cava (ligamentum venosum lies within uppermost attachment of hepatogastric ligament to liver)
   e. Esophageal impression to left of fissure for ligamentum venosum
B. Visceral (Fig. 2.16D)
1. Faces posteriorly, caudally, and toward left
2. Covered by peritoneum except at fossa for gallbladder and porta hepatis
   a. **Porta hepatis**: hilum of liver; fissure in left central part for blood vessels and hepatic ducts
   b. Right portion shows colic, renal, and duodenal impressions
3. Fossa for gallbladder and fissure for **round ligament of the liver (ligamentum teres hepatis)** anteriorly
4. Left portion: gastric impression and caudate lobe

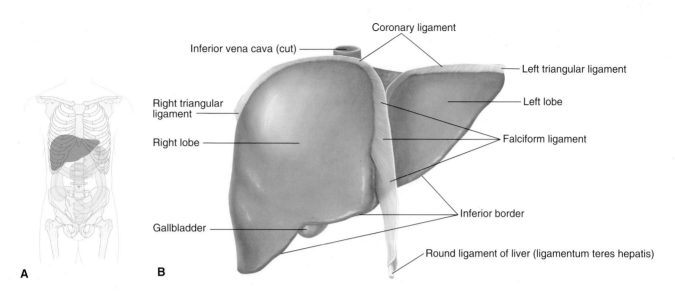

B

Coronary ligament

Inferior vena cava (cut)

Left triangular ligament

Right triangular ligament

Left lobe

Right lobe

Falciform ligament

Inferior border

Gallbladder

Round ligament of liver (ligamentum teres hepatis)

A

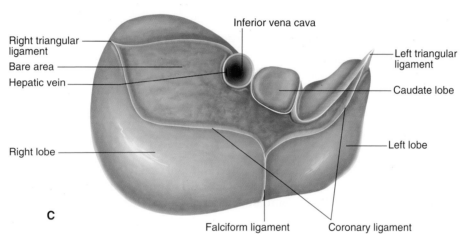

C

Inferior vena cava

Right triangular ligament

Left triangular ligament

Bare area

Hepatic vein

Caudate lobe

Right lobe

Left lobe

Falciform ligament

Coronary ligament

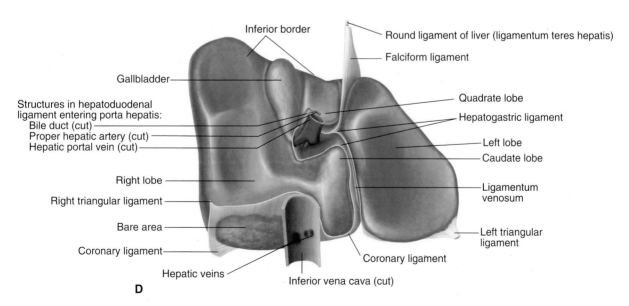

D

Inferior border

Round ligament of liver (ligamentum teres hepatis)

Gallbladder

Falciform ligament

Structures in hepatoduodenal ligament entering porta hepatis:
Bile duct (cut)
Proper hepatic artery (cut)
Hepatic portal vein (cut)

Quadrate lobe

Hepatogastric ligament

Left lobe

Right lobe

Caudate lobe

Right triangular ligament

Ligamentum venosum

Bare area

Coronary ligament

Left triangular ligament

Coronary ligament

Hepatic veins

Inferior vena cava (cut)

FIG. 2.16A–D. Liver: **A.** Location. **B.** Parts, Anterior View. **C.** Parts, Superior View. **D.** Parts, Inferior View.

II. Lobes of the Liver

A. Boundaries: delimited by an H-shaped arrangement of fossae and fissures on visceral surface
   1. To left lie fissure for round ligament of liver (ligamentum teres hepatis) anteriorly and fissure for ligamentum venosum posteriorly
   2. To right lie fossa for gallbladder anteriorly and sulcus for inferior vena cava posteriorly
   3. Porta hepatis: transverse part of H
B. Lobes
   1. **Right lobe**: largest; lies to right of fossa for gallbladder anteriorly and sulcus for inferior vena cava
   2. **Quadrate lobe**: lies between fossa for gallbladder and fissure for round ligament of liver, anterior to porta hepatis
   3. **Caudate lobe**: lies between sulcus for inferior vena cava and fissure for ductus venosus, posterior to porta; joined to right lobe by caudate process
   4. **Left lobe**: to left of fissure for ligamentum teres hepatis and fissure for ligamentum venosum

III. Liver Segments (Fig. 2.16E,F)

A. Further subdivisions of liver lobes into smaller segments based on liver vascular pattern
B. 8 segments defined by vascular branching

IV. Clinical Considerations

A. **Jaundice**
   1. Accumulation of bile pigment in bloodstream
   2. Frequently results from obstruction of duct system
B. Cancer: because of portal system, liver is frequent site for metastasis from almost any other body site (particularly GI tract)
C. **Cirrhosis** of liver: due to atrophy of parenchyma and hypertrophy of connective tissue
   1. Liver cells destroyed and replaced by fibrous tissue, which surrounds vessels and ducts making liver firm and impeding circulation through it
   2. Most common cause of portal hypertension and frequently seen with alcoholism
D. **Hepatomegaly**: enlarged liver associated with carcinoma, heart failure, fatty infiltration, or Hodgkin disease

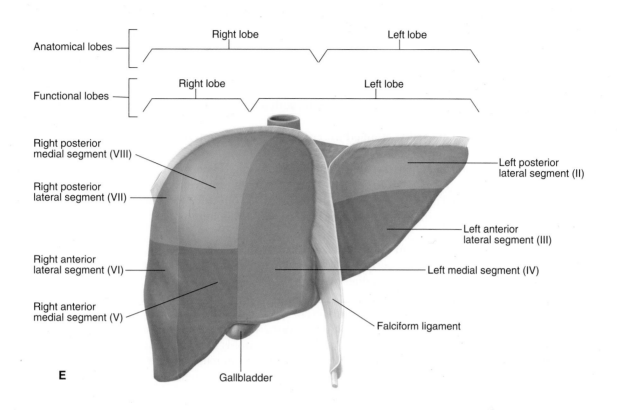

Anatomical lobes
Right lobe   Left lobe

Functional lobes
Right lobe   Left lobe

Right posterior medial segment (VIII)

Right posterior lateral segment (VII)

Right anterior lateral segment (VI)

Right anterior medial segment (V)

Left posterior lateral segment (II)

Left anterior lateral segment (III)

Left medial segment (IV)

Falciform ligament

Gallbladder

E

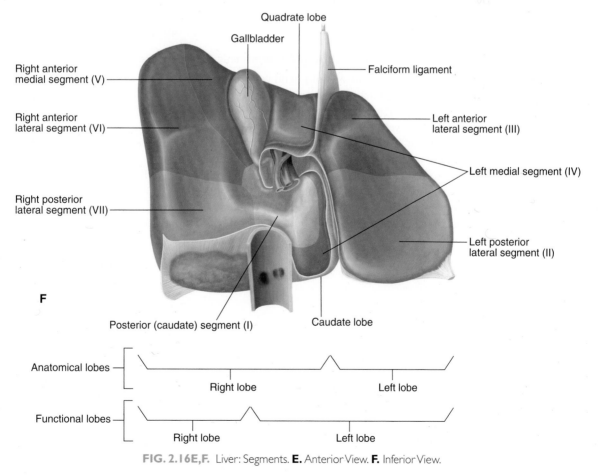

Quadrate lobe

Gallbladder

Right anterior medial segment (V)

Right anterior lateral segment (VI)

Right posterior lateral segment (VII)

Falciform ligament

Left anterior lateral segment (III)

Left medial segment (IV)

Left posterior lateral segment (II)

Posterior (caudate) segment (I)

Caudate lobe

Anatomical lobes
Right lobe   Left lobe

Functional lobes
Right lobe   Left lobe

F

FIG. 2.16E,F. Liver: Segments. **E.** Anterior View. **F.** Inferior View.

Liver Lobules, Blood Supply, Innervation, and Portal Circulation

I. Liver Lobule (Fig. 2.17A)

A. Polygonal shaped unit of structure, with scant connective tissue between adjoining lobules
B. Composition
  1. Hepatic cells: arranged in "cords" or "plates" with bile canaliculi compressed between 2 adjoining cells
  2. **Sinusoids**: narrow, endothelial-lined channels between liver cords
  3. Central vein: large venous channels running longitudinally, in center of lobule
  4. **Portal triad**: in connective tissue, usually at one angle of lobule, comprising 3 structures: hepatic duct, branch of portal vein, and branch of hepatic artery
C. Bile flow
  1. Bile formed in hepatic cells
  2. Drains toward periphery of lobule through canaliculi between cells
  3. Empties into small duct of triad
D. Circulation (Fig. 2.17B)
  1. Venous blood, carrying materials absorbed from alimentary canal, enters liver through right and left branches of portal vein, which it passes through to reach portal triad
  2. From branches, portal blood enters sinusoids to reach central vein of lobule
  3. Arterial blood enters through right and left hepatic arteries, branches of proper hepatic artery, carrying oxygenated blood through branches in portal triad, from which it enters sinusoids to reach central vein (Fig. 2.17C)
  4. **Central veins** from several lobules enter sublobular veins
  5. **Sublobular veins** unite into increasingly larger trunks, which finally converge to form 3 **hepatic veins** (right, middle, and left) that enter inferior vena cava

II. Collateral Portal Circulation (Portosystemic Anastomoses) (Fig. 2.17D)

A. Important clinically in cases of portal vein obstruction
B. 4 areas where portal and systemic circulation anastomose
  1. Gastroesophageal: esophageal tributaries of left gastric vein of portal system and esophageal veins of azygos system
  2. Anorectal: superior rectal tributary to inferior mesenteric vein of portal system and middle and inferior rectal veins of internal iliac system
  3. Paraumbilical: small paraumbilical veins within falciform ligament (tributaries of portal vein) and veins draining anterior abdominal wall
  4. Retroperitoneal: intestinal veins of portal system (right colic, ileocolic, left colic) with retroperitoneal (lumbar) tributaries of inferior vena cava

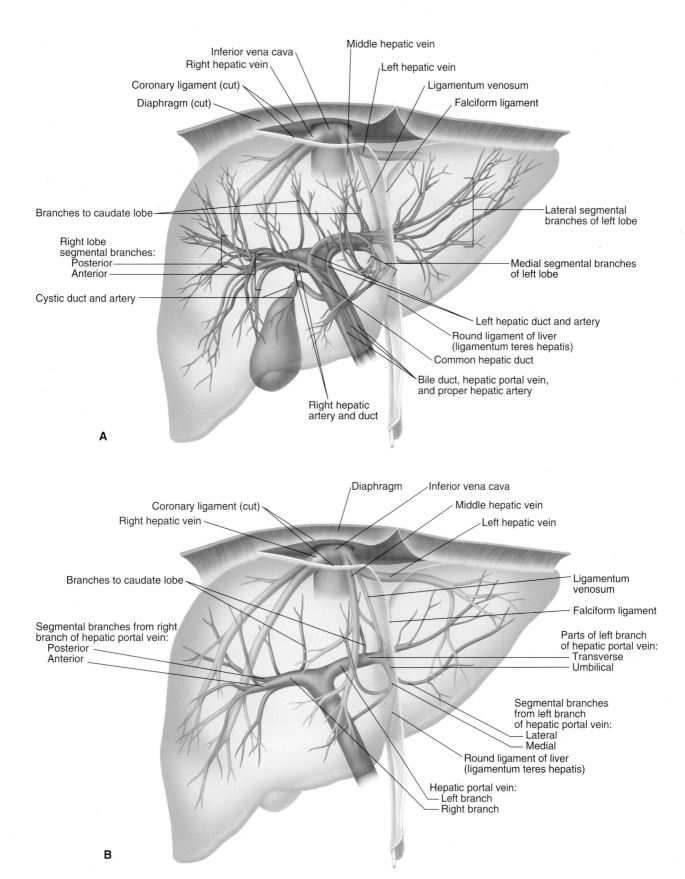

Inferior vena cava
Right hepatic vein
Coronary ligament (cut)
Diaphragm (cut)
Middle hepatic vein
Left hepatic vein
Ligamentum venosum
Falciform ligament

Branches to caudate lobe

Right lobe
segmental branches:
Posterior
Anterior

Cystic duct and artery

Lateral segmental
branches of left lobe

Medial segmental branches
of left lobe

Left hepatic duct and artery
Round ligament of liver
(ligamentum teres hepatis)
Common hepatic duct
Bile duct, hepatic portal vein,
and proper hepatic artery

Right hepatic
artery and duct

A

Diaphragm
Inferior vena cava
Coronary ligament (cut)
Right hepatic vein
Middle hepatic vein
Left hepatic vein

Branches to caudate lobe

Segmental branches from right
branch of hepatic portal vein:
Posterior
Anterior

Ligamentum
venosum

Falciform ligament

Parts of left branch
of hepatic portal vein:
Transverse
Umbilical

Segmental branches
from left branch
of hepatic portal vein:
Lateral
Medial

Round ligament of liver
(ligamentum teres hepatis)

Hepatic portal vein:
Left branch
Right branch

B

FIG. 2.17A,B. A. Liver Lobule and Portal Circulation. **B.** Portal and Hepatic Veins.

III. Lymphatic Drainage of the Liver

A. Liver is major lymph-producing organ, with about 1/3 to 1/2 of all body lymph entering thoracic duct from liver

B. Superficial lymphatics in subperitoneal fibrous capsule of liver and deep lymphatics in connective tissue accompany ramifications of portal triad and hepatic veins; most lymph is formed in perisinusoidal spaces (of Disse) and drains to deep lymphatics in surrounding intralobular portal triads

C. Superficial lymphatics from anterior part of diaphragmatic and visceral liver surface drain with deep vessels to hepatic lymph nodes scattered along hepatic vessels and ducts in lesser omentum; efferents from hepatic nodes drain into celiac lymph nodes, which then drain into cistern chyli

D. Superficial lymphatics from posterior part of diaphragmatic and visceral liver surface drain into phrenic lymph nodes or join deep lymphatics to follow hepatic veins, pass through diaphragm and drain into posterior mediastinal nodes; efferents join right lymphatic and thoracic ducts

IV. Nerves of the Liver

A. Numerous; both sympathetic and parasympathetic (vagal) fibers

B. Reach liver via an extensive hepatic plexus, largest derivative of celiac plexus

　1. Receives hepatic branch of anterior vagal trunk and small branches of right phrenic nerve to bare area

　2. Hepatic plexus accompanies hepatic artery and portal vein and their branches and enters liver at porta hepatis

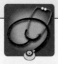

V. Clinical Considerations

A. **Portal hypertension**

　1. Abnormal increase in pressure in portal vein and its tributaries, often due to liver cirrhosis (scarring and fibrosis) which can lead to obstruction

　　a. Can produce enlarged varicose veins at portal/systemic anastomoses that may rupture, resulting in potentially fatal hemorrhage

　　b. **Portocaval shunt:** common way of reducing portal hypertension is to create a portosystemic shunt, either by anastomosing portal vein directly with inferior vena cava or anastomosing one of its tributaries into vena cava or into another systemic vein (e.g., splenic vein into left renal vein)

　2. With no valves in portal venous system, increased pressure causes retrograde flow into caval tributaries

　3. Veins in portosystemic anastomoses may be engorged, creating esophageal varicosities (**esophageal varices**), **hemorrhoids**, and varicosities on abdominal wall around umbilicus (**caput medusae**)

　4. Esophageal varices can rupture, resulting in severe hematemesis (vomiting of blood)

B. Liver biopsy: needle puncture commonly made through right 10th intercostal space in midaxillary line

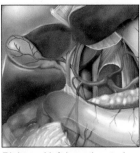

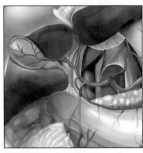

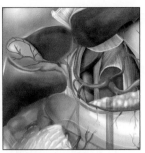

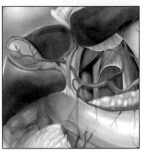

Right and left hepatic arteries arising from proper hepatic artery; right hepatic artery passing posterior to common hepatic duct (64%)

Right hepatic artery passing anterior to common hepatic duct (24%)

Right hepatic artery arising from superior mesenteric artery (12%)

Left hepatic artery arising from left gastric artery (11%)

C

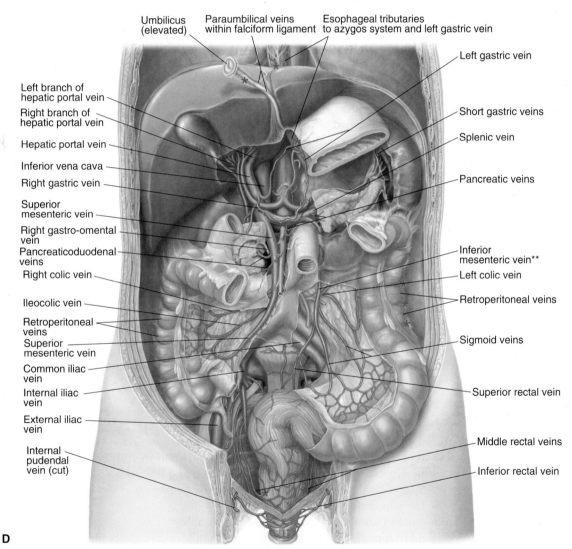

Umbilicus (elevated)

Paraumbilical veins within falciform ligament

Esophageal tributaries to azygos system and left gastric vein

Left gastric vein

Left branch of hepatic portal vein

Right branch of hepatic portal vein

Hepatic portal vein

Inferior vena cava

Right gastric vein

Superior mesenteric vein

Right gastro-omental vein

Pancreaticoduodenal veins

Right colic vein

Ileocolic vein

Retroperitoneal veins

Superior mesenteric vein

Common iliac vein

Internal iliac vein

External iliac vein

Internal pudendal vein (cut)

Short gastric veins

Splenic vein

Pancreatic veins

Inferior mesenteric vein**

Left colic vein

Retroperitoneal veins

Sigmoid veins

Superior rectal vein

Middle rectal veins

Inferior rectal vein

D

＊Denotes sites of portal–caval anastomosis in cases of portal hypertension:
  1. Esophageal tributaries of left gastric vein to esophageal tributaries of azygos system of veins
  2. Superior rectal vein to middle and inferior rectal veins
  3. Paraumbilical tributaries of left hepatic portal vein to superficial veins of anterior body wall
  4. Retroperitoneal veins to veins of posterior body wall

＊＊Inferior mesenteric vein can join the splenic vein (34%), the superior mesenteric vein (33%), or the junction of the splenic and superior mesenteric veins (32%)

FIG. 2.17C,D. **C.** Liver: Blood Supply Variations. **D.** Tributaries to the Portal Veins.

Gallbladder and Ducts

I. Surface Projection (Fig. 2.18A)

A. Fundus lies at right border of rectus muscle at end of 9th costal cartilage

II. Location

A. In fossa for gallbladder on visceral surface of liver
B. Joined to liver by connective tissue
C. Covered by peritoneum where it does not touch liver

III. Parts (Fig. 2.18B)

A. **Fundus**: directed inferiorly, anteriorly, and to right
B. **Body**: extends superiorly, posteriorly and to left
C. **Neck**: in form of S-shaped curve

IV. Relations

A. Fundus: touches anterior abdominal wall when full
B. Body: liver superiorly; transverse colon and descending duodenum inferiorly

V. Duct System (Fig. 2.18C)

A. **Cystic duct**
　1. About 4 cm long
　2. Runs posteriorly, inferiorly, and toward left from neck of gallbladder and joins common hepatic duct to form bile duct
　3. Contains spiral folds (valves of Heister)
B. **Common hepatic duct**
　1. Arises from union of **right** and **left hepatic ducts**, which leave through porta hepatis
　2. Runs caudally and to right in hepatoduodenal ligament to join cystic duct, forming bile duct
C. **Bile duct** (common bile duct)
　1. Approximately 7.5 cm long
　2. Runs caudally in free edge of hepatoduodenal ligament, with proper hepatic artery to its left and portal vein behind
　3. Passes posterior to first part of duodenum, then passes into head of pancreas
　4. Pancreatic duct unites with bile duct, forming **hepatopancreatic ampulla** and passing obliquely through wall of duodenum
　　a. Walls of terminal ends of ducts are thickened by smooth muscle, the sphincter of ampulla (of Oddi)
　　b. **Major duodenal papilla**: elevation into lumen of descending duodenum caused by sphincter; bile duct and pancreatic duct usually have common opening at major duodenal papilla

VI. Blood Supply and Innervation

A. Arteries (Fig. 2.18D)
　1. **Cystic artery**: usually from right hepatic artery within **cystohepatic triangle** (of Calot; formed by cystic duct, common hepatic duct, and liver)
　　a. Superficial branch: supplies free, inferior surface
　　b. Deep branch: to superior surface
　2. Origin and number of cystic arteries are variable
B. Veins: drain directly into liver capillaries through fossa of gallbladder
C. Lymphatics: drain into hepatic nodes from gallbladder and into hepatic and pancreaticoduodenal nodes from bile duct
D. Nerves
　1. Autonomics by way of celiac plexus
　2. Pain fibers from bile passages reach spinal cord via thoracic splanchnic nerves
　3. Pain is excruciating (due to distention or spasm) and felt in upper right quadrant or in epigastrium, but is often referred posteriorly to region of right scapula and is sometimes cardiac in type and distribution

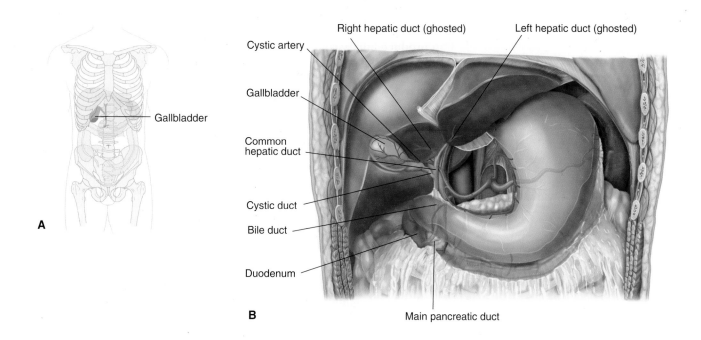

Cystic artery

Right hepatic duct (ghosted)

Left hepatic duct (ghosted)

Gallbladder

Common hepatic duct

Cystic duct

Bile duct

Duodenum

Main pancreatic duct

A

Gallbladder

B

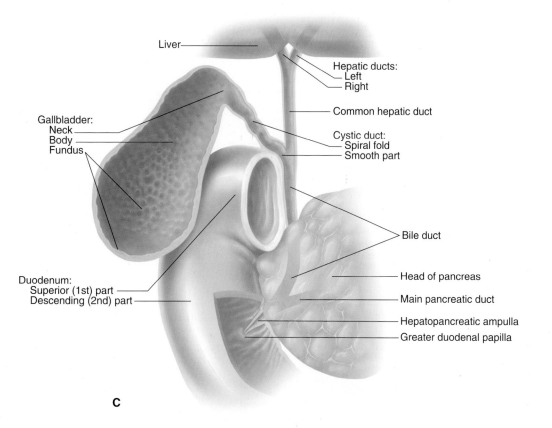

Liver

Hepatic ducts:
Left
Right

Common hepatic duct

Cystic duct:
Spiral fold
Smooth part

Gallbladder:
Neck
Body
Fundus

Bile duct

Head of pancreas

Main pancreatic duct

Duodenum:
Superior (1st) part
Descending (2nd) part

Hepatopancreatic ampulla

Greater duodenal papilla

C

FIG. 2.18A–C. Gallbladder. **A.** Location. **B.** Parts and Relations, Anterior View. **C.** Ducts, Anterior View.

VII. Clinical Considerations

A. **Gallstones**: obstruction of duct system as result of "stone" formation leads to pain and jaundice
   1. Common site for impaction of stones is distal end of hepatopancreatic ampulla because it is narrowest point of biliary passage
   2. Can produce biliary colic (pain in epigastric area)
   3. With relaxation of gallbladder, stone in cystic duct may pass back into gallbladder
B. Gallbladder is prone to recurrent bacterial infections, which are painful (initially in epigastrium)
C. **Cholecystitis** (inflammation of gallbladder)
   1. If cystic duct is blocked, bile accumulates and gallbladder enlarges; pain starts in epigastric region and later shifts to right hypochondriac region in junction of 9th costal cartilage and lateral border of rectus sheath
   2. Inflamed gallbladder may create pain in posterior thoracic wall and right shoulder (due to irritation of diaphragm)
D. If bile cannot leave gallbladder, it enters blood circulation and causes jaundice
E. **Laparoscopic cholecystectomy**: for people with severe biliary colic; careful dissection of cystohepatic triangle (of Calot) during surgery safeguards important structures
F. Cholecystoenterostomy: in certain cases of obstructive jaundice, anastomosis is created between gallbladder and some part of bowel (i.e., duodenum or jejunum)
H. **Endoscopic retrograde cholangiopancreatography (ERCP)**: imaging study involving injection of radiopaque dye through major duodenal papilla to explore biliary tree
I. Cholecystostomy: drainage of gallbladder without removal if removal is technically dangerous

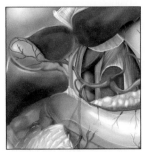

Cystic artery arising from right hepatic artery and passing posterior to common hepatic duct (76%)

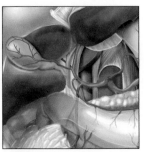

Cystic artery arising from right hepatic artery and passing anterior to common hepatic duct (13%)

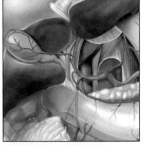

Cystic artery arising from left hepatic artery and passing anterior to common hepatic duct (6%)

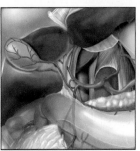

Cystic artery arising from gastroduodenal artery and passing anterior to common hepatic duct (3%)

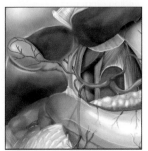

Cystic artery arising from proper hepatic artery and passing anterior to common hepatic duct (2%)

D

FIG. 2.18D. Gallbladder: Blood Supply.

Kidney: Parts and Relations

I. Relations (Fig. 2.19A–C)

A. **Right kidney**
1. Anterior
   a. Convex, faces anterolaterally
   b. Related to visceral surface of liver, right colic flexure, and 2nd part of duodenum
   c. Superior pole is related to suprarenal gland
2. Posterior
   a. More flattened
   b. Embedded in fat with no peritoneum
   c. Lies anterior to 12th rib, diaphragm, and lumbocostal arches, psoas and quadratus lumborum muscles, and tendon of transversus abdominis muscle
   d. Crosses upper lumbar arteries, T12, iliohypogastric, and ilioinguinal nerves
3. Lateral border: convex without important relations
4. Medial border
   a. Faces anteromedially
   b. Hilum centrally for renal vessels and ureter
   c. Above hilum, superior pole contacts suprarenal, and below hilum, contacts ureter

B. **Left kidney**
1. Anterior
   a. Convex, faces anterolaterally
   b. Related to spleen, body of pancreas and splenic vessels, stomach, left colic flexure, small intestine
   c. Superior pole is related to suprarenal gland
2. Posterior
   a. Less convex
   b. Embedded in fat with no peritoneum
   c. Crosses 11th and 12th ribs; in other respects, similar to right
3. Left border: similar to right
4. Medial: similar to right

II. Renal Fat and Fascia (Fig. 2.19D)

A. **Pararenal fat**: fat lying outside (primarily behind) renal fascia
B. **Renal fascia**
1. From extraperitoneal fascia
2. Splits near lateral border of kidney into 2 layers
   a. Anterior layer: over anterior surface and continues over renal vessels and aorta to join similar layer of other side
   b. Posterior layer: continues beneath kidney, does not cross midline but blends with psoas fascia
   c. Superiorly: layers fuse with each other to enclose suprarenal glands separately
   d. Laterally: layers fuse with transversalis fascia
   e. Inferiorly: layers do not fuse (kidneys can descend here); suprarenals do not descend with kidneys because they occupy separate compartment
C. **Perirenal fat**: fatty tissue lying outside of capsule and inside of renal fascia; fills renal sinus
D. **Renal capsule**: fibrous capsule closely applied to cortex

III. Support

A. Pararenal fat
B. Renal fascia
C. Renal vessels

IV. Nephron

A. Functional unit of kidney; 1 million or more per kidney
B. Parts
  1. **Glomerulus**: arterial capillary net
  2. **Bowman capsule**: surrounds capillary net
  3. **Proximal convoluted tubule**
  4. Loop of Henle: **distal convoluted tubule**

V. Duct System

A. Nephron joins duct system, which eventually opens at **renal papilla**, the apex of a renal pyramid, into **minor calyx**
B. Minor calyces unite to form 2 or 3 **major calyces**, which join to form **renal pelvis**, the expanded superior end of **ureter**

VI. General Structure (Fig. 2.19E)

A. **Medulla**: aggregated into 8 to 18 **renal pyramids**, striated in appearance; contains collecting ducts, portions of Henle loop, and parts of secretory tubules
B. Cortex lies beneath capsule, overlies bases of renal pyramids and dips down between them as **renal columns**
  1. Pars radiata: conical projections from bases of pyramids into cortex; contains ducts and parts of Henle loop
  2. Pars convoluta: surrounds radiate part; contains glomeruli, capsules, and convoluted parts of nephron
C. Kidney lobe
  1. Pyramid and associated cortex
  2. 5 to 6 are seen in fetus and may persist in adult (but unusual)
D. **Renal sinus**
  1. Large central cavity opening anteromedially at renal hilum
  2. Occupied by renal vessels, calyces and proximal renal pelvis, padded with perirenal fat
E. **Renal hilum**: anteromedial passageway to/from renal sinus for vessels and renal pelvis

VII. Clinical Considerations

A. Congenital anomalies
  1. **Pelvic kidney**
    a. Kidney at original site of development near pelvic brim
    b. Can be found on one or both sides
    c. Often found anterior to sacrum
    d. Arterial supply via common iliac artery
  2. **Horseshoe kidney**
    a. Caudal poles (rarely superior poles) of the 2 kidneys are joined
    b. Seen in about 1 in 600 fetuses
    c. Kidney located at level of L3–L5 vertebrae due to arrest by inferior mesenteric artery
    d. Produces no symptoms
  3. **Bifid ureter**
    a. Fairly common (3%); due to division of metanephric diverticulum (ureteric bud, primordium of renal pelvis, and ureter)
    b. May be unilateral or bilateral, and partial or complete, but separate opening into bladder is uncommon
B. **Polycystic kidneys**
  1. Heritable disease marked by cysts in both kidneys
  2. Infantile: autosomal recessive that may be congenital or appear at any time during childhood
  3. Adult form: autosomal dominant, marked by progressive deterioration of renal function

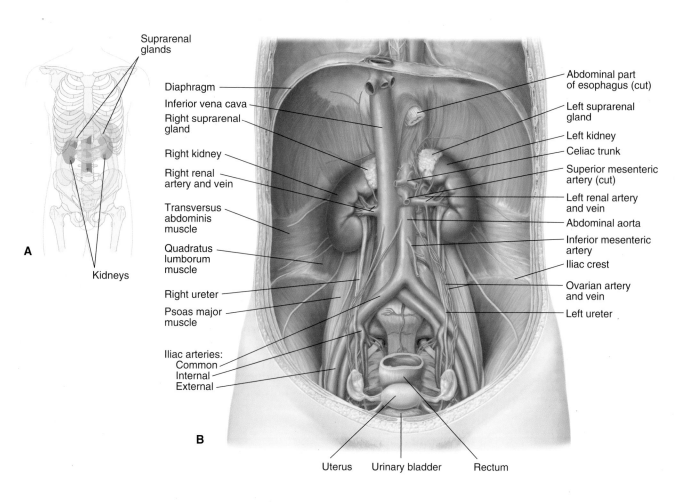

A

Suprarenal glands

Kidneys

Diaphragm
Inferior vena cava
Right suprarenal gland
Right kidney
Right renal artery and vein
Transversus abdominis muscle
Quadratus lumborum muscle
Right ureter
Psoas major muscle
Iliac arteries:
Common
Internal
External

Abdominal part of esophagus (cut)
Left suprarenal gland
Left kidney
Celiac trunk
Superior mesenteric artery (cut)
Left renal artery and vein
Abdominal aorta
Inferior mesenteric artery
Iliac crest
Ovarian artery and vein
Left ureter

B

Uterus   Urinary bladder   Rectum

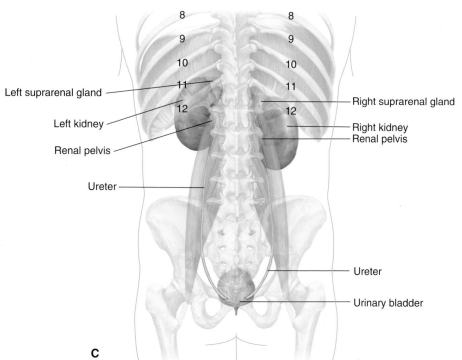

Left suprarenal gland
Left kidney
Renal pelvis
Ureter

Right suprarenal gland
Right kidney
Renal pelvis
Ureter
Urinary bladder

C

FIG. 2.19A–C. Kidneys. **A.** Location. **B.** Parts and Relations, Anterior View. **C.** Parts and Relations, Posterior View.

C. Perinephric abscess (pus around kidney)
 1. Extension determined by renal fascia, because fascia at hilum tends to prevent contralateral spread
 2. May spread inferiorly into pelvis due to loose fascia attachment
D. Nephroptosis: floating or hypermobile kidney; different from an ectopic kidney (which is congenital)
E. Renal transplantation
 1. Established procedure for treatment of selected cases of chronic renal failure
 2. Site usually in iliac fossa of greater pelvis
 3. Renal artery and vein are joined to external iliac artery and vein, and ureter is sutured into urinary bladder
F. Nephrosis: any kidney disease characterized by purely degenerative lesions of renal tubules
G. **Renal cysts**: solitary or multiple and often found during ultrasound examinations
H. Surgical approach to both kidney and suprarenal
 1. From back and side, by an incision below and parallel to 12th rib; if necessary, can be extended to front of abdomen, paralleling inguinal ligament
 2. Entire procedure can remain retroperitoneal and avoids cutting nerves as incision is parallel to their course
 3. Kidney structures can be separated from overlying structures (e.g., duodenum and pancreas) as kidney belongs to posterior body wall, whereas other organs have become only secondarily retroperitoneal

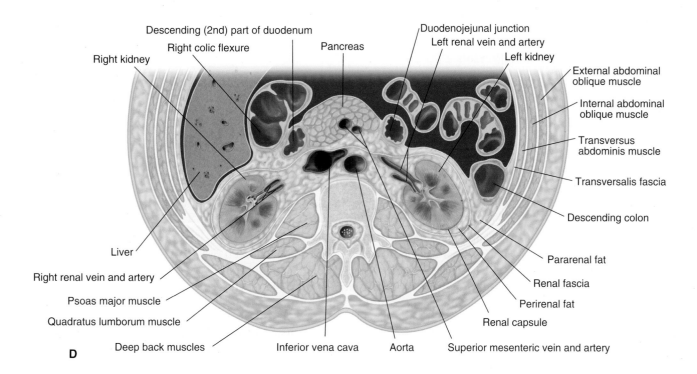

Descending (2nd) part of duodenum
Right colic flexure
Right kidney
Pancreas
Duodenojejunal junction
Left renal vein and artery
Left kidney
External abdominal oblique muscle
Internal abdominal oblique muscle
Transversus abdominis muscle
Transversalis fascia
Descending colon
Liver
Right renal vein and artery
Psoas major muscle
Quadratus lumborum muscle
Deep back muscles
Inferior vena cava
Aorta
Superior mesenteric vein and artery
Renal capsule
Perirenal fat
Renal fascia
Pararenal fat

D

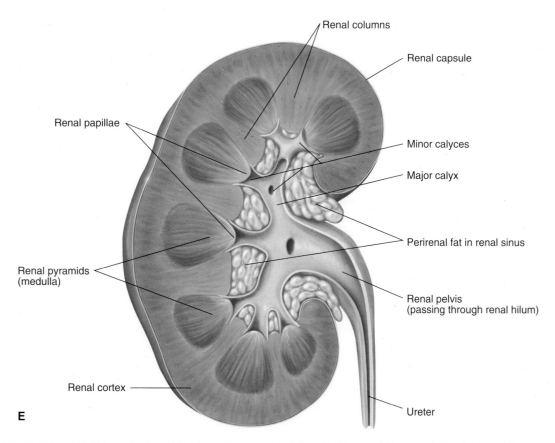

Renal columns
Renal capsule
Renal papillae
Minor calyces
Major calyx
Perirenal fat in renal sinus
Renal pyramids (medulla)
Renal pelvis (passing through renal hilum)
Renal cortex
Ureter

E

FIG. 2.19D,E. D. Kidneys: Parts and Relations, Cross-sectional View. **E.** Kidney and Suprarenal Glands: Internal Features.

Kidney: Blood Supply, Lymph Drainage, and Innervation

I. Renal Vessels (Fig. 2.20A)

A. Arteries
1. Arise from aorta at right angles at level of upper portion of L2 vertebral body
2. **Left renal artery**
   a. Slightly above level of right renal artery
   b. Lies posterior to renal vein, body of pancreas, and splenic vein
   c. Inferior mesenteric vein crosses it anteriorly
3. **Right renal artery**
   a. Longer than left
   b. Passes behind inferior vena cava and right renal vein with head of pancreas and descending duodenum overlying veins
4. Renal artery branches (Fig. 2.20B)
   a. **Interlobar arteries**: enter renal columns between pyramids
   b. **Arcuate arteries**: pass along bases of pyramids
   c. **Interlobular arteries**: branch from arcuate arteries, giving rise chiefly to afferent glomerular arteries and to some nutrient and perforating capsular arteries
   d. Capillary net of glomerulus coalesces to form efferent glomerular arteries
   e. These vessels break up into true capillary net around nephrons and also give rise to a few arteriolae rectae, which enter medulla and run toward pelvis

B. Veins
1. Begin in venous plexuses draining capillary bed around tubules
2. Open into venae rectae, then into interlobular veins, arcuate veins, interlobar veins, and finally renal vein
3. Stellate veins lie beneath capsule and drain part of area supplied by perforating capsular arteries; these veins drain into interlobular veins
4. Renal veins
   a. Terminate in inferior vena cava
   b. **Left renal vein**
      i. Longer than right
      ii. Crosses aorta anteriorly just below superior mesenteric artery and opens into inferior vena cava above right vein
      iii. Tributaries: left inferior phrenic, left gonadal, and left suprarenal
   c. **Right renal vein**
      i. Short, lies in front of renal artery
      ii. No extrarenal tributaries

C. Anastomoses between renal and systemic vessels occur in fat around kidney where perforating capsular arteries join branches from suprarenal, gonadal, superior and inferior mesenteric arteries

II. Relations of Structures at Hilum

A. Renal vein most anterior, artery intermediate, and renal pelvis most posterior
B. Branches of arteries and veins may pass posterior to renal pelvis

III. Nerve Supply

A. Extensive, from renal plexus (extension of celiac and intermesenteric plexuses that accompany renal artery) as well as from direct branches of thoracic and lumbar splanchnic nerves
B. Pain fibers, mainly from renal pelvis and upper part of ureter, enter spinal cord via splanchnic nerves

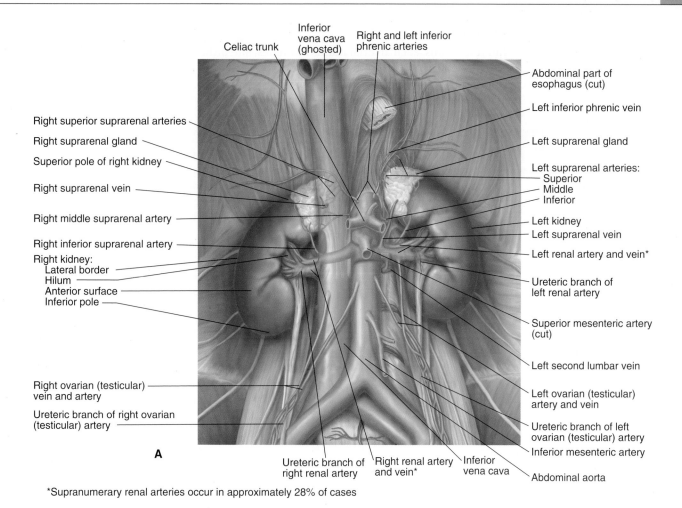

Inferior vena cava (ghosted)

Celiac trunk

Right and left inferior phrenic arteries

Abdominal part of esophagus (cut)

Left inferior phrenic vein

Right superior suprarenal arteries

Right suprarenal gland

Superior pole of right kidney

Right suprarenal vein

Right middle suprarenal artery

Right inferior suprarenal artery

Right kidney:
Lateral border
Hilum
Anterior surface
Inferior pole

Right ovarian (testicular) vein and artery

Ureteric branch of right ovarian (testicular) artery

Left suprarenal gland

Left suprarenal arteries:
Superior
Middle
Inferior

Left kidney

Left suprarenal vein

Left renal artery and vein*

Ureteric branch of left renal artery

Superior mesenteric artery (cut)

Left second lumbar vein

Left ovarian (testicular) artery and vein

Ureteric branch of left ovarian (testicular) artery

Inferior mesenteric artery

A

Ureteric branch of right renal artery

Right renal artery and vein*

Inferior vena cava

Abdominal aorta

*Supranumerary renal arteries occur in approximately 28% of cases

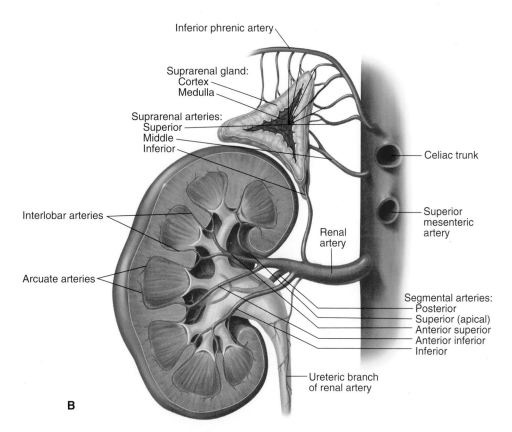

Inferior phrenic artery

Suprarenal gland:
Cortex
Medulla

Suprarenal arteries:
Superior
Middle
Inferior

Celiac trunk

Interlobar arteries

Superior mesenteric artery

Renal artery

Arcuate arteries

Segmental arteries:
Posterior
Superior (apical)
Anterior superior
Anterior inferior
Inferior

Ureteric branch of renal artery

B

FIG. 2.20A,B. Blood Supply, Lymph Drainage, and Innervation.

IV. Special Features

A. Within renal sinus, each arterial ramus branches, and although pattern varies, distribution considered constant enough to allow division of kidney into vascular segments that correspond to prevailing vascular pattern

B. 5 **segmental arteries** determine 5 renal segments

V. Clinical Considerations

A. **Supernumerary renal arteries**: extra renal arteries are common (nearly 30%), usually representing retained embryological supply

B. **Retroaortic left renal vein**: venous remodeling during development may result in left renal vein passing behind aorta, where it may be compressed

C. **Nutcracker syndrome**: left renal vein passes below origin of superior mesenteric artery, where it may be compressed

Ureters

I. Parts and Relations (Fig. 2.21A)

A. Origin: renal pelvis at level of body of L2 vertebra
B. Abdominal portion (Fig. 2.21B)
   1. Lies beneath peritoneum, embedded in subserous tissue on medial part of psoas major muscle
   2. Crossed by gonadal vessels
   3. Enters true pelvis, crossing bifurcation of common iliac vessels
      a. Right ureter
         i. Near origin, covered by descending duodenum, to right of inferior vena cava
         ii. Crossed by right colic and ileocolic vessels, mesentery, and terminal ileum
      b. Left ureter: crossed by left colic vessels and sigmoid mesocolon
C. Pelvic portion
   1. Female (Fig. 2.21C)
      a. Forms posteroinferior boundary of ovarian fossa
      b. Runs medially and anteriorly adjacent to lateral aspect of cervix and upper vagina to fundus of bladder
      c. Crossed superiorly by uterine artery, inferiorly by vaginal artery
   2. Male (Fig. 2.21D)
      a. Runs inferiorly on lateral pelvic wall along anterior border of greater sciatic notch, anterior to internal iliac artery, inferior to obturator, and superior to inferior vesical, and middle rectal arteries
      b. At level of lower part of sciatic notch, turns medially to reach posterolateral surface of bladder; here it passes superior to seminal vesicle
      c. Enters bladder by passing obliquely medially through posterior bladder wall; crossed superiorly by ductus deferens
D. Intramural portion
   1. Runs obliquely through bladder wall for 2 cm
   2. Opens at lateral angles of **trigone of bladder**

II. Constrictions: Areas of Diminished Diameter

A. Ureteropelvic junction
B. Crossing over common iliac bifurcation
C. At junction with bladder

III. Vessels and Nerves

A. Arteries: ureteric branches of renal, gonadal, superior and inferior vesical arteries
B. Veins: follow correspondingly named arteries and terminate in correspondingly named veins
C. Lymphatics: pass to lumbar and internal iliac nodes
D. Nerves
   1. Via autonomic innervation from sympathetic fibers (T11–L2) traveling through renal, aortic, or hypogastric plexuses
   2. Vagus contributes parasympathetic fibers to its upper part, sacral segments 2 to 4 to its lower part
   3. Most nerves to ureters are sensory, returning via segments T11–L2

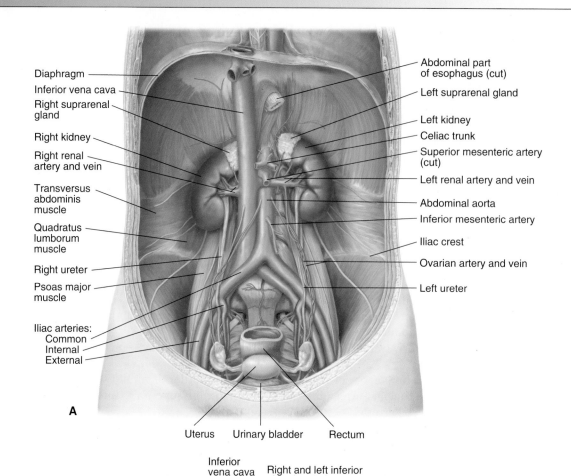

Diaphragm

Inferior vena cava

Right suprarenal gland

Right kidney

Right renal artery and vein

Transversus abdominis muscle

Quadratus lumborum muscle

Right ureter

Psoas major muscle

Iliac arteries:
Common
Internal
External

Abdominal part of esophagus (cut)

Left suprarenal gland

Left kidney

Celiac trunk

Superior mesenteric artery (cut)

Left renal artery and vein

Abdominal aorta

Inferior mesenteric artery

Iliac crest

Ovarian artery and vein

Left ureter

Uterus   Urinary bladder   Rectum

A

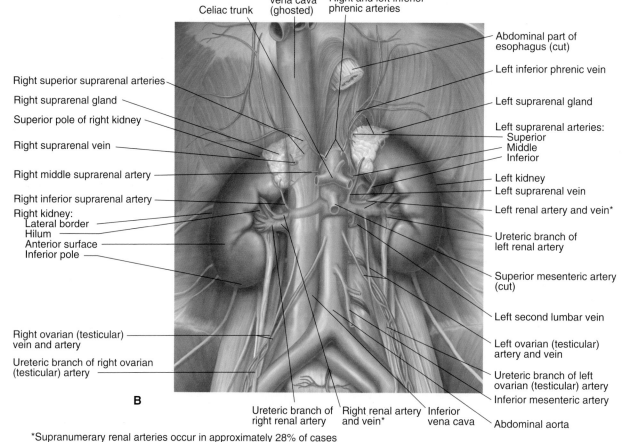

Celiac trunk

Inferior vena cava (ghosted)

Right and left inferior phrenic arteries

Right superior suprarenal arteries

Right suprarenal gland

Superior pole of right kidney

Right suprarenal vein

Right middle suprarenal artery

Right inferior suprarenal artery

Right kidney:
Lateral border
Hilum
Anterior surface
Inferior pole

Right ovarian (testicular) vein and artery

Ureteric branch of right ovarian (testicular) artery

Abdominal part of esophagus (cut)

Left inferior phrenic vein

Left suprarenal gland

Left suprarenal arteries:
Superior
Middle
Inferior

Left kidney

Left suprarenal vein

Left renal artery and vein*

Ureteric branch of left renal artery

Superior mesenteric artery (cut)

Left second lumbar vein

Left ovarian (testicular) artery and vein

Ureteric branch of left ovarian (testicular) artery

Inferior mesenteric artery

Abdominal aorta

Ureteric branch of right renal artery   Right renal artery and vein*   Inferior vena cava

B

*Supranumerary renal arteries occur in approximately 28% of cases

FIG. 2.21 A,B. A. Ureters, Anterior View. **B.** Upper Ureters, Anterior View.

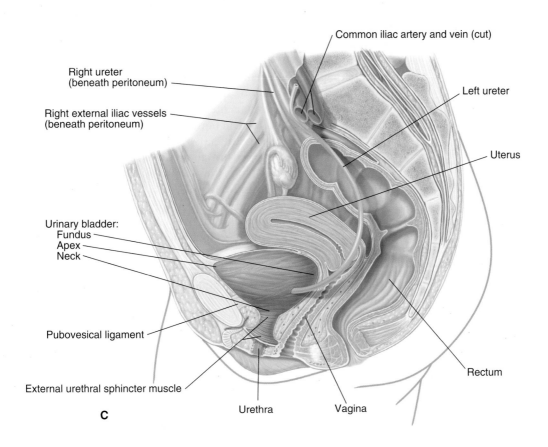

Common iliac artery and vein (cut)

Right ureter
(beneath peritoneum)

Left ureter

Right external iliac vessels
(beneath peritoneum)

Uterus

Urinary bladder:
Fundus
Apex
Neck

Pubovesical ligament

Rectum

External urethral sphincter muscle

Urethra

Vagina

C

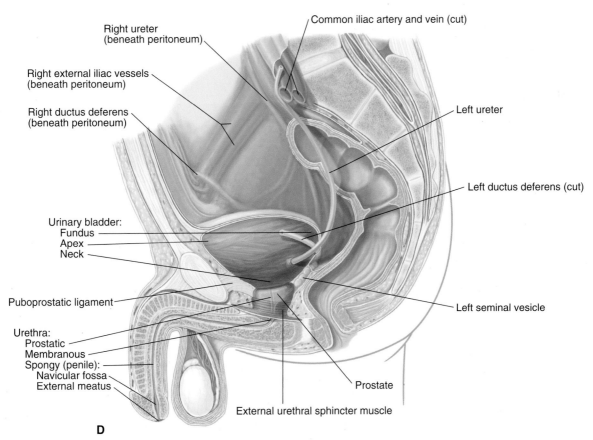

Common iliac artery and vein (cut)

Right ureter
(beneath peritoneum)

Right external iliac vessels
(beneath peritoneum)

Left ureter

Right ductus deferens
(beneath peritoneum)

Left ductus deferens (cut)

Urinary bladder:
Fundus
Apex
Neck

Puboprostatic ligament

Left seminal vesicle

Urethra:
Prostatic
Membranous
Spongy (penile):
Navicular fossa
External meatus

Prostate

External urethral sphincter muscle

D

FIG. 2.21C,D. Ureters in the Pelvis, Lateral View. **C.** Female. **D.** Male.

IV. Clinical Considerations

A. **Kidney stones**: may descend in ureter and become lodged, particularly in areas of ureteric constriction, resulting in extreme pain and urinary retention, which can damage kidney structure

   1. Stretching of ureteric wall or spasmotic contraction of muscles associated with stone passage results in acute pain (ureteric colic)
   2. Depending on level of obstruction, pain can be referred to lumbar or inguinal areas or external genitalia
      a. Pain can also be referred to cutaneous areas innervated by T11–L2, passing anteriorly from loin (lumbar region) to groin (inguinal region) as stone progresses down ureter
      b. Pain may be accompanied by nausea, vomiting, cramping, and diarrhea

B. Obstruction of ureter at any level leads to dilation of parts above it, including renal pelvis and calyces, resulting in **hydronephrosis**

C. Congenital anomalies

   1. Ureters may be double over part or extent
   2. Ectopic ureter: ureter may connect with urethra or vagina, causing incontinence

Suprarenal Gland

I. Position, Size, Shape, and Relations (Fig. 2.22A)

A. Location: at superior pole of kidney, at L1, within renal fascia
B. Size: length and width, 3–5 cm: thickness, 0.4–0.6 cm; weight, 3.5–6 g; heavier in male than in female
C. Shape and relations
  1. Right: pyramidal, with hilum below apex near anterior border
     a. Anterior: medially, inferior vena cava without peritoneum; laterally liver, without peritoneum above, with peritoneum below
     b. Posterior: diaphragm above; superior pole and anterior surface of right kidney below
  2. Left: semilunar in shape; hilum near caudal end of anterior surface; slightly larger than right
     a. Anterior: peritoneum of omental bursa above; pancreas and splenic vein, without peritoneum, below
     b. Posterior: medially, left crus of diaphragm; laterally, anterior surface of left kidney

II. Blood and Nerve Supply

A. Arteries (Fig. 2.22B)
  1. **Superior suprarenal arteries**: (approximately 20) from inferior phrenic artery (from aorta)
  2. **Middle suprarenal artery**: directly from aorta
  3. **Inferior suprarenal artery**: from renal artery (from aorta)
B. Veins
  1. **Suprarenal vein**: receives blood from all parts of gland and leaves through hilum
     a. Right: enters posterior surface of inferior vena cava; extremely short
     b. Left: enters left renal vein
C. Nerve supply: via celiac plexus and thoracic and lumbar splanchnic nerves; fibers are mostly preganglionic sympathetic fibers that go directly to cells of medulla

III. Parts

A. Cortex: derived from mesoderm
B. Medulla: derived from embryonic neural crest ectoderm
C. Capsule: tough, connective tissue

IV. Secretions

A. Cortex: cortisol, corticosterone, aldosterone, dehydro-3-epiandrosterone, progesterone, estradiol, and estrone
B. Medulla: epinephrine and norepinephrine

V. General Functions

A. Cortex
  1. Gluconeogenesis
  2. Enhances water diuresis, probably by increasing glomerular filtration
  3. Maintains electrolyte balance, thus maintaining blood volume and pressure
  4. Fat deposition
  5. Affects lymphocytes (lympholytic)
  6. Antiinflammatory and antiallergic
  7. Essential to life
B. Medulla
  1. Essential to "fight-or-flight" mechanism: raises blood pressure and increases heart rate
  2. Dilates bronchi and breaks down glycogen, thus elevating blood sugar

VI. Clinical Considerations

A. Chief pathology involves cortex only

B. Hyperactivity
   1. Cushing disease
   2. Adrenogenital syndrome
   3. Primary or secondary aldosteronism (abnormality of electrolyte balance caused by excessive secretion of aldosterone)
      a. Primary
         i. Due to oversecretion of aldosterone by suprarenal adenoma
         ii. Characterized typically by hypokalemia, alkalosis, muscular weakness, polyuria, polydypsia, and hypertension
      b. Secondary: extra suprarenal stimulation of aldosterone secretion associated with edematous states, as in nephritic syndrome, hepatic cirrhosis, heart failure, and malignant hypertension

C. Hypofunction
   1. Acute suprarenal insufficiency (Waterhouse-Friderichsen syndrome)
   2. Chronic suprarenal insufficiency (Addison disease)
   3. Symptoms: bronze-like skin pigmentation, severe prostration, progressive anemia; low blood pressure, diarrhea, and digestive disturbances due to adrenal hypofunction

D. Pheochromocytoma: tumor of medulla that produces paroxysmal or sustained hypertension, resulting from excess production of catecholamines

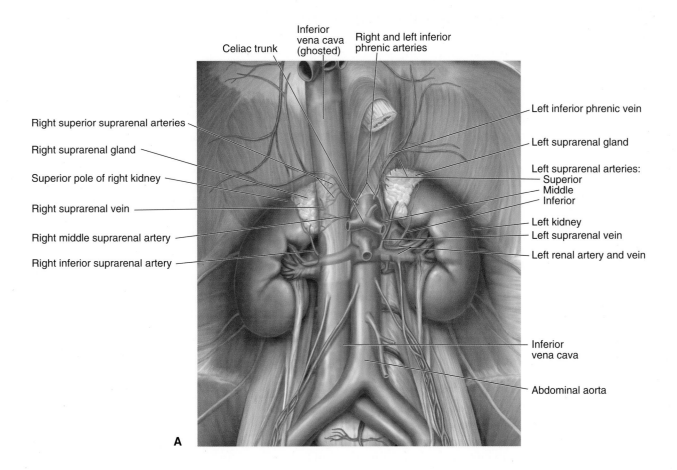

Celiac trunk

Inferior vena cava (ghosted)

Right and left inferior phrenic arteries

Right superior suprarenal arteries

Right suprarenal gland

Superior pole of right kidney

Right suprarenal vein

Right middle suprarenal artery

Right inferior suprarenal artery

Left inferior phrenic vein

Left suprarenal gland

Left suprarenal arteries:
Superior
Middle
Inferior

Left kidney

Left suprarenal vein

Left renal artery and vein

Inferior vena cava

Abdominal aorta

A

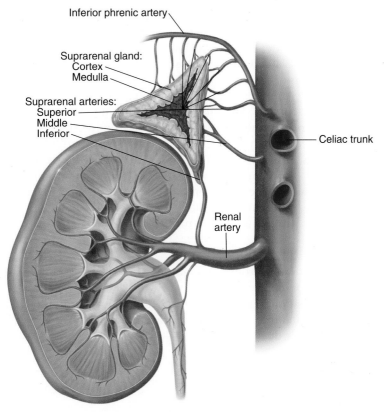

Inferior phrenic artery

Suprarenal gland:
Cortex
Medulla

Suprarenal arteries:
Superior
Middle
Inferior

Celiac trunk

Renal artery

B

FIG. 2.22A,B. Suprarenal Gland. **A.** Anterior View. **B.** Blood Supply.

Lymphatics of the Abdomen

I. Visceral Lymph Nodes (Fig. 2.23A,B)

A. Stomach: to gastric and pancreaticosplenic nodes, eventually to lateral aortic nodes around celiac trunk

B. Liver
   1. Convex surface: to posterior mediastinal nodes, superior gastric nodes, celiac group of lateral aortic nodes, and hepatic nodes
   2. Visceral surface: hepatic and posterior mediastinal nodes

C. Gallbladder: to hepatic and pancreaticoduodenal nodes; to hepatic nodes from bile duct

D. Duodenum: to pancreaticoduodenal nodes and then to celiac and superior mesenteric nodes

E. Jejunum and ileum: lacteal vessels to mesenteric nodes in mesentery and then to superior mesenteric group of preaortic nodes (Fig. 2.23C)

F. Colon
   1. Ascending and transverse: through right colic and middle colic nodes to mesenteric nodes to superior mesenteric group of preaortics
   2. Descending and sigmoid: left colic nodes along left colic and sigmoid arteries to inferior mesenteric group of preaortics (Fig. 2.23D)

G. Pancreas: to pancreaticosplenic nodes (then to celiac group of preaortics), to pancreaticoduodenal nodes, and to superior mesenteric group of preaortic nodes

II. Parietal Lymph Nodes

A. Epigastric nodes: along inferior epigastric vessels

B. **Lumbar nodes**
   1. **Right lateral aortic nodes**: anterior to inferior vena cava at level of renal vessels, posterior to inferior vena cava, on origins of right psoas muscle and right crus of diaphragm
      a. Afferents: from common iliac nodes; ovary, testis, uterus, kidney, suprarenal, and abdominal muscles
      b. Efferents: chiefly form **right lumbar trunk**, but some pass to pre- and retroaortic nodes or thoracic duct
   2. **Left lateral aortic nodes**: on left side of aorta, on origin of left psoas muscle and left crus of diaphragm
      a. Afferents and efferents similar to above but for left side
      b. Drain to **left lumbar trunk**, which usually receives intestinal trunk draining GI viscera
   3. **Preaortic nodes**: in front of aorta around origin of 3 major arterial branches and named accordingly: celiac, superior mesenteric, and inferior mesenteric nodes
      a. Afferents: few from lateral aortics, mainly from viscera supplied by related arteries
      b. Efferents: few to retroaortics, mainly to intestinal trunk
   4. **Retroaortic nodes**: on bodies of 3rd and 4th lumbar vertebrae behind aorta
      a. Afferents: from lateral and preaortic nodes
      b. Efferents: to cisterna chyli

III. Cisterna Chyli

A. Location: in front of second lumbar vertebra, behind and to right of aorta beneath right crus of diaphragm

B. Formation: right and left lumbar trunks and intestinal trunk

C. Termination: narrows down and passes through aortic hiatus of diaphragm to become **thoracic duct**

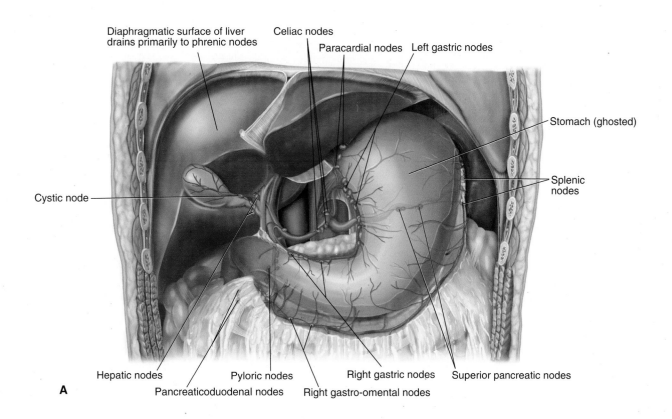

Diaphragmatic surface of liver
drains primarily to phrenic nodes

Celiac nodes

Paracardial nodes   Left gastric nodes

Stomach (ghosted)

Splenic nodes

Cystic node

Hepatic nodes   Pyloric nodes   Right gastric nodes   Superior pancreatic nodes

Pancreaticoduodenal nodes   Right gastro-omental nodes

A

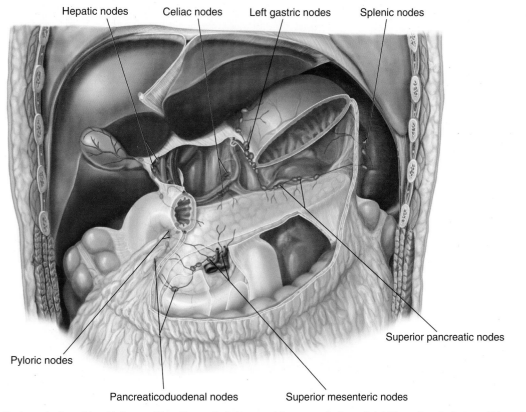

Hepatic nodes   Celiac nodes   Left gastric nodes   Splenic nodes

Superior pancreatic nodes

Pyloric nodes

B

Pancreaticoduodenal nodes   Superior mesenteric nodes

FIG. 2.23A,B. Lymphatics of the Abdomen: Liver, Stomach, Spleen, and Pancreas. **A.** Superficial Dissection. **B.** Deeper Dissection.

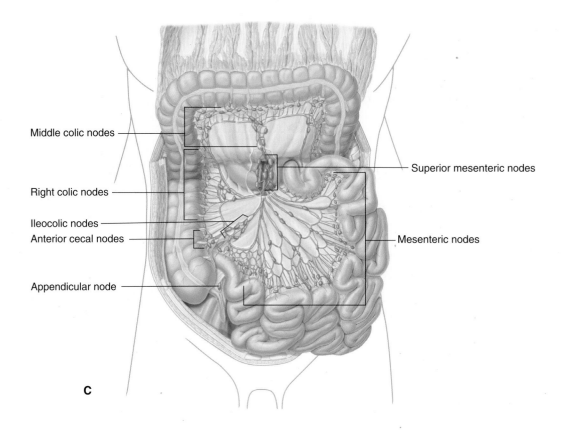

Middle colic nodes

Right colic nodes

Ileocolic nodes
Anterior cecal nodes

Appendicular node

Superior mesenteric nodes

Mesenteric nodes

C

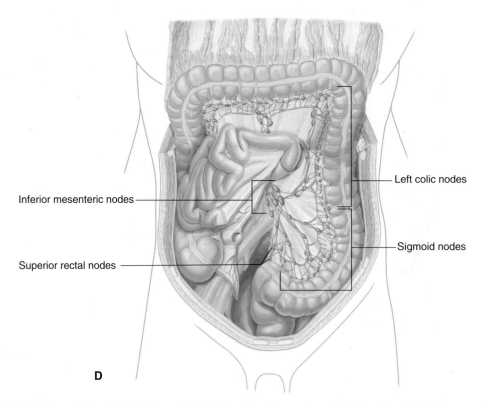

Inferior mesenteric nodes

Superior rectal nodes

Left colic nodes

Sigmoid nodes

D

FIG. 2.23C,D. Lymphatics of the Abdomen. **C.** Small Intestine, Cecum, Appendix, Ascending Colon, Transverse Colon.
D. Descending Colon, Sigmoid Colon, Rectum.

IV. Clinical Considerations

A. Surgeon may judge extent of metastases from a malignancy by examining nodes draining the area

B. For example, from sigmoid colon, first check for nodes in sigmoid mesocolon, and then examine inferior mesenteric group found at origin of inferior mesenteric artery

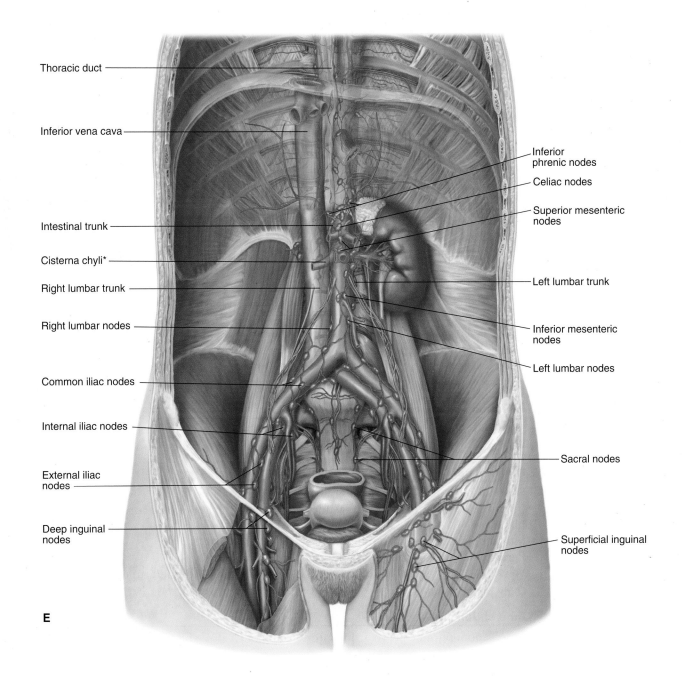

Thoracic duct

Inferior vena cava

Intestinal trunk

Cisterna chyli*

Right lumbar trunk

Right lumbar nodes

Common iliac nodes

Internal iliac nodes

External iliac nodes

Deep inguinal nodes

E

Inferior phrenic nodes

Celiac nodes

Superior mesenteric nodes

Left lumbar trunk

Inferior mesenteric nodes

Left lumbar nodes

Sacral nodes

Superficial inguinal nodes

*Cisterna chyli is present in approximately 25% of cases

FIG. 2.23E. Lymphatics of the Posterior Abdominal Wall and Abdominal Viscera.

Respiratory Diaphragm

I. Location, Configuration, and Composition (Fig. 2.24)

A. Serves as septum between thoracic and abdominal cavities
B. Dome shaped, with concavity facing inferiorly
C. Composed of skeletal muscle peripherally and dense collagenous connective tissue, the **central tendon**

II. Origin of Muscular Fibers

A. Sternal part: 2 muscular bands from posterior surface of xiphoid process
B. Costal part: from costal cartilages and ribs 7 to 12
C. Lumbar part: from lumbocostal arches and crura
   1. Lumbocostal ligaments (arches)
      a. **Medial arcuate ligament**
         i. Tendinous arch crossing psoas muscle
         ii. Attached medially to body of 1st (and 2nd) lumbar vertebrae and laterally to anterior transverse process of 1st (and 2nd) lumbar vertebrae
      b. **Lateral arcuate ligament**
         i. Tendinous arch crossing quadratus lumborum muscle
         ii. Attached medially to transverse process of 1st lumbar vertebra and laterally to tip of 12th rib
         iii. **Lumbocostal triangle**: inherent weak area of diaphragm located superior to lateral arcuate ligament
   2. Crura
      a. **Right crus**: larger than left and arises from bodies of lumbar vertebrae 1 to 3; most medial fibers cross in front of aorta to left side
         i. Forms esophageal hiatus by encircling esophagus
         ii. Forms suspensory muscle of duodenum by extending inferiorly toward left
      b. **Left crus**: arises from bodies of lumbar vertebrae 1 and 2
      c. **Median arcuate ligament:** unites crura across aorta, forming aortic hiatus

III. Insertion

A. Central tendon, where muscular fibers converge
B. Here, become tendinous beneath pericardial sac near central portion of diaphragm

IV. Blood Supply

A. Superior phrenic arteries: small branches of thoracic aorta
B. Inferior phrenic arteries: primary supply; branches from abdominal aorta just below aortic hiatus
C. Musculophrenic artery: supplies periphery of diaphragm
D. Pericardiacophrenic artery: supplies small portion centrally
E. Veins: accompany arteries; left inferior phrenic vein drains with left suprarenal vein to left renal vein; right inferior phrenic vein drains to inferior vena cava

V. Innervation and Action

A. Innervation: phrenic nerve, from anterior rami of C3, C4, and C5
B. Action
   1. Contraction of muscle causes descent of central tendon, which decreases pressure and increases volume of thoracic cavity
   2. Results in air being "pulled" into lungs

VI. Orifices in Diaphragm with Major Structures Passing Through

A. **Caval foramen**
   1. At level of 8th thoracic vertebra, to right of midline
   2. Transmits inferior vena cava and right phrenic nerve through central tendon

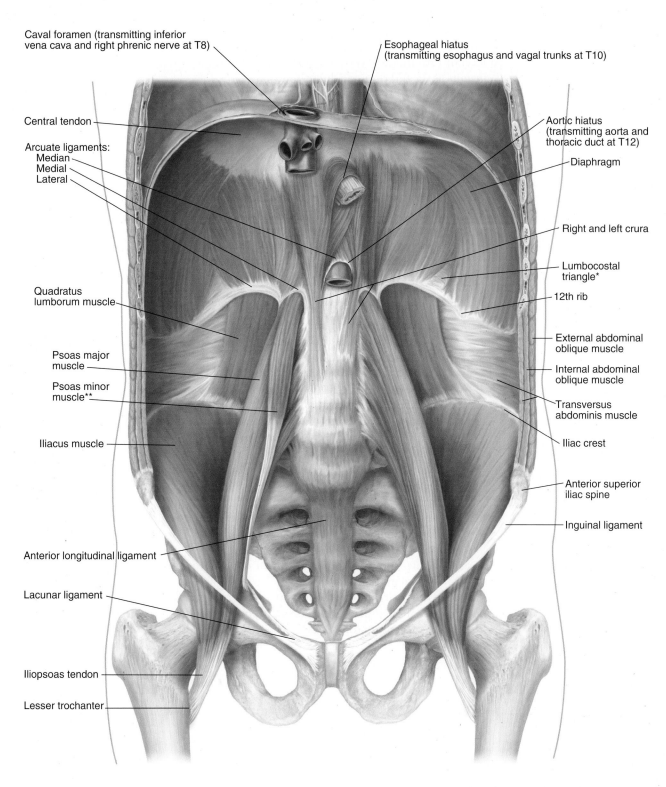

Caval foramen (transmitting inferior
vena cava and right phrenic nerve at T8)

Esophageal hiatus
(transmitting esophagus and vagal trunks at T10)

Central tendon

Aortic hiatus
(transmitting aorta and
thoracic duct at T12)

Arcuate ligaments:
Median
Medial
Lateral

Diaphragm

Right and left crura

Lumbocostal
triangle*

Quadratus
lumborum muscle

12th rib

External abdominal
oblique muscle

Psoas major
muscle

Internal abdominal
oblique muscle

Psoas minor
muscle**

Transversus
abdominis muscle

Iliacus muscle

Iliac crest

Anterior superior
iliac spine

Anterior longitudinal ligament

Inguinal ligament

Lacunar ligament

Iliopsoas tendon

Lesser trochanter

* Lumbocostal triangle is present in 80% of cases
** Psoas minor muscle is present in 50% of cases

FIG. 2.24. Respiratory Diaphragm.

B. **Esophageal hiatus**
1. At level of 10th thoracic vertebra
2. Transmits esophagus and anterior and posterior vagal trunks
3. Formed by fibers of right crus

C. **Aortic hiatus**
1. At level of 12th thoracic vertebra, just to left of midline
2. Transmits aorta and thoracic duct

D. Minor openings
1. Each crus: hiatus for greater, lesser, and least thoracic splanchnic nerves
2. Anteriorly: between sternal and costal parts of diaphragm for passage of superior epigastric artery

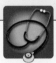

VII. Clinical Considerations

A. Diaphragmatic hernias: may be classified as congenital, acquired, or traumatic
1. Traumatic and many congenital hernias have no sacs and are not "true" hernias, but term is of common usage; traumatic diaphragmatic hernias often occur through left lumbocostal triangle
2. **Hiatal hernia**: abdominal viscera, especially stomach, may ascend through esophageal hiatus into thorax; majority of acquired (nontraumatic) hernias are located at esophageal hiatus and have sacs
3. **Congenital diaphragmatic hernia**
   a. Part of stomach and intestine may herniate through large posterolateral defect (foramen of Bochdalek, or pleuroperitoneal canal) in area of lumbocostal triangle
   b. 95% on left side (due to liver on right)
   c. Seen in 1 in 2,200 newborns; mortality rate = 76% due to left pulmonary hypoplasia

B. Inflammation affecting diaphragm can result in referred pain, which radiates to 2 different areas due to sensory nerve supply
1. Pain from diaphragmatic pleura or peritoneum is referred to skin of shoulder area supplied by C3–C5 (anterior rami that contribute to phrenic nerve)
2. Irritation of peripheral areas of diaphragm, innervated by inferior intercostal nerves, is referred to skin over costal margin of anterolateral abdominal wall

C. Hiccups (hiccough)
1. Sharp sound of inhalation with continuous involuntary spasms of glottis and diaphragm
2. Due to irritation of afferent or efferent nerve endings of phrenic nerve or of medullary centers in brainstem that control respiratory muscles (especially diaphragm)

Vessels of the Posterior Abdominal Wall

I. Abdominal Aorta (Fig. 2.25)

A. Enters abdomen anterior to T12 vertebral body by passing beneath median arcuate ligament uniting crura of diaphragm

B. Ends at L4 vertebral level by branching into common iliac arteries

C. Lies anterior to anterior longitudinal ligament near midline

D. Branches

   1. **Inferior phrenic arteries** (paired)

      a. Arise at T12 vertebral level

      b. Supply inferior surface of diaphragm

      c. Provide multiple small superior suprarenal branches

   2. **Celiac trunk**: at upper L1 vertebral level

   3. **1st lumbar arteries** (paired): at middle of L1 vertebral level

   4. **Middle suprarenal arteries** (paired): at middle of L1 vertebral level

   5. **Superior mesenteric artery**: at lower L1 vertebral level

   6. **Renal arteries** (paired): at upper L2 vertebral level

   7. **2nd lumbar arteries** (paired): at middle of L2 vertebral level

   8. **Gonadal (ovarian or testicular) arteries** (paired): at lower L2 vertebral level

   9. **3rd lumbar arteries** (paired): at middle of L3 vertebral level

  10. **Inferior mesenteric artery**: at middle of L3 vertebral level

  11. **4th lumbar arteries** (paired): at middle of L4 vertebral level

  12. **Median sacral artery**: at middle of L4 vertebral level from posterior surface

  13. **Common iliac arteries** (paired): at lower L4 vertebral level; terminal branches of aorta

II. Inferior Vena Cava

A. Begins at L5 vertebral level by union of common iliac veins

B. Ends by passing through caval foramen at T8 vertebral level to drain to right atrium

C. Lies to right of midline

   1. Inferiorly, lies to right of abdominal aorta

   2. Superiorly, lies embedded in sulcus on posterior surface of liver

D. Tributaries

   1. **Common iliac veins** (paired): unite at L5 vertebral level to form inferior vena cava

   2. **4th lumbar veins** (paired): at middle of L4 vertebral level

   3. **3th lumbar veins** (paired): at middle of L3 vertebral level

   4. **Right gonadal vein**: at L3 vertebral level

   5. **2nd lumbar veins** (paired): at middle of L2 vertebral level

   6. **Renal veins** (paired): at middle of L2 vertebral level

   7. **Right suprarenal vein**: at L1 vertebral level

   8. **Hepatic veins** (right, middle, and left): at T9 vertebral level

   9. **Inferior phrenic veins** (paired): at T8/9 vertebral level

III. Ascending Lumbar Veins (Paired)

A. Vertical anastomotic channels between adjacent lumbar veins

B. Lie posterior to psoas major muscles

C. Unite with subcostal veins to form azygos vein on right and hemiazygos vein on left

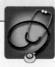

IV. Clinical Considerations

A. Abdominal aortic aneurysm (AAA)

1. Usually found immediately superior to aortic bifurcation; pulsations of large aneurysm can be detected near midline and pulsating mass can be moved from side to side; diagnosed by imaging (CT scan)

2. Acute rupture of aortic aneurysm results in severe pain in abdomen or back; unrecognized mortality rate is almost 90% due to severe blood loss

3. AAA bypass graft or endovascular catheterization procedure with stenting may be required to prevent rupture

B. Greenfield filter (IVC filter)

1. Metal filter designed to catch recurrent lower limb emboli

2. Inserted into hepatic portion of inferior vena cava

C. Control bleeding in pelvis or lower limb: compress (if patient is thin and relaxed) inferior part of abdominal aorta against body of L4 vertebra

D. Venous collateral circulation for abdomen and pelvis: 3 collateral routes by valveless veins of trunk can carry blood to heart when inferior vena cava is ligated or obstructed

1. Superior and inferior epigastric veins

2. Thoracoepigastric veins

3. Epidural venous plexus inside vertebral column (communicates with lumbar veins of inferior vena caval system and tributaries of azygos system of veins (part of caval system)

E. Aorta located posterior to pancreas and stomach; therefore, tumor can transmit aortic pulsations, which may be confused with AAA

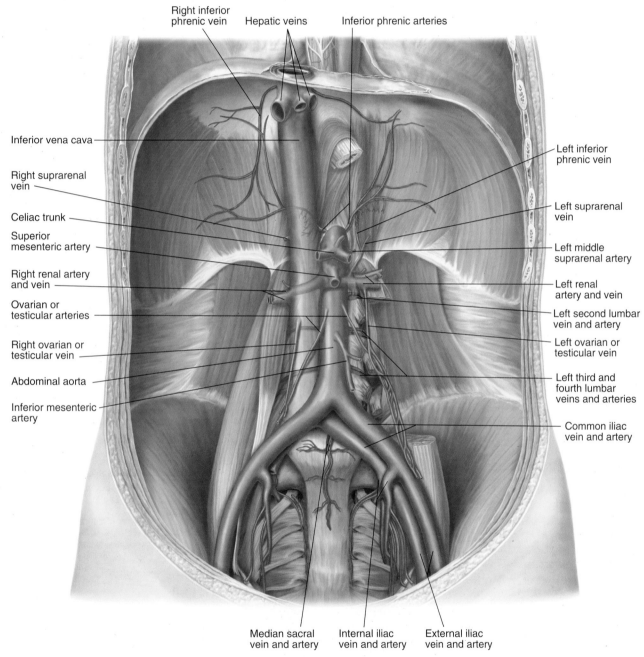

Right inferior phrenic vein

Hepatic veins

Inferior phrenic arteries

Inferior vena cava

Right suprarenal vein

Celiac trunk

Superior mesenteric artery

Right renal artery and vein

Ovarian or testicular arteries

Right ovarian or testicular vein

Abdominal aorta

Inferior mesenteric artery

Left inferior phrenic vein

Left suprarenal vein

Left middle suprarenal artery

Left renal artery and vein

Left second lumbar vein and artery

Left ovarian or testicular vein

Left third and fourth lumbar veins and arteries

Common iliac vein and artery

Median sacral vein and artery

Internal iliac vein and artery

External iliac vein and artery

FIG. 2.25. Vessels of the Posterior Abdominal Wall.

Nerves of the Posterior Abdominal Wall

I. Lumbar Plexus (Fig. 2.26A)

A. Anterior (ventral) rami of L1–L4

B. Branches
 1. **Iliohypogastric and ilioinguinal nerves**: from L1, lie anterior to quadratus lumborum
 2. **Genitofemoral nerve**: L1–L2; passes through psoas major muscle to pass inferiorly on its anterior surface
 3. **Lateral femoral cutaneous nerve**: L2–L3; passes obliquely across lower quadratus lumborum and iliacus muscles
 4. **Femoral nerve**: L2–L4; lies in groove between iliacus and psoas major muscles
 5. **Obturator nerve**: L2–L4; lies beneath psoas major muscle within abdomen, then medial to uppermost fibers of obturator internus muscle within pelvis
 6. Direct branches to quadratus lumborum, iliacus, and psoas major (and minor) muscles

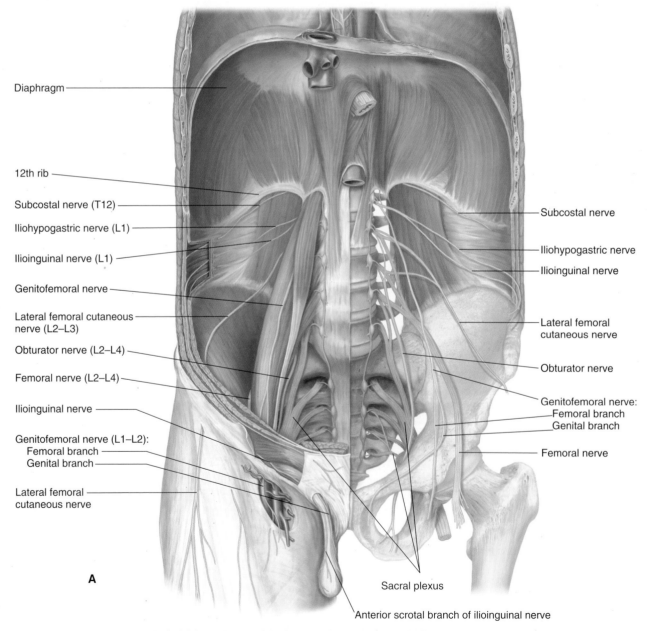

Diaphragm

12th rib

Subcostal nerve (T12)

Iliohypogastric nerve (L1)

Ilioinguinal nerve (L1)

Genitofemoral nerve

Lateral femoral cutaneous nerve (L2–L3)

Obturator nerve (L2–L4)

Femoral nerve (L2–L4)

Ilioinguinal nerve

Genitofemoral nerve (L1–L2):
 Femoral branch
 Genital branch

Lateral femoral cutaneous nerve

Subcostal nerve

Iliohypogastric nerve

Ilioinguinal nerve

Lateral femoral cutaneous nerve

Obturator nerve

Genitofemoral nerve:
 Femoral branch
 Genital branch

Femoral nerve

Sacral plexus

Anterior scrotal branch of ilioinguinal nerve

A

FIG. 2.26A. Nerves of the Posterior Abdominal Wall. **A.** Somatic Nerves.

II. Lumbar Sympathetic Trunk (Fig. 2.26B)

A. Enters abdomen by passing beneath medial arcuate ligament

B. Lies anterior to attachment of psoas major muscle

C. Usually consists of 4 ganglia connected by interganglionic rami

D. Connections

  1. **White rami communicantes**: pass from L1 and L2 anterior rami, deep to psoas major muscle, to reach sympathetic trunk

  2. **Gray rami communicantes**: pass to anterior rami of L1–L5 deep to psoas major muscle

  3. **Lumbar splanchnic nerves**: pass anteromedially to join autonomic plexuses on anterior surface of abdominal aorta

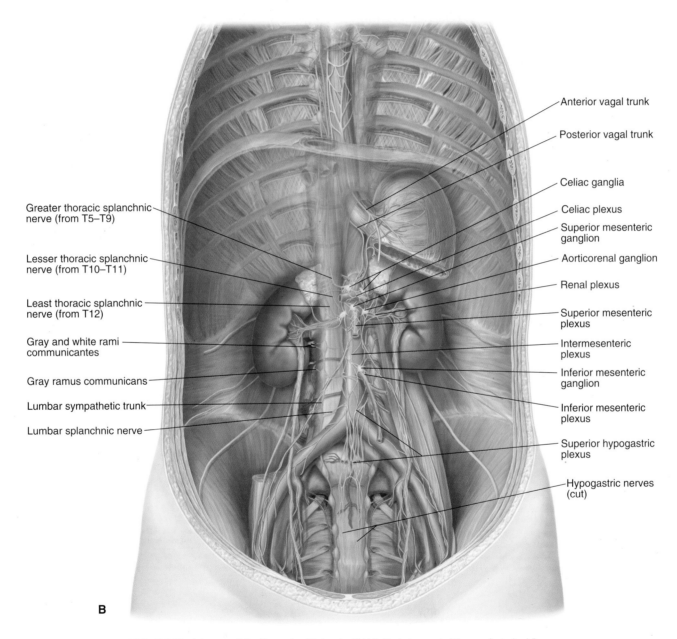

Greater thoracic splanchnic nerve (from T5–T9)

Lesser thoracic splanchnic nerve (from T10–T11)

Least thoracic splanchnic nerve (from T12)

Gray and white rami communicantes

Gray ramus communicans

Lumbar sympathetic trunk

Lumbar splanchnic nerve

Anterior vagal trunk

Posterior vagal trunk

Celiac ganglia

Celiac plexus

Superior mesenteric ganglion

Aorticorenal ganglion

Renal plexus

Superior mesenteric plexus

Intermesenteric plexus

Inferior mesenteric ganglion

Inferior mesenteric plexus

Superior hypogastric plexus

Hypogastric nerves (cut)

B

FIG. 2.26B. Nerves of the Posterior Abdominal Wall. **B.** Autonomic Nerves, Anterior View.

III. Review of the Autonomic Supply of the Abdomen (Fig. 2.26C,D)

- A. Sympathetic
    - 1. Thoracic splanchnic nerves
        - a. Pass through common hiatus in crus of diaphragm on each side
        - b. **Greater thoracic splanchnic nerve**
            - i. From T5–T9 sympathetic ganglia
            - ii. Passes to **celiac ganglion** on each side to synapse; postsynaptic fibers form **celiac plexus** on celiac trunk and its branches; some presynaptic fibers reach **superior mesenteric ganglion**
            - iii. Some fibers pass into suprarenal medulla without synapse, to synapse on cells there
        - c. **Lesser thoracic splanchnic nerve**
            - i. From T10–T11 sympathetic ganglia
            - ii. Passes to **aorticorenal ganglion** above origin of renal artery
            - iii. Postsynaptic fibers enter renal and **intermesenteric plexus**
        - d. **Least thoracic splanchnic nerve**
            - i. From T12 sympathetic ganglion (often absent)
            - ii. Passes into **renal plexus**
    - 2. **Lumbar splanchnic nerves**
        - a. L1 and L2 pass into celiac, superior mesenteric, and intermesenteric plexuses
        - b. L3 and L4 pass into superior hypogastric plexus
- B. Parasympathetic
    - 1. Vagal trunks
        - a. Anterior and posterior
            - i. Enter abdomen through esophageal hiatus
            - ii. Direct gastric and hepatic branches to stomach and liver/gallbladder
        - b. Celiac branches pass through celiac ganglia without synapsing to enter celiac and superior mesenteric plexuses
        - c. Presynaptic fibers synapse within viscera walls
        - d. Vagal fibers distribute as far distally as distribution of superior mesenteric artery (i.e., distally to proximal 2/3 of transverse colon, or the end of embryonic midgut)
    - 2. Pelvic splanchnic nerves
        - a. From spinal cord levels S2–S4
        - b. Leave anterior rami S2–S4 to join inferior hypogastric plexus
        - c. Some fibers travel superiorly across left pelvic brim within extraperitoneal connective tissue to reach embryonic hindgut (i.e., distal 1/3 of transverse colon, descending and sigmoid colon, and rectum and anal canal)
        - d. Presynaptic fibers synapse within viscera walls

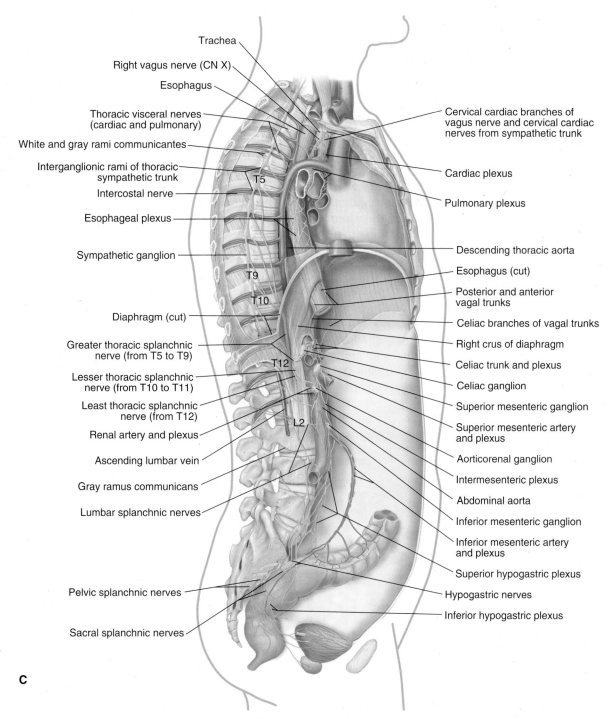

Trachea

Right vagus nerve (CN X)

Esophagus

Thoracic visceral nerves
(cardiac and pulmonary)

White and gray rami communicantes

Interganglionic rami of thoracic
sympathetic trunk

Intercostal nerve

Esophageal plexus

Sympathetic ganglion

Diaphragm (cut)

Greater thoracic splanchnic
nerve (from T5 to T9)

Lesser thoracic splanchnic
nerve (from T10 to T11)

Least thoracic splanchnic
nerve (from T12)

Renal artery and plexus

Ascending lumbar vein

Gray ramus communicans

Lumbar splanchnic nerves

Pelvic splanchnic nerves

Sacral splanchnic nerves

T5

T9

T10

T12

L2

Cervical cardiac branches of
vagus nerve and cervical cardiac
nerves from sympathetic trunk

Cardiac plexus

Pulmonary plexus

Descending thoracic aorta

Esophagus (cut)

Posterior and anterior
vagal trunks

Celiac branches of vagal trunks

Right crus of diaphragm

Celiac trunk and plexus

Celiac ganglion

Superior mesenteric ganglion

Superior mesenteric artery
and plexus

Aorticorenal ganglion

Intermesenteric plexus

Abdominal aorta

Inferior mesenteric ganglion

Inferior mesenteric artery
and plexus

Superior hypogastric plexus

Hypogastric nerves

Inferior hypogastric plexus

C

FIG. 2.26C. Nerves of the Posterior Abdominal Wall, Autonomic Nerves. **C.** Right Lateral View.

C. Autonomic plexuses of abdomen
1. Perivascular plexuses: fibers travel on vessel walls
   a. Celiac plexus: both sympathetic and parasympathetic fibers
   b. **Superior mesenteric plexus**: both sympathetic and parasympathetic fibers
   c. Renal plexus: both sympathetic and parasympathetic fibers
   d. **Inferior mesenteric plexus**: sympathetic fibers only; parasympathetic fibers travel within fusion fascia
2. Communicating plexuses
   a. **Intermesenteric plexus**
      i. Lies anteriorly on aorta between superior and inferior mesenteric arteries
      ii. Continuous with superior mesenteric, renal, and inferior mesenteric plexuses
      iii. Receives upper lumbar splanchnic contributions
      iv. Carries sympathetic fibers only
   b. **Superior hypogastric plexus**
      i. Lies anteriorly on aorta below inferior mesenteric arteries, passes over aortic bifurcation into pelvis to become paired hypogastric nerve bundles, then inferior hypogastric plexus on sides of rectum
      ii. Continuous with intermesenteric plexus
      iii. Receives lower lumbar splanchnic contributions
      iv. Carries sympathetic fibers only

IV. Clinical Considerations

A. Nerve sparing AAA bypass grafting
1. Superior hypogastric plexus carries most of sympathetic supply to pelvic viscera and may be damaged in AAA graft placement
2. Retrograde ejaculation is one potential consequence of damage
B. **Congenital megacolon (Hirschsprung disease)**: lack of neural crest migration into hindgut (usually) leads to immotile gut due to lack of innervation
C. Partial lumbar sympathectomy: may be used to treat arterial disease in lower limb by removing 2 or more lumbar sympathetic ganglia by division of their rami communicantes (care must be taken to preserve genitofemoral nerve, lumbar lymphatics, and ureter)

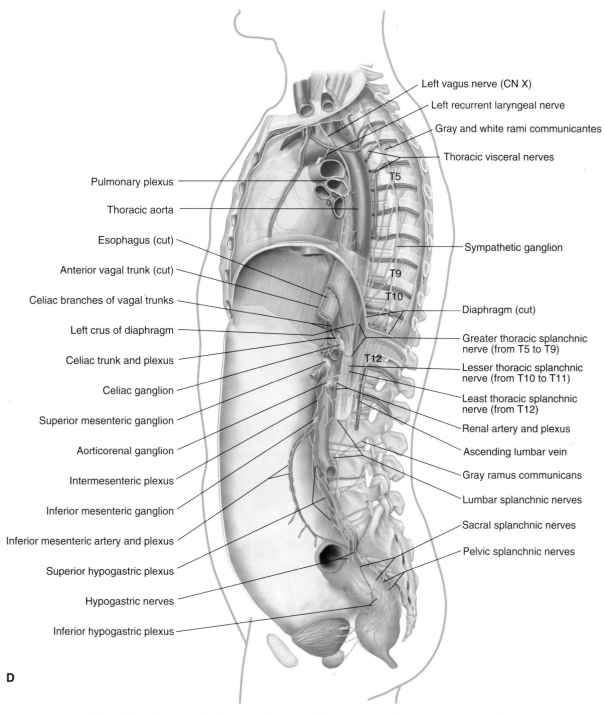

Left vagus nerve (CN X)

Left recurrent laryngeal nerve

Gray and white rami communicantes

Thoracic visceral nerves

T5

Pulmonary plexus

Thoracic aorta

Esophagus (cut)

Anterior vagal trunk (cut)

Celiac branches of vagal trunks

Left crus of diaphragm

Celiac trunk and plexus

Celiac ganglion

Superior mesenteric ganglion

Aorticorenal ganglion

Intermesenteric plexus

Inferior mesenteric ganglion

Inferior mesenteric artery and plexus

Superior hypogastric plexus

Hypogastric nerves

Inferior hypogastric plexus

Sympathetic ganglion

T9

T10

Diaphragm (cut)

Greater thoracic splanchnic nerve (from T5 to T9)

Lesser thoracic splanchnic nerve (from T10 to T11)

T12

Least thoracic splanchnic nerve (from T12)

Renal artery and plexus

Ascending lumbar vein

Gray ramus communicans

Lumbar splanchnic nerves

Sacral splanchnic nerves

Pelvic splanchnic nerves

D

FIG. 2.26D. Nerves of the Posterior Abdominal Wall, Autonomic Nerves. **D.** Left Lateral View.

Cross-sectional Anatomy of the Abdomen

I. T10 Vertebral Level (Fig. 2.27A–C)

A. Liver occupies right

B. Stomach and spleen lie to left

C. Inferior border of lung may hang into costodiaphragmatic recess posteriorly

II. L1 Vertebral Level (Fig. 2.27D–F)

A. Liver occupies right side anterior to kidney

B. Duodenum and pancreas somewhat central on abdominal aorta and IVC

C. Transverse colon and jejunum variably seen

D. Kidneys just superior to renal hilum are seen

III. L3 Vertebral Level (Fig. 2.27G–I)

A. Ascending and descending colon frame small bowel coils

B. May see 3rd part of duodenum

C. IVC lies on right side of abdominal aorta

D. Ureters lie anteriorly on bulging psoas major muscles

IV. L5/S1 Vertebral Level (Fig. 2.27J–L)

A. Ascending colon or cecum lies anterior to iliacus muscle

B. Descending colon to left side posteriorly

C. Coils of small bowel, with jejunum primarily left and ileum primarily right, lie anteriorly

D. Iliac alae and iliacus muscles lie posterior to colon

E. IVC may be seen forming, whereas abdominal aorta has bifurcated into common iliac arteries

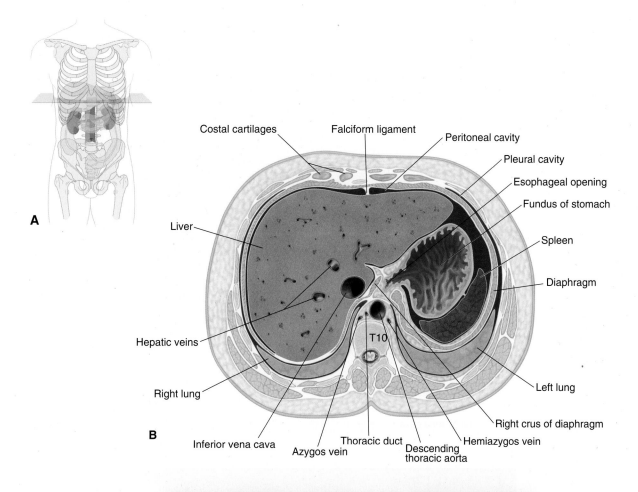

A. Plane of Cross Section through Vertebral Level T10.

B. Cross Section through Vertebral Level T10.

Costal cartilages

Falciform ligament

Peritoneal cavity

Pleural cavity

Esophageal opening

Fundus of stomach

Spleen

Diaphragm

Liver

Left lung

Hepatic veins

Right crus of diaphragm

Right lung

Hemiazygos vein

Inferior vena cava

Azygos vein

Thoracic duct

Descending thoracic aorta

T10

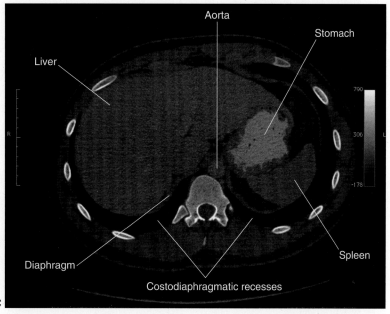

Aorta

Stomach

Liver

Diaphragm

Costodiaphragmatic recesses

Spleen

FIG. 2.27A–C. **A.** Plane of Cross Section through Vertebral Level T10. **B.** Cross Section through Vertebral Level T10. **C.** Computed Tomography Scan through Vertebral Level T10.

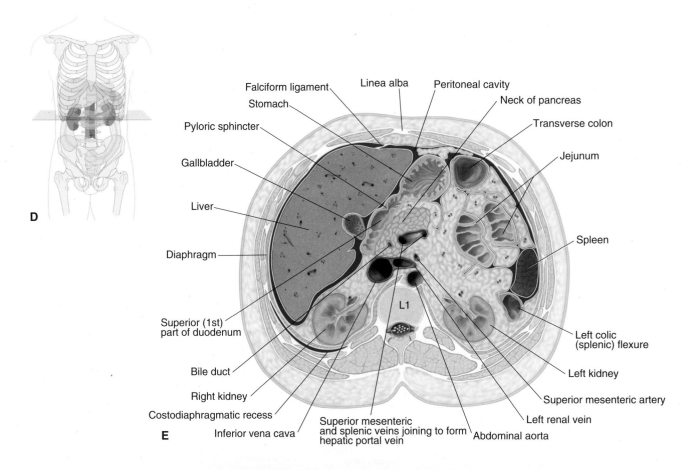

D

E

Falciform ligament

Linea alba

Peritoneal cavity

Stomach

Neck of pancreas

Pyloric sphincter

Transverse colon

Gallbladder

Jejunum

Liver

Spleen

Diaphragm

L1

Superior (1st)
part of duodenum

Left colic
(splenic) flexure

Bile duct

Left kidney

Right kidney

Superior mesenteric artery

Costodiaphragmatic recess

Left renal vein

Inferior vena cava

Superior mesenteric
and splenic veins joining to form
hepatic portal vein

Abdominal aorta

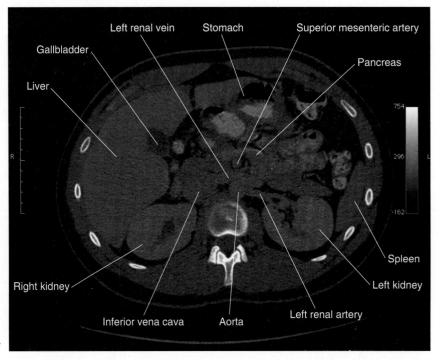

F

Left renal vein

Stomach

Superior mesenteric artery

Gallbladder

Pancreas

Liver

754

296

L

-162

Right kidney

Inferior vena cava

Aorta

Left renal artery

Left kidney

Spleen

R

FIG. 2.27D–F. D. Plane of Cross Section through Vertebral Level L1. **E.** Cross Section through Vertebral Level L1.
F. Computed Tomography Scan through Vertebral Level L1.

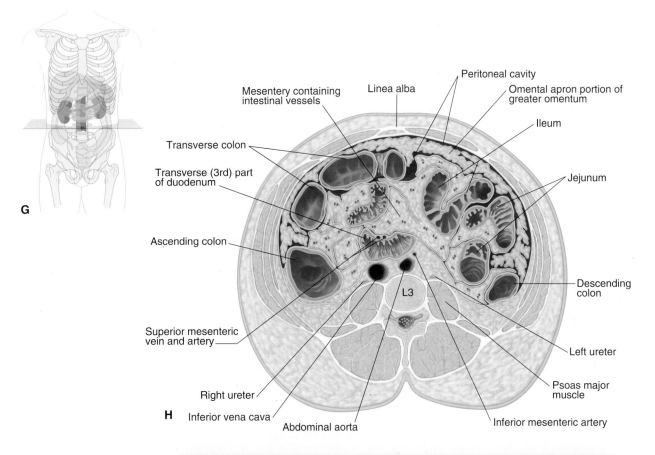

Mesentery containing intestinal vessels

Linea alba

Peritoneal cavity

Omental apron portion of greater omentum

Ileum

Transverse colon

Jejunum

Transverse (3rd) part of duodenum

Ascending colon

Descending colon

Superior mesenteric vein and artery

Left ureter

Right ureter

Psoas major muscle

H

Inferior vena cava

Abdominal aorta

Inferior mesenteric artery

L3

G

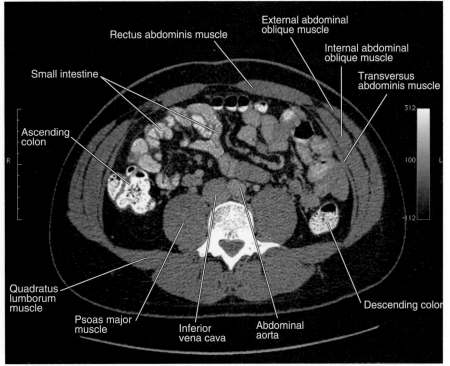

Rectus abdominis muscle

External abdominal oblique muscle

Internal abdominal oblique muscle

Small intestine

Transversus abdominis muscle

Ascending colon

Quadratus lumborum muscle

Psoas major muscle

Inferior vena cava

Abdominal aorta

Descending colon

I

R

L

312

100

-112

FIG. 2.27G–I. G. Plane of Cross Section through Vertebral Level L3. **H.** Cross Section through Vertebral Level L3. **I.** Computed Tomography Scan through Vertebral Level L3.

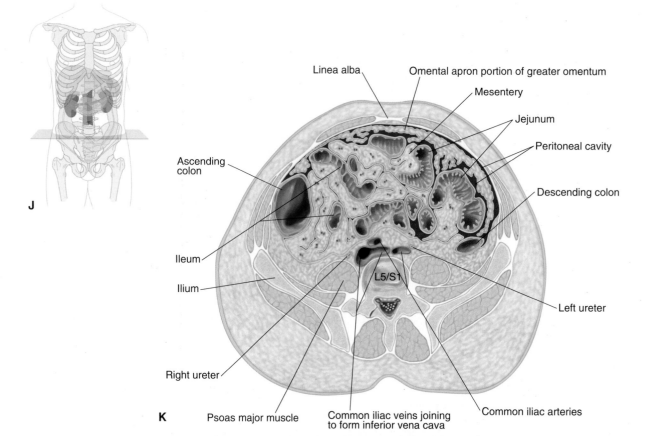

J

Linea alba
Omental apron portion of greater omentum
Mesentery
Jejunum
Peritoneal cavity
Descending colon
Ascending colon
Ileum
Ilium
L5/S1
Left ureter
Right ureter
Psoas major muscle
Common iliac veins joining to form inferior vena cava
Common iliac arteries

K

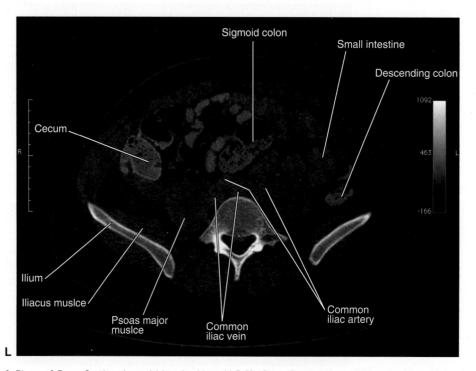

Sigmoid colon
Small intestine
Descending colon
1092
463
L
-166
Cecum
R
Ilium
Iliacus muslce
Psoas major muslce
Common iliac vein
Common iliac artery

L

FIG. 2.27J–L. J. Plane of Cross Section through Vertebral Level L5. **K.** Cross Section through Vertebral Level L5. **L.** Computed Tomography Scan through Vertebral Level L5.

Pelvis & Perineum

Surface Anatomy of the Pelvis and Perineum

I. Palpable Features and Surface Anatomy of the Pelvis (Fig. 3.1A–D)

A. **Iliac crest**
  1. Arching upper limit of iliac ala
  2. Highest point lies at level of spine of L4 vertebra
  3. Ends anteriorly and posteriorly as superior iliac spines
B. **Anterior superior iliac spine**
C. **Posterior superior iliac spine**
  1. Often visible as skin dimple
  2. Lies at level of 2nd sacral spine
D. **Natal cleft**: midline cleft between gluteal muscles
E. **Gluteal fold**: lower border of gluteus maximus
F. **Ischial tuberosity**: palpable near middle of gluteal fold when thigh is flexed
G. **Ischiopubic ramus**
  1. Union of inferior pubic ramus and ischial ramus
  2. Subcutaneous throughout its length
  3. Marks lateral boundary of urogenital triangle

Palpable bony structures

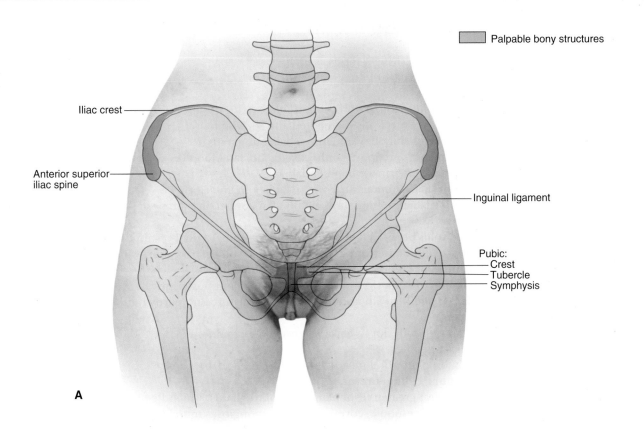

Iliac crest

Anterior superior iliac spine

Inguinal ligament

Pubic:
- Crest
- Tubercle
- Symphysis

A

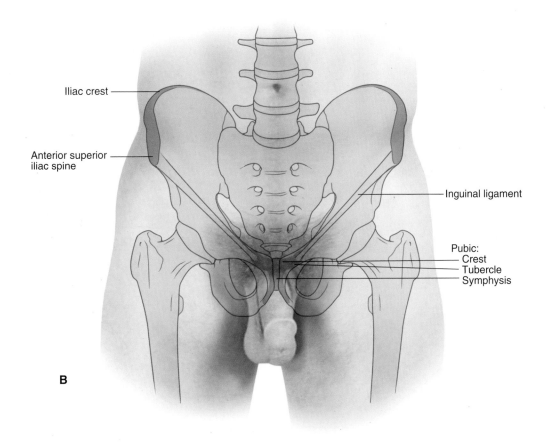

Iliac crest

Anterior superior iliac spine

Inguinal ligament

Pubic:
- Crest
- Tubercle
- Symphysis

B

FIG. 3.1A,B. Palpable Features of the Pelvis, Anterior View **A.** Female. **B.** Male.

II. External Genitalia in Female (Fig. 3.1E)

A. **Mons pubis**
1. Eminence overlying symphysis pubis
2. Composed mainly of fat, covered with hair

B. **Labia majora**
1. Bilateral longitudinal folds of skin that extend posteroinferiorly from mons
2. Skin of outer surface is pigmented and set with hair
3. Inner layer is smooth with large sebaceous glands
4. Between layers are loose connective tissue, fat, blood vessels, nerves, and glands
5. **Pudendal cleft** (rima): between labia
6. **Anterior labial commissure**: where labia join anteriorly
7. **Posterior labial commissure**: mainly skin connecting the posterior ends of labia

C. **Labia minora**
1. Paired folds between labia majora, surrounding vaginal vestibule
2. **Prepuce**: most anterior part of labia, which split to pass above clitoris
3. **Frenulum of clitoris**: meeting of labia below clitoris
4. **Frenulum of labia** (fourchette): where labia join posteriorly

D. **Clitoris**: located beneath anterior labial commissure and partly hidden by prepuce

E. **Vestibule**
1. Area posteroinferior to clitoris between labia minora
2. Several openings
   a. External urethral meatus
   b. Vagina, behind urethra
   c. Ducts of **greater vestibular (Bartholin) glands**, which lie at posteroinferior ends of bulbs of vestibule, covered by bulbospongiosus muscles
3. **Hymen**: membrane of variable size and form partly blocking vaginal orifice prior to initial penetration

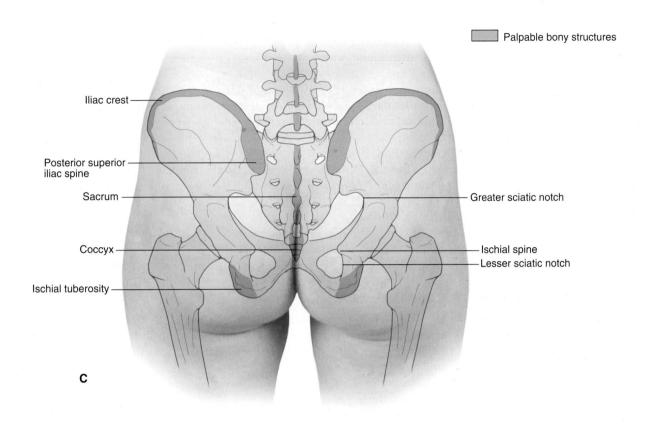

Palpable bony structures

Iliac crest

Posterior superior iliac spine

Sacrum

Coccyx

Ischial tuberosity

Greater sciatic notch

Ischial spine
Lesser sciatic notch

C

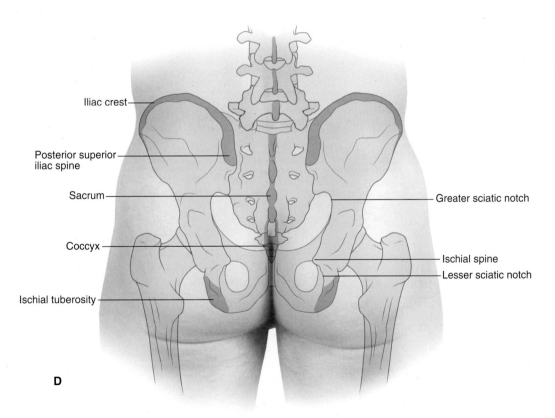

Iliac crest

Posterior superior iliac spine

Sacrum

Coccyx

Ischial tuberosity

Greater sciatic notch

Ischial spine
Lesser sciatic notch

D

FIG. 3.1C,D. Palpable Features of the Pelvis, Posterior View. **C.** Female. **D.** Male.

III. External Genitalia in Male (Fig. 3.1F)

A. **Scrotum**
1. Cutaneous sac containing testes
2. Divided by median raphe, which is continuous on penis and along midline to anus
3. Composed of 2 layers
   a. Skin: thin and pigmented, with hair and sebaceous glands
   b. **Dartos** (tunica dartos scroti): superficial fascia containing scattered smooth muscle; closely bound to skin but only loosely attached to deeper layers

B. **Penis**
1. **Glans** caps distal end
   a. Penetrated by vertical slitlike external urethral meatus
   b. Joins shaft at flared corona of glans, which lies beneath prepuce in uncircumsized penis
2. **Prepuce**
   a. Redundant skin partially covering glans
   b. Gathered on ventral midline at **frenulum**
3. **Shaft**: pendulous portion extending from attachment at root to glans

IV. Clinical Considerations

A. Cysts or abscesses of greater vestibular glands (Bartholin) can occur
B. **Imperforate hymen**: failure of an opening to occur in hymen, which may not be recognized until puberty when menstrual fluid dilates vagina, creating pressure (hematocolpos)
C. **Episiotomy**: incision in vulva made to prevent uncontrolled tissue damage to perineum during parturition

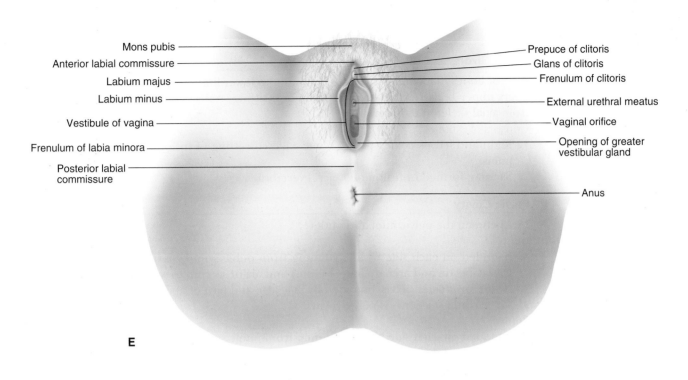

Mons pubis

Anterior labial commissure

Labium majus

Labium minus

Vestibule of vagina

Frenulum of labia minora

Posterior labial commissure

Prepuce of clitoris

Glans of clitoris

Frenulum of clitoris

External urethral meatus

Vaginal orifice

Opening of greater vestibular gland

Anus

E

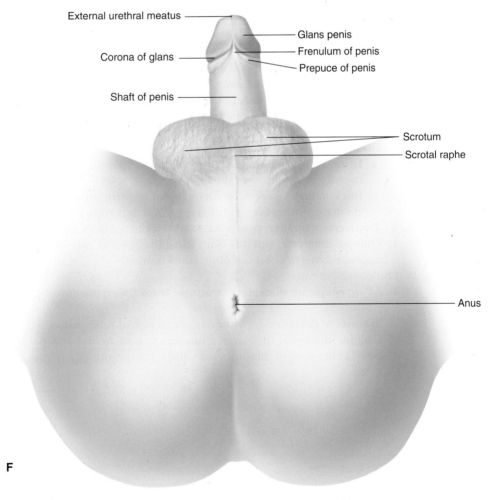

External urethral meatus

Corona of glans

Shaft of penis

Glans penis

Frenulum of penis

Prepuce of penis

Scrotum

Scrotal raphe

Anus

F

FIG. 3.1E,F. External Genitalia, Inferior View. **E.** Female. **F.** Male.

Bony Pelvis

I. Pelvic Girdle

A. Ring of bones that connects vertebral column to lower limbs

B. Bears upper body weight when standing and sitting, transferring weight of upper body from axial skeleton to lower limbs

C. Consists of 3 bones

   1. Right and left **os coxae**, or hip bone: each consisting of fusion of **ilium, ischium**, and **pubis**

   2. **Sacrum**: formed by fusion of 5 sacral vertebrae

II. Pelvic Cavity

A. Lies between the pelvic inlet and outlet

B. Inlet

   1. Bounded on each side by line running from pubic symphysis along **iliopectineal line** (pubic pectin and arcuate line of ilium) and ala of sacrum to sacral promontory

   2. "False" or greater pelvis, bounded by iliac alae and part of abdominal cavity, lies above

   3. "True" or lesser pelvis is pelvic cavity

C. Outlet

   1. Bounded on each side by line running from pubic symphysis along ischiopubic ramus (inferior pubic ramus and ischial ramus) and sacrotuberous ligaments to coccyx

   2. Closed by pelvic diaphragm

III. Pelvic Measurements (Fig. 3.2A–D)

A. Inlet measurements

   1. **Anteroposterior (AP)** or **conjugate diameter**: passes from upper margin of pubic symphysis to middle of sacral promontory

   2. **Obstetric conjugate diameter**

      a. Measured from back of pubic symphysis to sacral promontory

      b. Shorter than AP diameter and is minimal distance between promontory and symphysis

   3. **Diagonal conjugate diameter**

      a. Distance between lower pubic symphysis margin and sacral promontory; only one measured by palpation through vagina

      b. Inlet diameter said to be adequate for parturition when promontory cannot be felt via vagina; otherwise, pelvis is regarded as contracted

   4. **Transverse diameter**: passes across widest part of inlet (side to side)

   5. **Oblique diameter**: extends from sacroiliac joint of one side to iliopubic eminence of opposite side (or center of obturator foramen)

B. Outlet measurements

   1. **AP** or **conjugate diameter**: measured from lower margin of pubic symphysis to tip of coccyx

   2. **Transverse diameter**: measured between ischial tuberosities

   3. **Oblique diameter**: measured from junction of ischial and pubic rami of one side to point of crossing of sacrotuberous and sacrospinous ligaments of opposite side

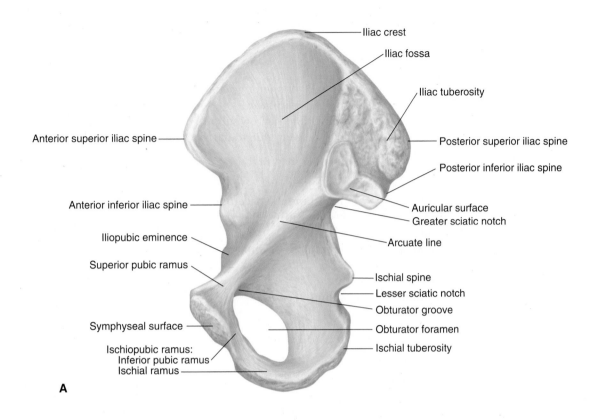

Iliac crest

Iliac fossa

Iliac tuberosity

Anterior superior iliac spine

Posterior superior iliac spine

Posterior inferior iliac spine

Anterior inferior iliac spine

Auricular surface

Greater sciatic notch

Iliopubic eminence

Arcuate line

Superior pubic ramus

Ischial spine

Lesser sciatic notch

Obturator groove

Symphyseal surface

Obturator foramen

Ischiopubic ramus:
Inferior pubic ramus
Ischial ramus

Ischial tuberosity

A

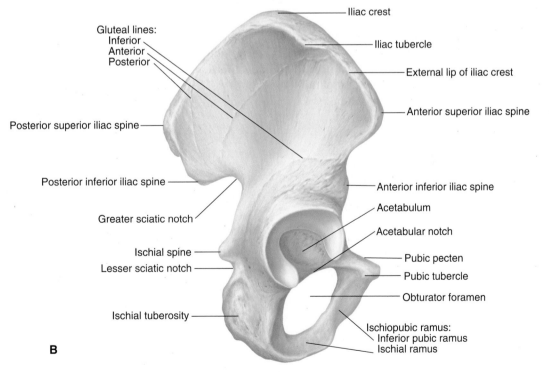

Iliac crest

Gluteal lines:
Inferior
Anterior
Posterior

Iliac tubercle

External lip of iliac crest

Posterior superior iliac spine

Anterior superior iliac spine

Posterior inferior iliac spine

Anterior inferior iliac spine

Acetabulum

Greater sciatic notch

Acetabular notch

Ischial spine

Pubic pecten

Lesser sciatic notch

Pubic tubercle

Obturator foramen

Ischial tuberosity

Ischiopubic ramus:
Inferior pubic ramus
Ischial ramus

B

FIG. 3.2A,B. Os Coxae. **A.** Medial View. **B.** Lateral View.

IV. Pelvic Classifications

A. Bony pelvis may be reliable indicator of sex, particularly in forensic medicine

B. Diameter, shapes, and measurements are especially applicable in females insofar as size and shape of inlet affect parturition

C. Classes

1. **Anthropoid** (apelike)
   a. 23%
   b. Long narrow oval with AP diameter greater than transverse
   c. Long sacrum with deep pelvic cavity
   d. Prominent ischial spines and narrow subpubic angle
   e. May cause difficulty in delivery due to narrow transverse diameter

2. **Gynecoid**
   a. About 50%
   b. Wide, circular inlet
   c. Wide subpubic arch and widely spaced ischial spines
   d. Provides reasonably uneventful delivery

3. **Android**
   a. About 20%; twice as common in white as in nonwhite females
   b. Heart-shaped inlet
   c. Narrow subpubic angle
   d. Prominent ischial spines
   e. Resembles male pelvis

4. **Platypelloid**
   a. 2.5%
   b. Flattened type
   c. Short sacrum
   d. AP diameter is short, and transverse is long
   e. May be difficult for fetal head to engage inlet, and cesarean section may be necessary

V. Axis of Birth Canal

A. Path followed by fetal head in course through pelvis

B. Extends downward and backward in axis of inlet as far as ischial spines (level of uterovaginal angle), where it turns forward and downward at almost 90° angle and continues in axis of vagina (approximately parallel to inlet)

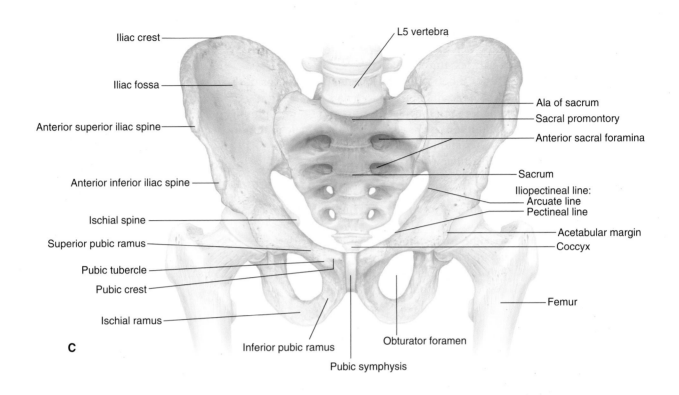

Iliac crest

Iliac fossa

Anterior superior iliac spine

Anterior inferior iliac spine

Ischial spine

Superior pubic ramus

Pubic tubercle

Pubic crest

Ischial ramus

Inferior pubic ramus

Pubic symphysis

L5 vertebra

Ala of sacrum

Sacral promontory

Anterior sacral foramina

Sacrum

Iliopectineal line:
Arcuate line
Pectineal line

Acetabular margin

Coccyx

Femur

Obturator foramen

C

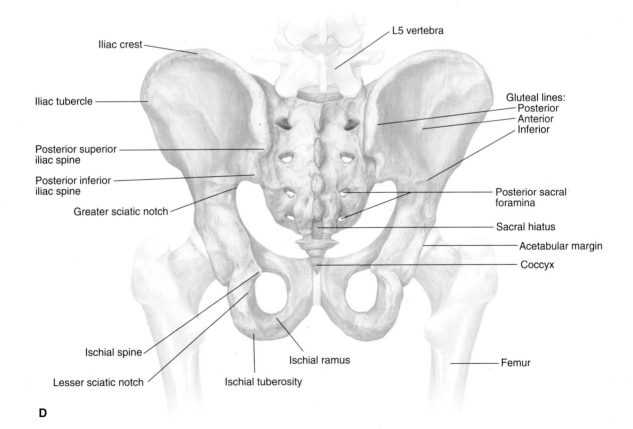

Iliac crest

Iliac tubercle

Posterior superior iliac spine

Posterior inferior iliac spine

Greater sciatic notch

Ischial spine

Lesser sciatic notch

Ischial tuberosity

Ischial ramus

L5 vertebra

Gluteal lines:
Posterior
Anterior
Inferior

Posterior sacral foramina

Sacral hiatus

Acetabular margin

Coccyx

Femur

D

FIG. 3.2C,D. Articulated Bony Pelvis, Male. **C.** Anterior View. **D.** Posterior View.

VI. Comparison of Female and Male Pelvis (Fig. 3.2E–J)

A. Female
   1. Bones are thinner and lighter
   2. Muscle markings not as prominent
   3. Cavity less funnel shaped
   4. Distance between ischial spines and tuberosities is greater
   5. Greater sciatic notch is wider
   6. Smaller sacral surfaces for articulation with ilium and with 5th lumbar vertebra
   7. Subpubic angle is close to 90° in female and more acute in male
   8. Greater and lesser pelvis: shallow and wide
   9. Pelvic inlet: wide, oval, and rounded
   10. Pelvic outlet: comparatively large

B. Male
   1. In addition to above, male ischial spines are heavier and project farther into pelvic outlet
   2. Sacrum usually more concave anteriorly
   3. Greater and lesser pelvis: narrow and deep
   4. Pelvic inlet: narrow and heart-shaped
   5. Pelvic outlet: comparatively small

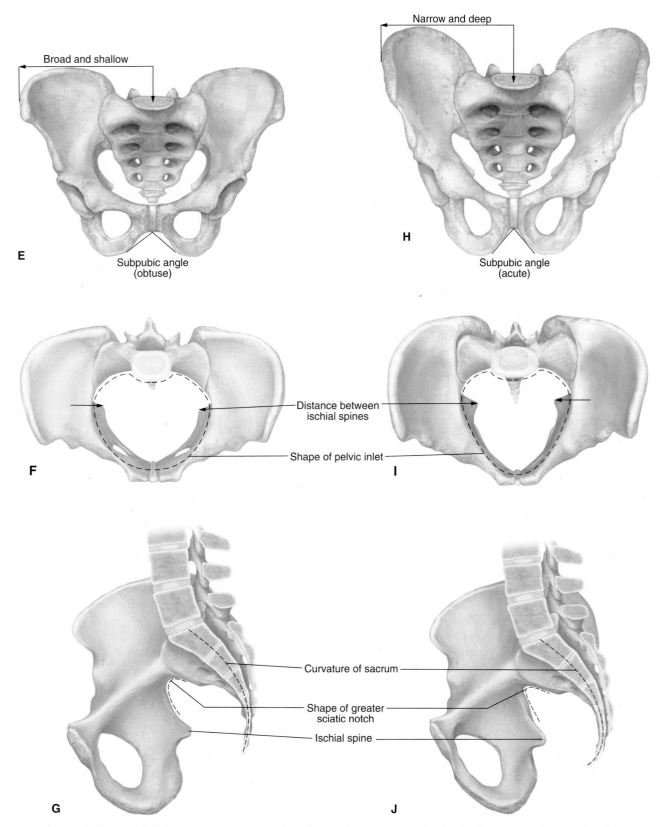

FIG. 3.2E–J. Bony Pelvis. **E.** Female, Anterior View. **F.** Female, Superior View. **G.** Female, Hemisection. **H.** Male, Anterior View. **I.** Male, Superior View. **J.** Male, Hemisection.

Pelvic Viscera and Pelvic Peritoneum

I. Pelvic Viscera of Both Sexes (Fig. 3.3A–D)

A. **Bladder**
   1. Posterior to body of pubis and pubic symphysis
   2. Superior surface covered with peritoneum, which is not bound strongly to pubic bone and permits bladder to expand between peritoneum and anterior abdominal wall

B. **Rectum** and **anal canal**
   1. Anterior to sacrum and coccyx
   2. Supported by pelvic diaphragm

II. Female Pelvic Viscera

A. **Vagina**
   1. Lies between bladder and urethra anteriorly and rectum and anal canal posteriorly
   2. Surrounded by endopelvic fascia
   3. Attached to cervix of uterus superiorly
   4. Opens at vulva or vaginal vestibule inferiorly

B. **Uterus**
   1. Lies above vagina, typically anteverted above bladder
   2. Covered with peritoneum except laterally

C. **Uterine tubes**
   1. Connected to lateral aspect of uterus below fundus
   2. Open into uterine cavity and pelvic cavity adjacent to ovaries

D. **Ovaries**
   1. Lie within ovarian fossa on lateral pelvic wall
   2. Connected by peritoneum to uterine tubes

III. Male Pelvic Viscera

A. **Ductus deferens** (vas deferens)
   1. Paired: each enters abdominopelvic cavity through deep inguinal ring
   2. Passes onto posterior aspect of bladder and becomes ampullated

B. **Seminal vesicle**
   1. Paired: posterior to bladder and anterior to rectum
   2. Surrounded by endopelvic fascia

IV. Pelvic Peritoneum

A. Continuous from abdominal cavity into pelvic cavity, but peritoneal cavity does not reach inferior limit of pelvic cavity, so pelvic viscera are only partially covered by peritoneum and lie largely below it

B. Beneath peritoneum, pelvic viscera are embedded in extraperitoneal connective tissue called **endopelvic fascia**

C. In both sexes
   1. Superior surface of bladder is covered with peritoneum
   2. Rectum
      a. Upper 1/3 covered anteriorly and laterally by peritoneum; **pararectal fossae** lie laterally
      b. Middle 1/3 covered only anteriorly
      c. Lower 1/3 is retroperitoneal

D. In female
   1. Peritoneum passes from bladder onto anterior surface of uterus, creating small **vesicouterine pouch**

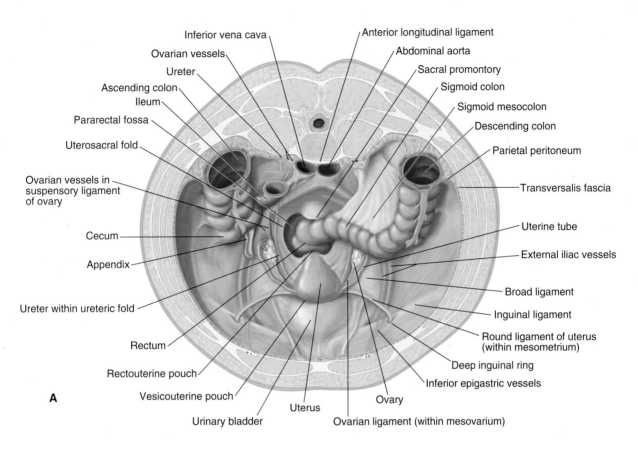

Inferior vena cava
Ovarian vessels
Ureter
Ascending colon
Ileum
Pararectal fossa
Uterosacral fold
Ovarian vessels in suspensory ligament of ovary
Cecum
Appendix
Ureter within ureteric fold
Rectum
Rectouterine pouch
Vesicouterine pouch
Urinary bladder
Uterus
Ovary
Ovarian ligament (within mesovarium)

Anterior longitudinal ligament
Abdominal aorta
Sacral promontory
Sigmoid colon
Sigmoid mesocolon
Descending colon
Parietal peritoneum
Transversalis fascia
Uterine tube
External iliac vessels
Broad ligament
Inguinal ligament
Round ligament of uterus (within mesometrium)
Deep inguinal ring
Inferior epigastric vessels

A

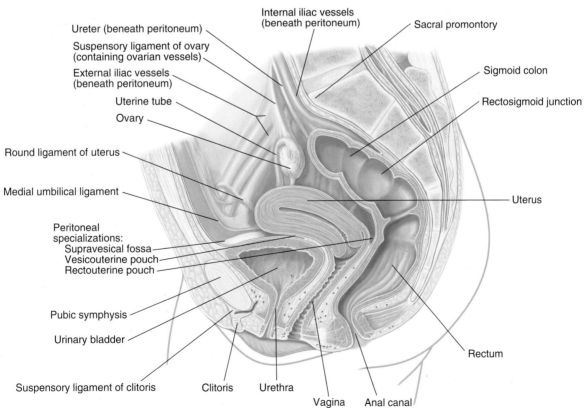

Ureter (beneath peritoneum)
Suspensory ligament of ovary (containing ovarian vessels)
External iliac vessels (beneath peritoneum)
Uterine tube
Ovary
Round ligament of uterus
Medial umbilical ligament
Peritoneal specializations:
Supravesical fossa
Vesicouterine pouch
Rectouterine pouch
Pubic symphysis
Urinary bladder
Suspensory ligament of clitoris
Clitoris
Urethra
Vagina
Anal canal

Internal iliac vessels (beneath peritoneum)
Sacral promontory
Sigmoid colon
Rectosigmoid junction
Uterus
Rectum

B

FIG. 3.3A,B. Pelvic Peritoneum, Female Pelvis. **A.** Superior View. **B.** Sagittal View.

2. Passes over uterus, uterine tubes, and ovaries as **broad ligament**, which is divided into 3 parts
   a. **Mesosalpinx**: 2 fused layers hanging below uterine tube on either side
   b. **Mesovarium**: fused layers continuous with mesosalpinx that surround ovary
   c. **Mesometrium**: splits into anterior and posterior layers on each side that connect uterus laterally to lateral pelvic wall
3. Passes from uterus to cover anteriorly upper 2/3 of rectum
   a. Dips inferiorly to touch posterior fornix of vagina
   b. Forms **rectouterine pouch** (**pouch of Douglas**)
E. In male
   1. Peritoneum posterior to bladder passes onto rectum
   2. May contact superior extremities of seminal vesicles
   3. **Rectovesical pouch** formed between bladder and rectum

V. Endopelvic Fascia and Ligaments

A. In both sexes
   1. Endopelvic fascia lies beneath pelvic peritoneum
   2. Surrounds and supports pelvic viscera
   3. May form ligamentous sheets
   4. Rectal fusion fascia
      a. Lies on either side of rectum on lower 2/3 of rectum below peritoneal reflection
      b. Lies anterior to rectum in lower 1/3
B. In female
   1. **Round ligament of uterus** and **ovarian ligament**
      a. **Round ligament of uterus**: lies under anterior lamina of broad ligament in course to deep inguinal ring
      b. **Ovarian ligament**: attaches laterally to ovary and contained within mesovarium
      c. Both attached to side of uterus under peritoneum just below uterine tube
      d. Both are remnants of gubernaculum
   2. **Pubovesical ligaments**: endopelvic fascia; attach bladder to pelvic diaphragm fibers arising on posterior surface of pubis
   3. **Rectouterine fold**: variable shelf-like fold in the posterior lamina of mesometrium which passes from isthmus of uterus to posterior wall of pelvis lateral to rectum
   4. **Rectovaginal septum**: lies between rectum and upper half of posterior vaginal wall
C. In male
   1. **Puboprostatic ligaments**: endopelvic fascia; attach bladder neck and prostate to pubic origin of pelvic diaphragm
   2. **Sacrogenital fold**: shelf-like peritoneal fold passing from posterior surface of bladder to posterior wall of pelvis lateral to rectum
   3. **Rectovesical septum**: lies between rectum and posterior surface of bladder, ductus deferentes, seminal vesicles, and posterior surface of prostate gland

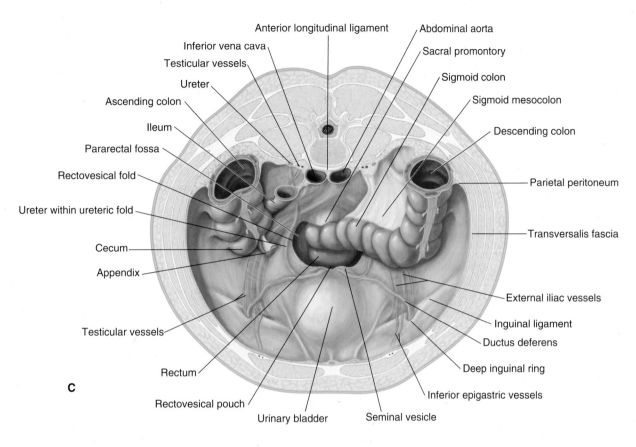

Anterior longitudinal ligament
Inferior vena cava
Testicular vessels
Ureter
Ascending colon
Ileum
Pararectal fossa
Rectovesical fold
Ureter within ureteric fold
Cecum
Appendix
Testicular vessels
Rectum
Rectovesical pouch
Urinary bladder
Seminal vesicle
Abdominal aorta
Sacral promontory
Sigmoid colon
Sigmoid mesocolon
Descending colon
Parietal peritoneum
Transversalis fascia
External iliac vessels
Inguinal ligament
Ductus deferens
Deep inguinal ring
Inferior epigastric vessels

C

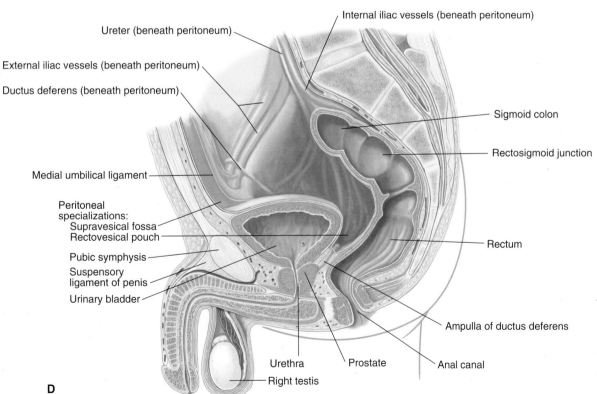

Ureter (beneath peritoneum)
External iliac vessels (beneath peritoneum)
Ductus deferens (beneath peritoneum)
Medial umbilical ligament
Peritoneal specializations:
Supravesical fossa
Rectovesical pouch
Pubic symphysis
Suspensory ligament of penis
Urinary bladder
Internal iliac vessels (beneath peritoneum)
Sigmoid colon
Rectosigmoid junction
Rectum
Ampulla of ductus deferens
Anal canal
Urethra
Prostate
Right testis

D

FIG. 3.3C,D. Pelvic Peritoneum, Male Pelvis. **C.** Superior View. **D.** Sagittal View.

Urinary Bladder and Urethra

I. Bladder: Surfaces and Relations (Fig. 3.4A,B)

A. **Fundus**, or **base** (posterior)
   1. Triangular, directed caudally and posteriorly
   2. Separated from rectum by vagina or seminal vesicles, ductus deferentes, and rectovesical septum

B. **Apex**
   1. Directed toward pubic symphysis
   2. **Median umbilical ligament** (urachus): continues up onto abdominal wall from apex to umbilicus

C. Superior surface
   1. Bounded laterally by lateral borders that delimit it from inferior surface
   2. Bounded posteriorly by line connecting ureters
   3. Covered by peritoneum and related to anterior surface of uterus or sigmoid colon and coils of ileum in male

D. Inferolateral surface
   1. Directed inferior and lacks peritoneum
   2. Separated from pubis by **prevesical cleft (space of Retzius)**

E. **Neck**
   1. Triangular, in contact with sphincter urethrae muscle (female) or base of prostate
   2. Contains urethral orifice

II. Bladder Support

A. Pubovesical (female) or puboprostatic (male) ligaments: between pubis and bladder or prostate

B. **Rectovesical ligaments**
   1. From bladder to sides of rectum and sacrum
   2. Within rectouterine or sacrogenital folds

C. **Median umbilical ligament (urachus)**: from apex of bladder to abdominal wall

III. Peritoneal Folds

A. **Median umbilical fold**: contains median umbilical ligament

B. **Medial umbilical folds**
   1. Contain **medial umbilical ligaments**, remnants of distal portions of umbilical arteries
   2. Lateral boundaries of **supravesicular fossae**

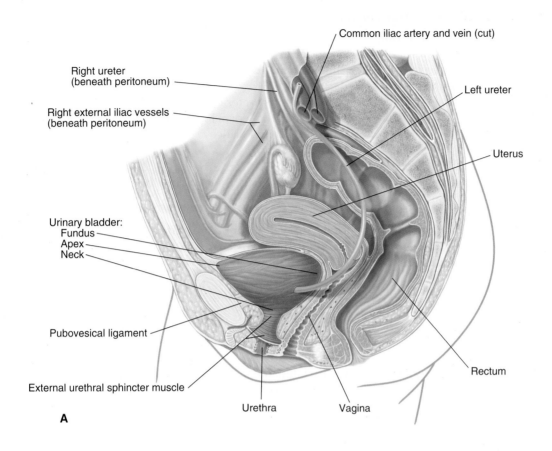

Common iliac artery and vein (cut)

Right ureter
(beneath peritoneum)

Right external iliac vessels
(beneath peritoneum)

Left ureter

Uterus

Urinary bladder:
Fundus
Apex
Neck

Pubovesical ligament

Rectum

External urethral sphincter muscle

Urethra   Vagina

A

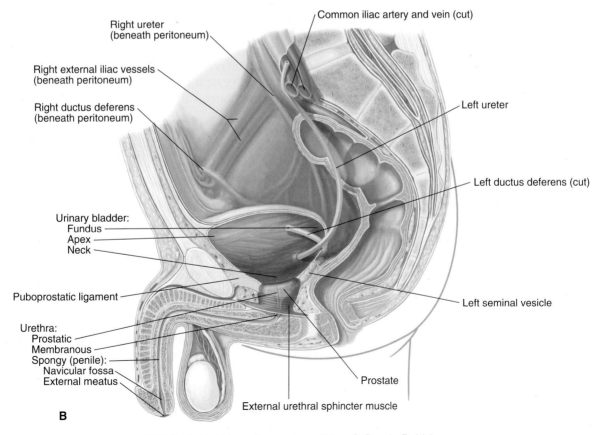

Common iliac artery and vein (cut)

Right ureter
(beneath peritoneum)

Right external iliac vessels
(beneath peritoneum)

Right ductus deferens
(beneath peritoneum)

Left ureter

Left ductus deferens (cut)

Urinary bladder:
Fundus
Apex
Neck

Puboprostatic ligament

Left seminal vesicle

Urethra:
Prostatic
Membranous
Spongy (penile):
Navicular fossa
External meatus

Prostate

External urethral sphincter muscle

B

FIG. 3.4A,B. Urinary Bladder, Lateral View. **A.** Female. **B.** Male.

IV. Special Features of Interior (Fig. 3.4C,D)

A. **Interureteric ridge**
  1. Transverse ridge on posterior inner wall of bladder
  2. Ureteric orifices are slitlike openings at superolateral ends of ridge
B. **Trigone**
  1. Smooth triangular area below interureteric ridge and above internal urethral orifice
  2. **Uvula of bladder** (male): formed by median lobe of prostate pressing on posteroinferior bladder wall behind internal urethral orifice

V. Bladder Musculature

A. Smooth muscle, plexiform in arrangement, forming meshwork
B. **Detrusor urinae muscle**: bladder wall muscle
C. **Internal urethral sphincter**
  1. Traditionally recognized, although no annular sphincter exists
  2. Neck of bladder and urethral wall characterized by circularly disposed elastic tissue that aids in maintaining a collapsed lumen in urethra

VI. Urethra

A. Female urethra
  1. About 4 cm long
  2. External orifice opens posteroinferior to glans of clitoris and anterior to vaginal orifice
  3. Lies in front of lower half of vagina
  4. Surrounded by voluntary sphincter urethrae muscle; some muscle fibers enclosing urethra and vagina together as **urethrovaginal sphincter**
  5. Perforates perineal membrane
B. Male urethra
  1. About 20 cm
  2. 3 parts
    a. **Prostatic urethra**
      i. 3–4 cm long
      ii. **Urethral crest**: sagittal ridge posteriorly
      iii. **Prostatic sinuses**: on either side of crest; where most prostatic ducts open
      iv. **Seminal colliculus**: small eminence near midpoint of crest
        a) Small slit leads into a blind pouch called the **prostatic utricle,** remnant of paramesonephric duct
        b) **Ejaculatory ducts** open onto seminal colliculus beside prostatic utricle
    b. **Membranous urethra**
      i. About 1 cm long; shortest part of urethra
      ii. Surrounded by sphincter urethrae muscle
      iii. Passes through perineal membrane
      iv. Wall of membranous portion is thin
    c. **Spongy or penile urethra**
      i. About 15 cm long
      ii. Enters bulb of penis at underside of perineal membrane, traverses full length of corpus spongiosum, and terminates at external urethral orifice
      iii. **Bulbourethral glands:** lie behind and to either side of membranous portion of urethra; their ducts perforate perineal membrane to enter spongy portion of urethra
      iv. Lumen, about 5 mm in diameter through most of length of penis; larger in bulb and again widened in glans penis as **fossa navicularis**

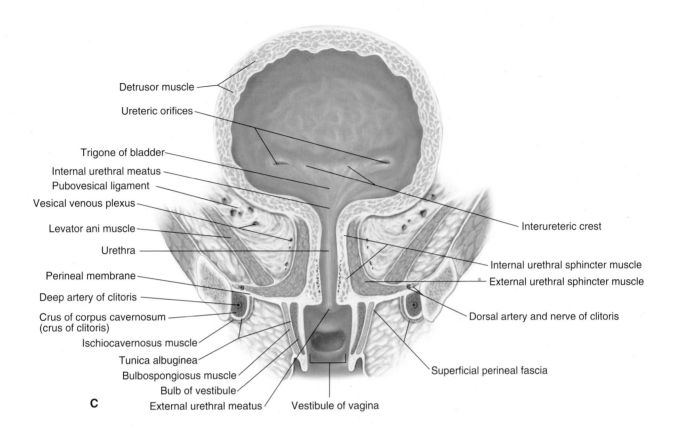

Detrusor muscle

Ureteric orifices

Trigone of bladder

Internal urethral meatus

Pubovesical ligament

Vesical venous plexus

Levator ani muscle

Urethra

Perineal membrane

Deep artery of clitoris

Crus of corpus cavernosum
(crus of clitoris)

Ischiocavernosus muscle

Tunica albuginea

Bulbospongiosus muscle

Bulb of vestibule

External urethral meatus

Interureteric crest

Internal urethral sphincter muscle

External urethral sphincter muscle

Dorsal artery and nerve of clitoris

Superficial perineal fascia

Vestibule of vagina

C

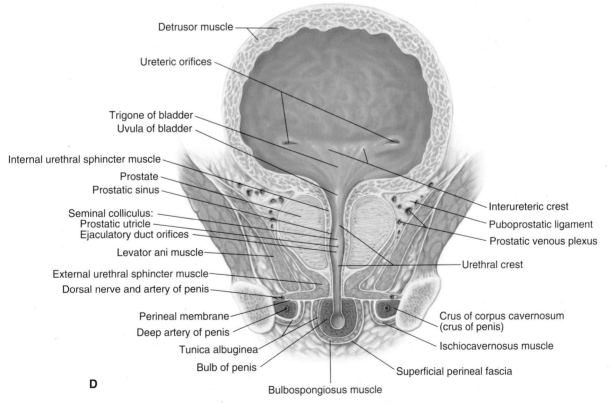

Detrusor muscle

Ureteric orifices

Trigone of bladder

Uvula of bladder

Internal urethral sphincter muscle

Prostate

Prostatic sinus

Seminal colliculus:
Prostatic utricle
Ejaculatory duct orifices

Levator ani muscle

External urethral sphincter muscle

Dorsal nerve and artery of penis

Perineal membrane

Deep artery of penis

Tunica albuginea

Bulb of penis

Interureteric crest

Puboprostatic ligament

Prostatic venous plexus

Urethral crest

Crus of corpus cavernosum
(crus of penis)

Ischiocavernosus muscle

Superficial perineal fascia

Bulbospongiosus muscle

D

FIG. 3.4C,D. Urinary Bladder, Coronal Section, Anterior View. **C.** Female. **D.** Male.

VII. Clinical Considerations

A. Distended bladder

1. When filled, it contains about 500 cc of urine
2. When excessively distended, rises to level of umbilicus lifting several cm of parietal peritoneum from abdominal wall
3. Can be punctured (**suprapubic cystostomy**) without entering peritoneal cavity

B. Cancers develop in lining epithelium and are usually multiple and superficial; with time, they invade muscular coat

C. Urinary stress incontinence

1. Common in multiparous women, resulting in loss of urinary control
2. Increase in intraabdominal pressure (e.g., from heavy lifting, sneezing, coughing, or laughter) can lead to urine leakage
3. Thought to be due to changes in bladder position and alteration of support mechanisms, especially levator ani muscles and pubovesical ligaments
4. May be associated with urinary bladder or uterine prolapse

D. Cystoscopy: interior of bladder and its orifices can be examined with cystoscope passed through urethra and by variety of imaging techniques (e.g., ultrasound)

E. Cystostomy: for temporary drainage of urinary tract due to urethral obstruction or stone removal

F. Cystectomy

1. Partial: for chronic ulcers, diverticuli, fistulae, benign tumors, or localized cancer
2. Total: in some cases of cancer of bladder or other pelvic viscera or in bladder extrophy

G. Vesicovisceral fistulae: rare; may be due to trauma, infection, or neoplastic disease

1. In female, occurs most commonly between bladder and vagina (**vesicovaginal**); vesicouterine fistulae are rare
2. In male, may occur between bladder and rectum (**vesicorectal**)

H. Instrumentation of male urethra

1. External urethral opening is narrowest part of urethra and least distensible portion; instrument passing through this opening should pass through any other parts of lumen
2. Membranous urethra is next narrowest portion but is distensible
3. Immediately below perineal membrane, superior surface of urethra is unprotected for short distance; wall is thin, distensible, and vulnerable to rough instrumentation
4. Prostate enlargement (**benign prostatic hypertrophy [BPH]**) may cause urethral obstruction

I. Disorders of spongy or penile urethra

1. **Hypospadias**
   a. Common congenital anomaly of penis (1 per 300 newborns) with external opening on urethra; results from failure of urogenital folds to fuse on ventral surface of penis and to complete formation of spongy urethra
   b. In all cases, prepuce is deformed and frenulum is absent
   c. Types
      i. Glandular type: external urethral opening is on ventral aspect of glans penis
      ii. Penile type: defect is in body of penis
      iii. Penoscrotal or scrotal type; opening is in perineum
2. **Epispadias**
   a. Abnormal urethral opening on dorsum of penis
   b. Very rare condition, often associated with abnormalities of anterior abdominal wall
3. Rupture of spongy urethra in bulb of penis
   a. Common in "straddle injuries" (i.e., while riding a bike)
   b. Urine escapes into superficial perineal space and passes from there inferiorly into scrotum and superiorly beneath subcutaneous connective tissue of anterior abdominal wall

Ductus Deferens, Seminal Vesicles, and Prostate

I. Ductus Deferens (Vas Deferens) (Fig. 3.5A,B)

A. Excretory duct of testis
B. Course
   1. Ascends along posterior border of testis
   2. As part of spermatic cord, passes through superficial inguinal ring and inguinal canal to deep inguinal ring
   3. Enters abdominal cavity at deep inguinal ring, bends around inferior epigastric artery; curves inferomedially
   4. Crosses anterosuperior to external iliac vessels to enter pelvis
   5. Descends on medial side of medial umbilical ligament and obturator vessels and nerve
   6. Crosses ureter superiorly to pass to its medial side and run on fundus of bladder between seminal vesicles to base of prostate, where its terminal part widens into an **ampulla**
   7. Ampulla is joined by duct of seminal vesicle to form **ejaculatory duct**, which runs through prostate to open into prostatic urethra at seminal colliculus

II. Seminal Vesicle

A. Bilateral lobulated sacs consisting of irregular pouches
B. Relations
   1. Anterior surface against fundus of bladder
   2. Posterior surface separated from rectum by rectovesical fascia
   3. Superiorly, related to ureter and ductus deferens above it
   4. Medially, ampulla of ductus deferens
   5. Inferiorly, joins ductus deferens at posterior surface of prostate to form **ejaculatory duct**

III. Prostate

A. Cone-shaped glandular body, size of a chestnut, containing much connective tissue and smooth muscle
B. Parts and relations
   1. Base: faces superiorly against neck of bladder
   2. Apex: directed inferiorly into urogenital hiatus; rests on perineal membrane
   3. Posterior surface: separated from rectum by rectovesical septum
   4. Anterior surface: separated from symphysis pubis by a venous plexus and endopelvic fascia; urethra opens through this surface just above apex
   5. Inferolateral surfaces separated from levator ani muscles by venous plexus
C. Lobes
   1. Lateral (right and left): occupy almost entire base of gland, lateral and anterior to urethra
   2. Median (middle): glandular, posterior to urethra but anterior to ejaculatory ducts; contains subtrigonal and cervical glands (Albarran)
   3. Posterior: posterior to urethra and ejaculatory ducts and behind middle lobe
   4. Anterior: small, nonglandular area in front of urethra
D. **Prostatic urethra**
   1. **Urethral crest**: longitudinal ridge on posterior wall
   2. **Prostatic sinus**: depression on sides of crest into which prostatic ducts open
   3. **Seminal colliculus**: summit of urethral crest on which open **ejaculatory ducts** and a median blind-ending sac, the **prostatic utricle**
E. Prostate support
   1. **Puboprostatic ligaments** from **arcus tendineus fasciae pelvis**, thickened superior fascia of pelvic diaphragm
   2. Perineal membrane
   3. **Sphincter urethrae muscle**, which surrounds prostate

IV. Clinical Considerations

A. Benign prostatic hypertrophy (BPH)

1. Extremely common in advancing age
2. May cause problems with voiding and urinary continence
3. Frequent cause of hematuria in men; may be due to leakage of blood from enlarged veins due to benign hypertrophy

B. Prostate cancer

1. Anterior lobe: adenomas rare; no urethral encroachment
2. Posterior lobe: adenomas rare; lobe encountered in digital examination
3. Lateral lobe: hypertrophy causes urinary obstruction
4. Median lobe: important clinically; enlargement of mucous glands leads to obstruction; adenomas frequent, encroaching into urethra, blocking internal orifice
5. In advanced disease, cells metastasize to iliac and sacral lymph nodes and bones

C. Prostatitis

1. Acute bacterial prostatitis: uncommon; can result in dysuria and obstruction with voiding and onset of chills, fever, and pain in back and perineum
2. Chronic bacterial prostatitis: common cause of recurrent urinary tract infection

D. Prostatectomy: may lead to impotence; all or part of gland may be removed via **transurethral resection of the prostate (TURP)**

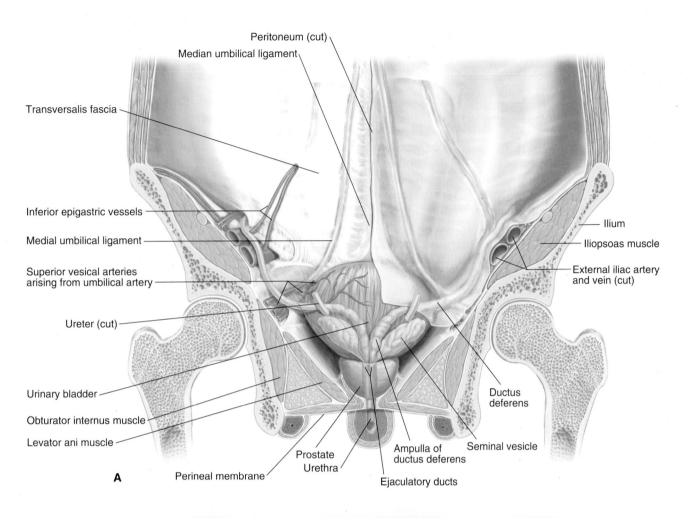

Peritoneum (cut)

Median umbilical ligament

Transversalis fascia

Inferior epigastric vessels

Medial umbilical ligament

Superior vesical arteries
arising from umbilical artery

Ureter (cut)

Urinary bladder

Obturator internus muscle

Levator ani muscle

Perineal membrane

Prostate
Urethra

Ampulla of
ductus deferens

Ejaculatory ducts

Seminal vesicle

Ductus
deferens

External iliac artery
and vein (cut)

Iliopsoas muscle

Ilium

A

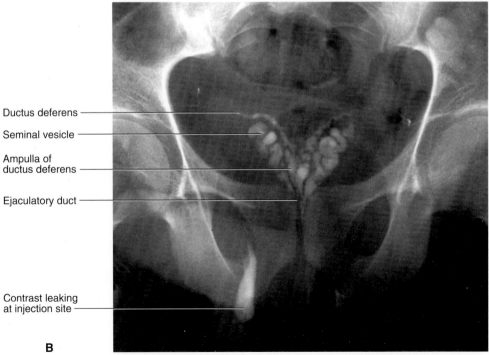

Ductus deferens

Seminal vesicle

Ampulla of
ductus deferens

Ejaculatory duct

Contrast leaking
at injection site

B

FIG. 3.5A,B. Male Internal Genitalia. **A.** Posterior View. **B.** Vasogram.

Urinary Bladder and Prostate: Blood Supply and Innervation

I. Arteries (Fig. 3.6A,B)

A. Bladder
   1. **Superior vesical branches**: several branches from umbilical artery, which is 1st branch of anterior division of internal iliac artery
   2. **Inferior vesical branches**
      a. In female: arise from vaginal artery from internal iliac
      b. In male: arise from distal portion of anterior division of internal iliac artery
B. Prostate: inferior vesical and middle rectal

II. Veins

A. Bladder: **vesical plexus** to internal iliac veins; receives deep dorsal vein of clitoris; communicates with prostatic plexus
B. Prostate: **prostatic plexus**; receives deep dorsal vein of penis; drains to internal iliac veins

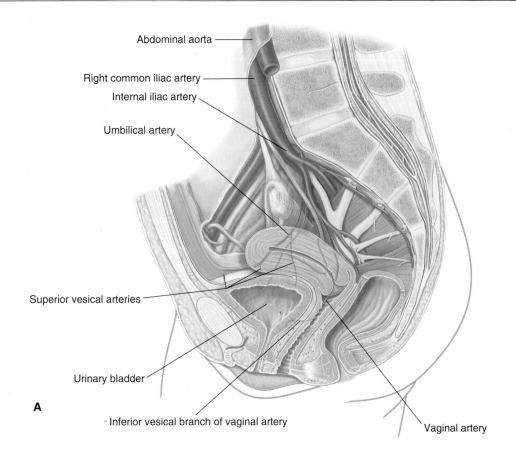

Abdominal aorta

Right common iliac artery

Internal iliac artery

Umbilical artery

Superior vesical arteries

Urinary bladder

A

Inferior vesical branch of vaginal artery

Vaginal artery

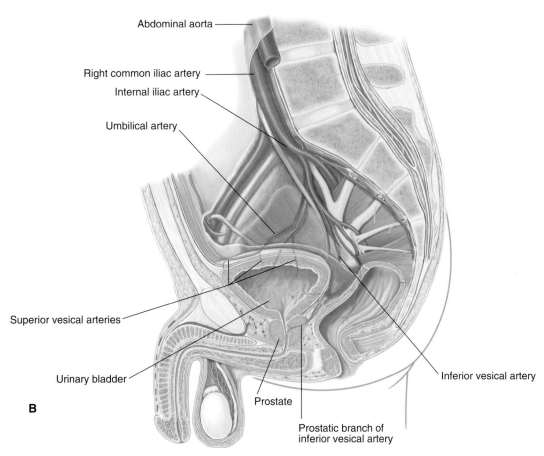

Abdominal aorta

Right common iliac artery

Internal iliac artery

Umbilical artery

Superior vesical arteries

Urinary bladder

B

Prostate

Prostatic branch of inferior vesical artery

Inferior vesical artery

FIG. 3.6A,B. Blood Supply to the Urinary Bladder, Sagittal View. **A.** Female. **B.** Male.

III. Nerves of the Bladder and Prostate (Fig. 3.6C,D)

A. Autonomic fibers from inferior hypogastric plexus to vesical and prostatic plexuses

B. Sympathetic innervation

   1. Presynaptic fibers: from lower thoracic and upper lumbar levels (T11–S2)
   2. Postsynaptic fibers: from superior hypogastric plexus via hypogastric nerves into inferior hypogastric plexus; some postsynaptic fibers are derived from sacral sympathetic trunk
   3. Innervates muscle of trigone and blood vessels

C. Parasympathetic innervation

   1. Presynaptic fibers: from pelvic splanchnic nerves from anterior rami S2–S4 into inferior hypogastric plexus
   2. Postsynaptic fibers: extremely short; ganglia located in bladder wall
   3. Serves emptying reflex, causing contraction of musculature of bladder wall (detrusor urinae muscle) and inhibitory to internal urethral sphincter in male; with toilet training, this reflex is suppressed when undesirable to void

D. Afferent innervation

   1. Conducted along both sympathetic and parasympathetic fibers
   2. Pain due to overstretched bladder travels with sympathetic fibers
   3. Proprioceptive impulses from bladder wall, initiated by stretching of muscle layers as bladder fills, travel over parasympathetic fibers whose stimulation results in reflex bladder emptying

E. Urinary retention

   1. Both sympathetic and somatic
      a. Sympathetic fibers: to internal urethral sphincter
      b. Somatic fibers from pudendal nerve (S2–S4) to sphincter urethrae muscle
   2. Bladder expands from within pelvis in extraperitoneal fat; overdistended, it can rise to level of umbilicus

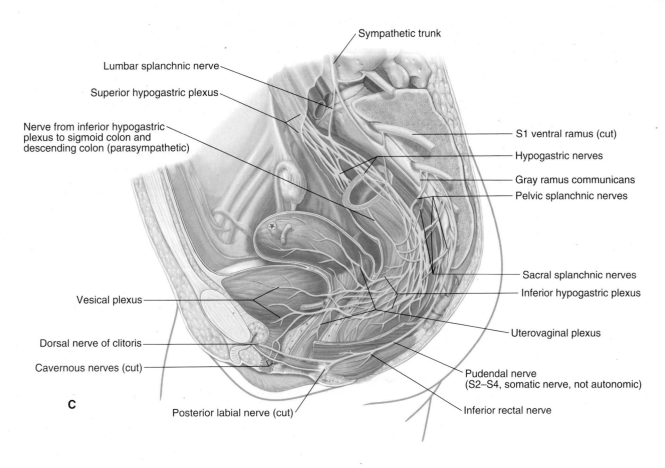

Sympathetic trunk

Lumbar splanchnic nerve

Superior hypogastric plexus

Nerve from inferior hypogastric
plexus to sigmoid colon and
descending colon (parasympathetic)

S1 ventral ramus (cut)

Hypogastric nerves

Gray ramus communicans

Pelvic splanchnic nerves

Sacral splanchnic nerves

Inferior hypogastric plexus

Vesical plexus

Uterovaginal plexus

Dorsal nerve of clitoris

Cavernous nerves (cut)

Pudendal nerve
(S2–S4, somatic nerve, not autonomic)

Inferior rectal nerve

C

Posterior labial nerve (cut)

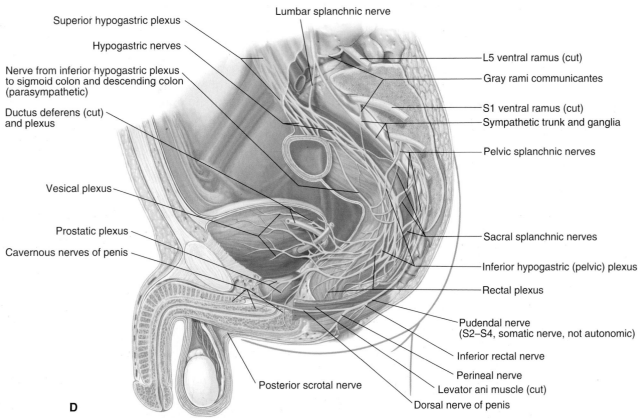

Superior hypogastric plexus

Lumbar splanchnic nerve

Hypogastric nerves

Nerve from inferior hypogastric plexus
to sigmoid colon and descending colon
(parasympathetic)

Ductus deferens (cut)
and plexus

L5 ventral ramus (cut)

Gray rami communicantes

S1 ventral ramus (cut)

Sympathetic trunk and ganglia

Pelvic splanchnic nerves

Vesical plexus

Prostatic plexus

Cavernous nerves of penis

Sacral splanchnic nerves

Inferior hypogastric (pelvic) plexus

Rectal plexus

Pudendal nerve
(S2–S4, somatic nerve, not autonomic)

Inferior rectal nerve

Perineal nerve

Levator ani muscle (cut)

Posterior scrotal nerve

Dorsal nerve of penis

D

FIG. 3.6C,D. Innervation of the Urinary Bladder, Sagittal View. **C.** Female. **D.** Male.

Ovary, Uterine Tubes, and Uterus: Parts and Relations

I. Ovary (Fig. 3.7A–D)

A. Germinal and endocrine gland

B. Location and relations

    1. In **ovarian fossa** on lateral wall of pelvis, with external iliac vessels above, ureter (which forms ovarian fossa) posteroinferiorly, and covered by fimbria of uterine tube superiorly

    2. Contained within a posterior projection of broad ligament called mesovarium

C. Surfaces and borders

    1. Lateral and medial surfaces

    2. Upper (tubal) extremity

    3. Lower (uterine) extremity

    4. Anterior (mesovarian) border

    5. Posterior (free) border

D. Supports

    1. Suspensory ligament of ovary

        a. Peritoneal fold running over external iliac vessels to reach upper extremity of ovary

        b. Contains ovarian vessels and endopelvic fascia

    2. Mesovarium

        a. Posterior projection from broad ligament

        b. Continuous with mesosalpinx anterosuperiorly and mesometrium anteroinferiorly

    3. Ovarian ligament

        a. Remnant of gubernaculum

        b. Continuous with round ligament of uterus where they both attach to uterus laterally below uterine tube

        c. Contained within mesovarium

II. Uterine Tube

A. Duct to carry ova from ovary to uterus

B. Location and relations

    1. Lies within **mesosalpinx**, the free upper border of broad ligament

    2. Curves posterolaterally from side of uterus to ovary in ovarian fossa

C. Parts

    1. Infundibulum: with abdominal ostium surrounded by **fimbria**; contacts ovary superiorly

    2. Ampulla

        a. Wide middle part

        b. Usual site of fertilization of ovum

    3. Isthmus: constricted medial part, which enters uterus

    4. Intramural portion (interstitial or intrauterine part): passes through uterine wall to open into uterine cavity

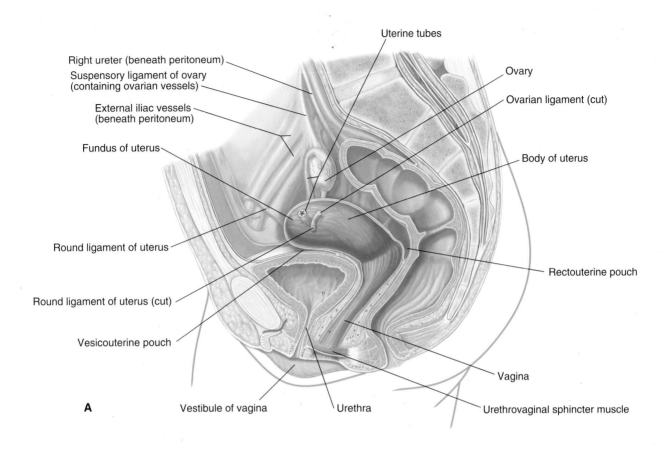

Uterine tubes

Right ureter (beneath peritoneum)

Suspensory ligament of ovary (containing ovarian vessels)

Ovary

External iliac vessels (beneath peritoneum)

Ovarian ligament (cut)

Fundus of uterus

Body of uterus

Round ligament of uterus

Rectouterine pouch

Round ligament of uterus (cut)

Vesicouterine pouch

Vestibule of vagina

Urethra

Vagina

Urethrovaginal sphincter muscle

A

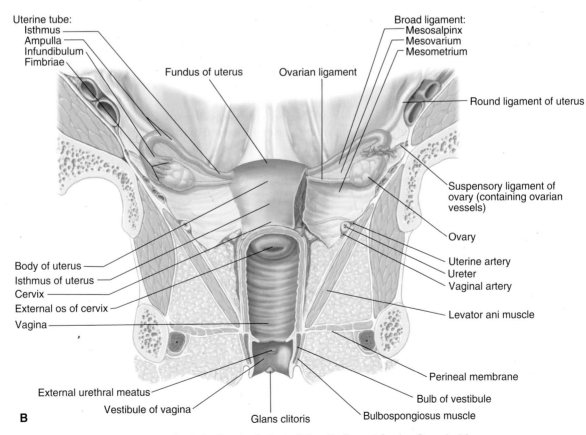

Uterine tube:
Isthmus
Ampulla
Infundibulum
Fimbriae

Fundus of uterus

Ovarian ligament

Broad ligament:
Mesosalpinx
Mesovarium
Mesometrium

Round ligament of uterus

Suspensory ligament of ovary (containing ovarian vessels)

Ovary

Uterine artery
Ureter
Vaginal artery

Body of uterus
Isthmus of uterus
Cervix
External os of cervix
Vagina

Levator ani muscle

Perineal membrane

External urethral meatus

Vestibule of vagina

Glans clitoris

Bulb of vestibule

Bulbospongiosus muscle

B

FIG. 3.7A,B. Internal Genitalia, Female. **A.** Sagittal View. **B.** Coronal Section, Posterior View.

III. Uterus

A. Organ adapted for development of fertilized ovum

B. Parts

1. **Body**

   a. Anterior (vesical) surface: lies on superior surface of bladder (**anteverted**), covered with peritoneum, which is reflected onto bladder, forming **vesicouterine pouch**

   b. Posterior (intestinal) surface: related to sigmoid colon and coils of ileum, covered with peritoneum

   c. Lateral surfaces

      i. Beneath mesometrium portion of broad ligament

      ii. Round ligament of uterus and ovarian ligament attach here inferior to uterine tube passing into uterus

2. **Fundus**

   a. Rounded portion anterosuperior to uterine tubes

   b. Directed anteriorly and superiorly, related to coils of ileum

3. **Isthmus**

   a. Constriction below body of uterus

   b. Demarcates body from cervix

   c. Indicates position of **internal os**

   d. Uterus is normally flexed (concave) anteriorly (**anteflexed**) at isthmus

4. **Cervix**

   a. Narrow portion below isthmus projecting into vagina

   b. 2 parts

      i. Supravaginal

         a) Separated from bladder anteriorly by parametrium (endopelvic fascia below mesometrium)

         b) Posteriorly covered with peritoneum and separated from rectum by coils of ileum

      ii. Vaginal

         a) Projects into vagina

         b) Ostium (**external os**): opening of cervix into vagina

         c) Surrounded by **fornices** (anterior, posterior, and lateral) of vagina; posterior fornix is deepest

5. Uterine walls consist of 3 layers

   a. Outer serous layer (peritoneum or **perimetrium**)

   b. Middle smooth muscle layer (**myometrium**), where main branches of blood vessels and nerves are located

   c. Inner vascular and mucous layer (**endometrium**), which is partly sloughed off each month during menstruation

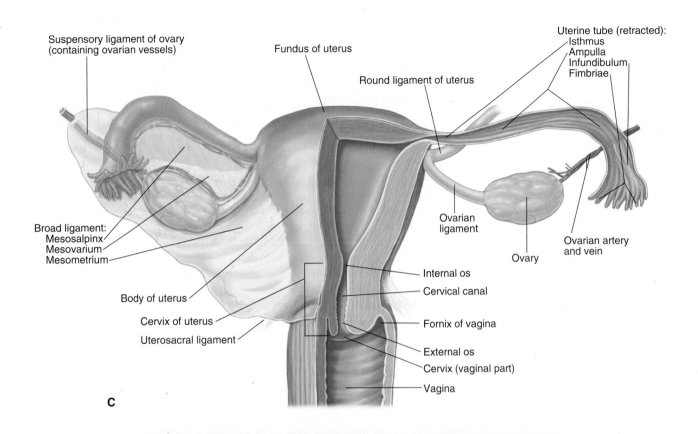

Suspensory ligament of ovary
(containing ovarian vessels)

Fundus of uterus

Round ligament of uterus

Uterine tube (retracted):
Isthmus
Ampulla
Infundibulum
Fimbriae

Broad ligament:
Mesosalpinx
Mesovarium
Mesometrium

Body of uterus

Cervix of uterus

Uterosacral ligament

Ovarian
ligament

Ovary

Ovarian artery
and vein

Internal os

Cervical canal

Fornix of vagina

External os

Cervix (vaginal part)

Vagina

C

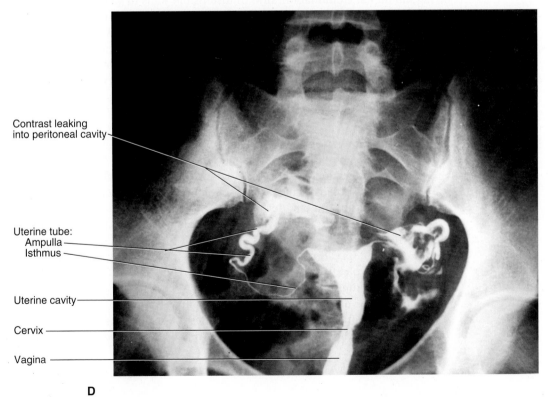

Contrast leaking
into peritoneal cavity

Uterine tube:
Ampulla
Isthmus

Uterine cavity

Cervix

Vagina

D

FIG. 3.7C,D. Internal Genitalia, Female. **C.** Details, Posterior View. **D.** Hysterosalpingogram.

IV. Clinical Considerations

A. **Ovarian cyst**: single or multiple; may occur as result of lack of ovulation of follicle and its continued growth

B. **Salpingitis**: inflammation of uterine tube(s); may be due to infection in peritoneal cavity and can result in infertility

C. **Salpingectomy**: removal of uterine tube(s)

D. **Tubal (ectopic) pregnancy**

  1. Most frequent type of ectopic pregnancy; fertilized ovum implants in mucosa of uterine tube (usually ampulla)

  2. Rupture of tubal pregnancy on right side may be mistaken for acute appendicitis

  3. Tubal rupture may lead to severe hemorrhage and peritonitis and endanger the mother

E. Relations of body of uterus are markedly changed by pregnancy, progressive enlargement bringing the uterus high into abdominal cavity

  1. Nonpregnant uterus cannot normally be felt via abdominal wall

  2. In pregnancy, uterine growth is initially slow, but it is palpable over pelvic brim by about 12 weeks of gestation, is at umbilicus by 20 weeks, and late in pregnancy can reach costal margin

G. **Laparoscopic tubal ligation**: surgical procedure of birth control via short suprapubic incision on pubic hairline

H. Bimanual uterus examination (palpation)

  1. Examiner passes 2 gloved fingers superiorly in vagina, while other hand is pressed posteroinferiorly on pubic region of anterior abdominal wall to determine size, shape, and position of uterus

  2. Softened uterine isthmus (**Hegar sign**) that feels separated from the body may be early sign of pregnancy

I. Vaginal digital examination: due to distensible walls of vagina, ischial spines, sacral promontory, and/or rectum are palpable, as are pulsations of uterine arteries and irregular ovaries (due to cysts) through lateral parts of fornix

J. Infection of vagina, uterus and tubes may result in peritonitis because tract communicates with peritoneal cavity through abdominal ostia of uterine tubes

K. **Hysterosalpingography**: uterine tube patency may be determined by injecting water-soluble radiopaque material or CO_2 gas into uterus; if patent, material passes through tubes into peritoneal cavity

L. **Cervical cancer**

  1. **Pap (Papanicolaou) smear**: cervical tissue study for detection of premalignant conditions

  2. Direct visualization: vagina distended with vaginal speculum to view cervix

  3. Cancer can spread by contiguity to bladder; there is no peritoneum between anterior cervix and bladder base

    a. Cancer spread can be lymphogenous metastasis to external and internal iliac or sacral lymph nodes

    b. Cancer spread can be bloodborne via iliac veins or internal vertebral venous plexus

M. Some developmental abnormalities

  1. **Bicornuate uterus** (duplication or doubled uterine cavities): due to incomplete fusion of embryonic paramesonephric ducts

  2. **Unicornuate uterus**: receiving uterine tube only from right or left side

Vagina and Support Mechanisms of the Uterus

I. Vagina

A. Extends from vaginal vestibule to cervix of uterus

B. Inclines posterosuperiorly, forming 100°–110° angle with uterus; posterior wall is 2.5–3.0 cm longer than anterior

C. Relations

1. Superiorly: surrounds cervix with anterior, lateral, and pronounced posterior fornix
2. Anteriorly: fundus of bladder and urethra
3. Posteriorly
   a. Posterior fornix contacts loops of ileum and sigmoid colon in rectouterine pouch
   b. Below pouch are rectovaginal fascia, rectal ampulla, and perineal body
4. Laterally: mesometrium portion of broad ligament, pelvic ureters (close to lateral fornices and, as these reach bladder, lie anterior to anterior fornix), uterine and vaginal vessels, pelvic surface of levator ani muscle, sphincter urethrae muscle
5. Inferiorly: vaginal vestibule is framed by bulbs of vestibule and bulbospongiosus muscles

II. Uterine Support (Fig. 3.8A–D)

A. Uterus held in place by various types of structures including muscles, ligaments, peritoneum, and fascia

B. Normal shape is **anteflexed**, or concave anteriorly, at isthmus

C. Normal position is **anteverted**
1. Lies superior to bladder
2. Makes an angle of 100°–110° with vagina

D. Muscular support
1. Pelvic diaphragm is most important support
2. Levator ani muscles and fascia support it from below

E. Peritoneal support
1. **Broad ligaments**
   a. Folds of peritoneum extending from lateral pelvic wall to attach to and cover uterus (**mesometrium**), uterine tubes (**mesosalpinx**), and ovaries (**mesovarium**)
   b. Helps to maintain normal position of ovaries and uterine tubes, less supportive of uterus
   c. Mesometrium covers endopelvic fascia (extraperitoneal connective tissue and smooth muscle or **parametrium**), including cardinal or transverse cervical ligament
2. Other peritoneal ligaments are folds covering endopelvic fascial bands
   a. **Transverse vesical fold**: continuous with anterior lamina of mesometrium
   b. **Uterosacral folds**: from cervix to rectum; contain uterosacral ligaments

F. **Endopelvic fascia**
1. **Cardinal or transverse cervical ligaments**
   a. Endopelvic fascia around vagina and cervix, which extends laterally across pelvis within lowest part of mesometrium to attach to deep fascia covering levator ani muscles
   b. Uterine and vaginal vessels lie in it, and ureter passes through it
2. **Uterosacral ligaments**: endopelvic fascia attached to cervix, running posteriorly to join deep fascia over sacrum

G. **Round ligament of uterus**
1. Remnant of gubernaculum
2. Fibrous cord attached to superior lateral border of uterus on either side; passes over external iliac vessels and inguinal ligament to leave abdomen through deep inguinal ring; traverses inguinal canal and anchored in labium majus
3. Helps to hold uterus in anteverted position over bladder

III. Clinical Considerations (Fig. 3.8E–G)

A. **Cystocele**: bulging of bladder into anterior vaginal wall

B. **Rectocele**: bulging of rectum into posterior vaginal wall

C. Abnormal uterine position

  1. **Retroflexion**: uterus flexed posteriorly at isthmus, may be asymptomatic

  2. **Retroversion**: angle between uterus and vagina increases, may lead to uterine prolapse

  3. **Uterine prolapse**: supports of uterus become stretched and lax; cervix descends, for varying degrees, into vagina or may extend into vestibule

D. **Hysterectomy**: removal of uterus

  1. May be partial, in which at least part of cervix is left, or complete (panhysterectomy)

  2. Uterine tubes and ovaries usually left in place

  3. Ureters must be preserved near cervix when ligating uterine arteries

  4. Vaginal hysterectomy: for repair of procidentia (prolapse) associated with cystocele and rectocele

E. Access through rectouterine pouch

  1. Relation of posterior fornix to the bottom of the rectouterine pouch makes possible palpation of pelvic viscera, drainage of abdominal fluids, and inspection of pelvic viscera without abdominal incisions

  2. **Posterior colpotomy** (vaginal incision): in treatment of pelvic abscess

  3. **Culdoscopy**: culdoscope (endoscope) inserted through incision in posterior vaginal fornix into peritoneal cavity to examine ovaries or uterine tubes or to drain pelvic abscess or fluid in rectouterine pouch (**culdocentesis**)

F. **Recto-** and **vesicovaginal fistulae**: abnormal connection between rectum and vagina or bladder and vagina; may result from injuries during childbirth or from faulty development

G. Interior of vagina can be distended for examination using vaginal speculum

H. Manual examination using gloved digits in vagina and/or rectum to palpate cervix, ischial spines, and sacral promontory

I. **Vaginismus**

  1. Emotional (psychosomatic) disorder leading to initial distention of bulbospongiosus and transverse perineal muscles leading to involuntary spasms of perivaginal and levator ani muscles

  2. Mild cases can cause dyspareunia (painful intercourse), whereas severe cases can prevent vaginal entry

Anteflexed

Anteverted

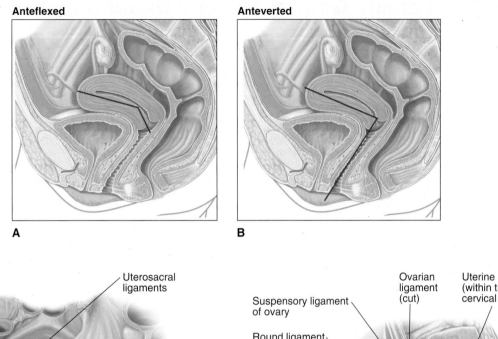

A

B

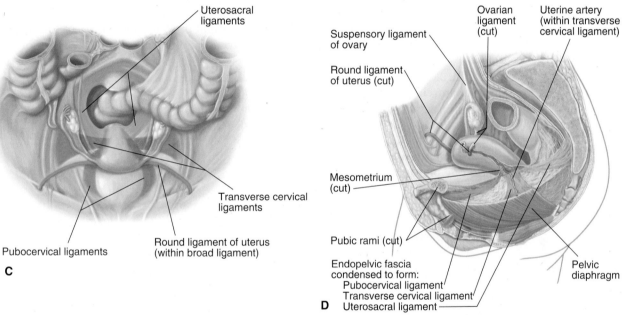

Uterosacral
ligaments

Ovarian
ligament
(cut)

Uterine artery
(within transverse
cervical ligament)

Suspensory ligament
of ovary

Round ligament
of uterus (cut)

Mesometrium
(cut)

Pubic rami (cut)

Transverse cervical
ligaments

Endopelvic fascia
condensed to form:
   Pubocervical ligament
   Transverse cervical ligament
   Uterosacral ligament

Pelvic
diaphragm

Pubocervical ligaments

Round ligament of uterus
(within broad ligament)

C

D

Retroflexed

Retroverted

Prolapsed

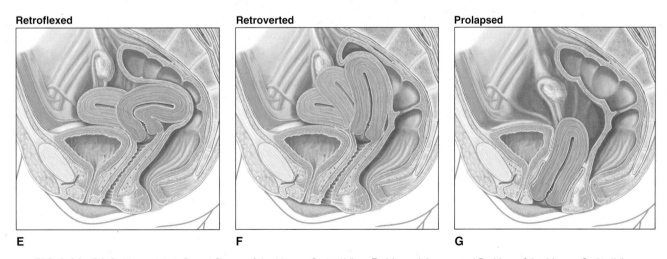

E

F

G

FIG. 3.8A–G. A. Normal Anteflexed Shape of the Uterus, Sagittal View. **B.** Normal Anteverted Position of the Uterus, Sagittal View. **C.** Supporting Structures of the Uterus, Superior View. **D.** Supporting Structures of the Uterus, Parasagittal View. **E.** Retroflexed Shape of the Uterus, Sagittal View. **F.** Retroverted Position of the Uterus, Sagittal View. **G.** Prolapsed Uterus, Sagittal View.

Female Genital System: Blood Supply and Innervation

I. Arteries (Fig. 3.9A)

A. Ovarian artery
1. From aorta near L2 vertebral level; descends in suspensory ligament of ovary, sending branches to ovary and uterine tube
2. Anastomoses with branches of uterine artery

B. Uterine artery
1. From anterior division of internal iliac
2. Crosses anterosuperior to ureter to reach side of uterus near isthmus through broad ligament, where it ascends to level of uterine tube
3. Supplies cervix, body of uterus, uterine tube, and upper vagina

C. Vaginal artery
1. From anterior division of internal iliac (comparable to inferior vesical in male)
2. Passes posteroinferior to ureter to reach side of vagina near fornices
3. Anastomoses with branches of uterine artery and provides inferior vesical branches
4. Forms longitudinal **azygos arteries** of vagina, in midline anteriorly and posteriorly

II. Veins

A. Ovarian vein
1. Drains ovary as a plexus, forming venae commitantes of ovarian artery, which ultimately coalesce to form ovarian vein on each side
2. Terminates in inferior vena cava at level of L2 (on right) or left renal vein (on left)
3. Communicates with uterine plexus, shares drainage of uterine tube

B. Uterine plexus
1. Drains uterus on each side primarily
2. Forms uterine veins, which end in internal iliac veins
3. Communicates with vaginal plexus and ovarian plexus

C. Vaginal plexus
1. Drains vagina; forms vaginal veins to internal iliac veins
2. Communicates with vesical, rectal, and uterine plexuses

III. Nerves (Fig. 3.9B)

A. Ovary and uterine tube: receive fibers from inferior hypogastric and ovarian plexuses

B. Uterus and vagina: uterovaginal portion of inferior hypogastric plexus
1. Uterine pain (labor pains or menstrual cramps) is felt in hypogastrium and posteriorly in lumbar area at and below level of iliac crest (i.e., hypogastric nerves, spinal cord segments T10–L1)
2. Most pain fibers from vagina travel with sacral parasympathetic fibers, as do those from cervix, and enter cord via pelvic splanchnic nerves (from S2–S4)
3. Lower 2–3 cm of vagina innervated by pudendal nerves (S2–S4)

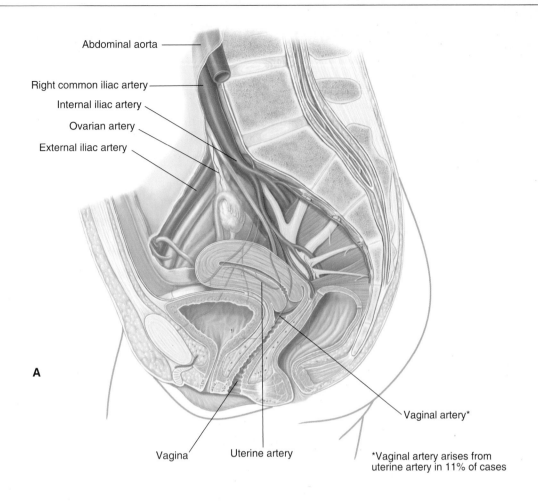

Abdominal aorta

Right common iliac artery

Internal iliac artery

Ovarian artery

External iliac artery

A

Vaginal artery*

Vagina   Uterine artery

*Vaginal artery arises from
uterine artery in 11% of cases

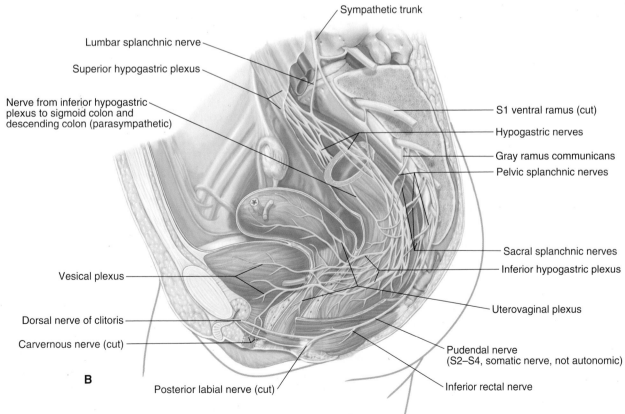

Sympathetic trunk

Lumbar splanchnic nerve

Superior hypogastric plexus

Nerve from inferior hypogastric
plexus to sigmoid colon and
descending colon (parasympathetic)

S1 ventral ramus (cut)

Hypogastric nerves

Gray ramus communicans

Pelvic splanchnic nerves

Sacral splanchnic nerves

Inferior hypogastric plexus

Uterovaginal plexus

Vesical plexus

Dorsal nerve of clitoris

Carvernous nerve (cut)

Pudendal nerve
(S2–S4, somatic nerve, not autonomic)

B

Posterior labial nerve (cut)

Inferior rectal nerve

FIG. 3.9A,B. Female Pelvis, Sagittal View. **A.** Blood Supply. **B.** Innervation.

Rectum and Anal Canal: Parts and Relations

I. Rectum (Fig. 3.10A,B)

A. Course and extent
   1. From 3rd sacral segment to slightly below tip of coccyx; bends abruptly posteriorly to become anal canal
   2. Total length: 12 cm
B. Curvature: follows anterior concavity of sacrum
C. Diameter
   1. Superior end: similar to sigmoid colon
   2. Inferior end: dilated to form rectal ampulla
D. Special structural characteristics (Fig. 3.10C,D)
   1. **Transverse rectal folds** (Houston valves): 3 transverse folds that project into lumen
      a. Upper: from left posterior wall near upper end
      b. Middle: largest; 3 cm below upper, extends inward from right anterior wall
      c. Lower: from left posterior wall
   2. Unlike colon, rectum has broad outer longitudinal muscle bands anteriorly and posteriorly
E. Peritoneal relationship
   1. Upper 2/3: has some peritoneum; most superior portion has peritoneum anteriorly and laterally
   2. Middle 1/3: has peritoneum anteriorly
   3. Lower 1/3: has no peritoneum
F. Relations
   1. Posteriorly: median and lateral sacral vessels; sympathetic trunks; anterior rami of S2–S5 and coccygeal nerves; piriformis, coccygeus and levator ani muscles; lower sacrum and coccyx
   2. Anteriorly
      a. Female
         i. Upper 2/3 covered by peritoneum and in relation to uterus, upper vagina, sigmoid colon and ileum
         ii. Lower 1/3 related to middle of vagina
      b. Male
         i. Upper 2/3 covered by peritoneum and related to sigmoid colon and ileum
         ii. Lower 1/3 related to bladder, seminal vesicles, ampulla of ductus deferens, and prostate
   3. Laterally: related to ileum and sigmoid colon, coccygeus and levator ani muscles

II. Anal Canal

A. Continuous with ampulla of rectum
B. Course and extent
   1. Origin: at level of apex of prostate, directed posteriorly and caudally
   2. Length: 2.5–4.0 cm (1.5 in)
C. Relations
   1. Surrounded by internal and external anal sphincters; supported by levator ani muscle
   2. Posteriorly: anococcygeal raphe and coccyx; puborectalis muscle forms sling that kinks anorectal junction forward and defines beginning of anal canal
   3. Anteriorly
      a. Female: perineal body, perineal membrane, and lower part of vagina
      b. Male: central tendinous point, perineal membrane, membranous urethra, and bulb of penis
   4. Laterally: external anal sphincter muscle and contents of ischioanal fossae
D. Special features
   1. **Anal columns**: vertical folds containing veins of rectal plexus
   2. **Anal sinuses**: pockets between columns inferiorly
   3. **Anal valves**: folds connecting adjacent columns at their inferior ends, forming anal sinuses

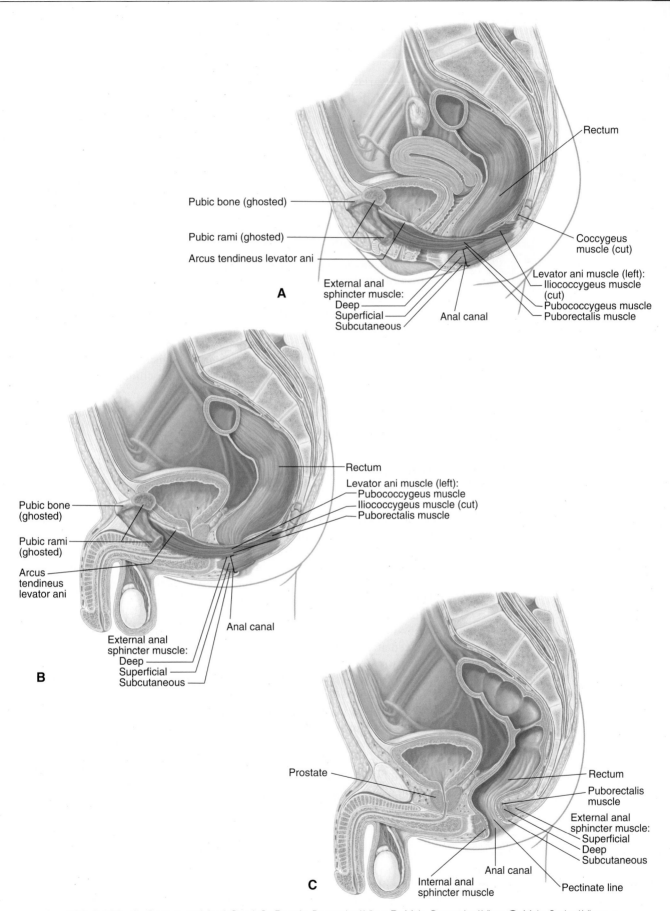

Rectum

Pubic bone (ghosted)

Pubic rami (ghosted)

Arcus tendineus levator ani

External anal sphincter muscle:
Deep
Superficial
Subcutaneous

Coccygeus muscle (cut)

Levator ani muscle (left):
Iliococcygeus muscle (cut)
Pubococcygeus muscle
Puborectalis muscle

Anal canal

A

Rectum

Levator ani muscle (left):
Pubococcygeus muscle
Iliococcygeus muscle (cut)
Puborectalis muscle

Pubic bone (ghosted)

Pubic rami (ghosted)

Arcus tendineus levator ani

Anal canal

External anal sphincter muscle:
Deep
Superficial
Subcutaneous

B

Prostate

Rectum

Puborectalis muscle

External anal sphincter muscle:
Superficial
Deep
Subcutaneous

Internal anal sphincter muscle

Anal canal

Pectinate line

C

FIG. 3.10A–C. Rectum and Anal Canal. **A.** Female, Parasagittal View. **B.** Male, Parasagittal View. **C.** Male, Sagittal View.

III. Anal Sphincters

A. **Internal anal sphincter**: thickening of inner circular layer of intrinsic smooth muscle coat of gut wall

B. **External anal sphincter**: striated, voluntary muscle
   1. Subcutaneous part: portion immediately around anal orifice
   2. Superficial part: main portion; arises from perineal body or central tendinous point, splits to encircle canal, and inserts in anococcygeal raphe and coccyx
   3. Deep part: true sphincter; encircles anus

C. **Puborectalis muscle**
   1. Not a true sphincter but essential for fecal continence
   2. Passes lateral to anorectal junction to sling posteriorly; some fibers blend with uppermost fibers of external anal sphincter muscle

IV. Clinical Considerations (Fig. 3.10E)

A. **Digital rectal examination** (**DRE**): can palpate structures related to rectum (i.e., prostate and seminal vesicles in males and cervix in females)
   1. In both sexes, sacrum, coccyx, ischial spines, and tuberosities are palpable as well as an inflamed appendix that has descended into lesser pelvis (in pararectal fossa)
   2. In females, rectouterine pouch is palpable; in males, rectovesical pouch
   3. In males, enlarged internal iliac nodes, pathological thickening of ureters, and swelling of ischioanal fossae (in cases of ischioanal abscesses) are palpable

B. **Proctoscopy**: allows examination of internal aspect of rectum as well as biopsies of lesions

C. **Resection of rectum**: often necessary in rectal cancer

D. **Sigmoidoscopy**: allows examination of rectum to sigmoid colon

E. **Rectal polyps**: protruding growths from mucous membrane
   1. Sessile: have narrow stalks attached to rectal mucosa; palpated by digital examination or visualized by proctoscopic examination
   2. Pedunculated: stemlike part
   3. All considered potentially malignant

F. **Anal fissures**: in chronically constipated patients, anal valves and mucosa can be torn by hard feces to create anal fissures (slitlike lesions)
   1. Usually located in posterior midline, inferior to anal valves
   2. Painful due to sensory fibers of inferior rectal nerves

G. **Anal abscesses**
   1. Ischioanal: located in ischioanal fossae with pus; painful
      a. Seen after **cryptitis** (an inflammation of the anal sinuses)
      b. Frequently an extension from pelvirectal abscesses
      c. Can follow tear in anal mucous membrane following anal fissures or penetrating wound in anal region
   2. Perianal: follow infection of anal fissure with spread to ischioanal fossa and form ischioanal abscesses or spread into pelvis to form pelvirectal abscess

H. **Anal fistula**: from spread of anal infection and cryptitis; one end opens into anal canal, other into abscess in ischioanal fossa or into perianal skin

I. **Fecal incontinence**: may be due to injury of pudendal nerve as result of stretching of nerve(s) during traumatic childbirth

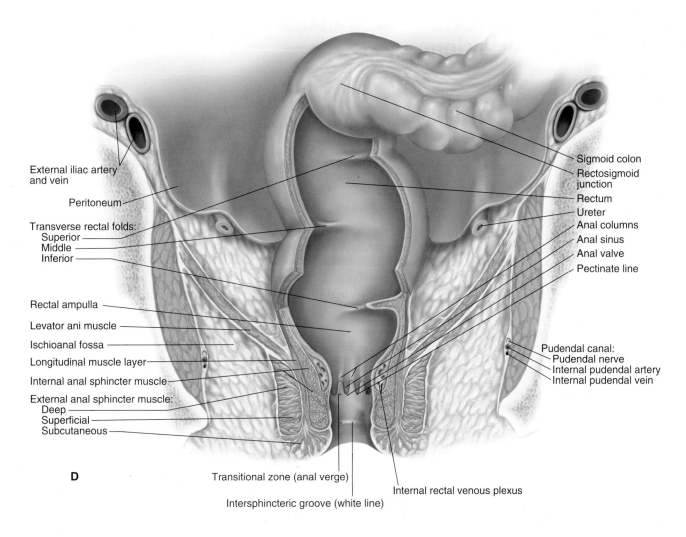

External iliac artery and vein

Peritoneum

Transverse rectal folds:
 Superior
 Middle
 Inferior

Rectal ampulla

Levator ani muscle

Ischioanal fossa

Longitudinal muscle layer

Internal anal sphincter muscle

External anal sphincter muscle:
 Deep
 Superficial
 Subcutaneous

Sigmoid colon

Rectosigmoid junction

Rectum

Ureter

Anal columns

Anal sinus

Anal valve

Pectinate line

Pudendal canal:
 Pudendal nerve
 Internal pudendal artery
 Internal pudendal vein

Transitional zone (anal verge)

Intersphincteric groove (white line)

Internal rectal venous plexus

D

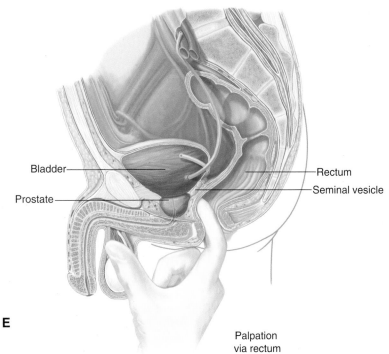

Bladder

Prostate

Rectum

Seminal vesicle

E

Palpation via rectum

FIG. 3.10D,E. D. Rectum and Anal Canal, Coronal Section, Anterior View. **E.** Digital Rectal Exam.

Rectum and Anal Canal: Blood Supply and Innervation

I. Arteries (Fig. 3.11A)

A. **Superior rectal artery**
 1. From inferior mesenteric artery
 2. 2 branches descend on either side of rectum; above anus, each gives rise to several small branches, which pass caudally, regularly spaced, to level of internal sphincter, at which point they form loops around caudal rectum and anastomose with other vessels

B. **Middle rectal artery**
 1. From internal iliac artery
 2. Approaches rectum from side immediately above pelvic diaphragm; joins loops at caudal end of rectum and upper anal canal

C. **Inferior rectal artery**
 1. 2–3 branches from internal pudendal artery
 2. Pass medially through ischioanal fossa to muscle around anal canal and skin around anus

II. Veins

A. **Rectal plexus**: network of vessels around anal canal; usually, at superior border of canal, some veins dilated

B. Drainage
 1. Chiefly through 6 ascending vessels, which begin in anal columns between muscularis and mucosa; they unite to form **superior rectal vein**, a tributary of inferior mesenteric vein
 2. **Middle rectal vein**: from plexus, with tributaries from bladder, vagina, prostate, and seminal vesicle, swings laterally on pelvic surface of levator ani to internal iliac vein
 3. **Inferior rectal vein**: from lower plexus into internal pudendal vein and then into internal iliac vein

III. Nerves (Fig. 3.11B)

A. Derived from inferior mesenteric and hypogastric plexuses (see Autonomics of the Pelvis for detailed explanation)

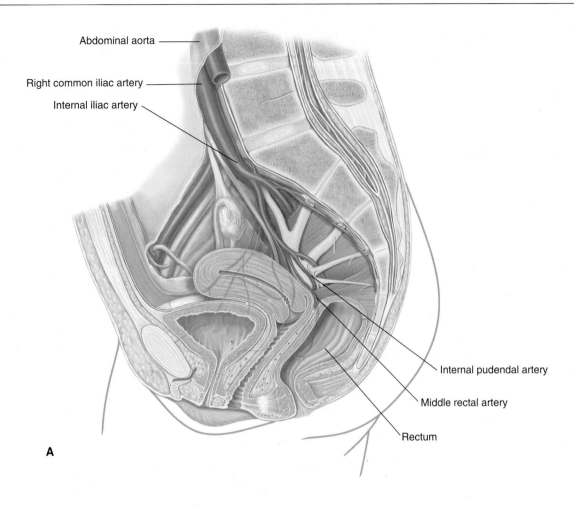

Abdominal aorta

Right common iliac artery

Internal iliac artery

Internal pudendal artery

Middle rectal artery

Rectum

A

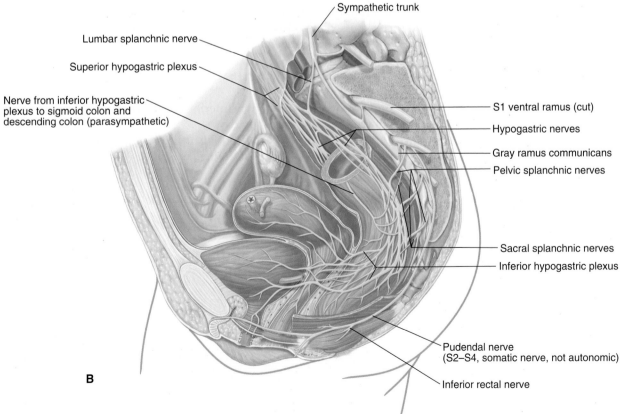

Sympathetic trunk

Lumbar splanchnic nerve

Superior hypogastric plexus

Nerve from inferior hypogastric plexus to sigmoid colon and descending colon (parasympathetic)

S1 ventral ramus (cut)

Hypogastric nerves

Gray ramus communicans

Pelvic splanchnic nerves

Sacral splanchnic nerves

Inferior hypogastric plexus

Pudendal nerve (S2–S4, somatic nerve, not autonomic)

Inferior rectal nerve

B

FIG. 3.11A,B. Rectum and Anal Canal, Female, Parasagittal View. **A.** Blood Supply. **B.** Innervation.

IV. Clinical Considerations

A. Landmarks of anal canal

1. **Anorectal junction**: above anal columns and sinuses, marking beginning of anal canal; kinked anteriorly by puborectal sling

2. **Pectinate (dentate) line**
   a. At anal valves at bottom of anal columns; mucocutaneous junction
   b. Internal hemorrhoids develop above and external hemorrhoids below this line
   c. Lymphatic dividing line between flow of lymph upward into pelvis, primarily to internal iliac nodes, or downward to superficial inguinal nodes
   d. Change from columnar and cuboidal epithelium in upper part canal and stratified epithelium in lower part occurs near this line and is important because carcinomas from the 2 types of epithelium differ
   e. Just below a change in nerve supply, with afferent innervation above through fibers of pelvic plexus (visceral type) and below through somatic nerve fibers in pudendal nerve; thus, an incision or needle above line is painless, whereas area below line is highly sensitive

3. **Anocutaneous line (white line of Hilton)**: marks lower end of GI tract and interval between external and internal anal sphincters

B. **Hemorrhoids**

1. If blood pressure in internal and external venous plexuses increases (i.e., in frequent straining), veins become dilated and tortuous, forming hemorrhoids or piles; may be internal (in anal columns) or external (below pectinate line)

2. **Internal hemorrhoids**
   a. Generally not painful (varicose veins of internal rectal plexus located above pectinate line and covered by anal mucosa)
   b. Bleeding is characteristically bright red due to plentiful arteriovenous anastomoses
   c. Internal hemorrhoids prolapsing into or through anal canal are often compressed by contraction of sphincters which impede their blood flow and may tend to ulcerate or strangulate

3. **External hemorrhoids**
   a. Thromboses or blood clots in veins of external rectal venous plexus and covered with skin
   b. Can be painful (supplied by inferior rectal nerves with somatic fibers), but tend to resolve in a few days
   c. Tend to be due to predisposing causes (i.e., chronic constipation, prolonged toilet sitting, straining, pregnancy, and any disorder that impedes venous return)

Pelvic Wall and Pelvic Diaphragm Muscles

I. Muscles of Lateral Pelvic Walls (Fig. 3.12A–D)

A. Obturator internus muscle
1. Arises from inner margins of obturator foramen and obturator membrane
2. Bends 90° around lesser sciatic notch to pass through lesser sciatic foramen and reach medial surface of greater trochanter of femur
3. Helps to form obturator canal inferior to superior pubic ramus
4. **Obturator fascia** forms 2 important structures
   a. **Arcus tendineus levator ani**: tendinous origin for part of levator ani muscle; runs across medial surface of obturator internus from posterior aspect of pubis to medial surface of ischial spine
   b. **Pudendal (Alcock) canal**: split in deep fascia on lower portion of muscle as it arises from medial surface of ischium; contains pudendal nerve and internal pudendal vessels
5. Innervation: nerve to obturator internus (L5, S1, S2)
6. Major action: rotates thigh laterally; assists in holding head of femur in acetabulum

B. Piriformis muscle
1. Arises from anterolateral surface of sacrum
2. Passes laterally through greater sciatic foramen to insert onto medial surface of greater trochanter of femur
3. Anterior rami of sacral plexus lie on anterior surface
4. Superior gluteal neurovascular bundle passes through greater sciatic foramen superior to piriformis; other neurovascular structures pass inferior to piriformis
5. Innervation: anterior rami of S1 and S2
6. Major actions: rotates thigh laterally; abducts thigh; assists in holding head of femur in acetabulum

II. Pelvic Diaphragm (Fig. 3.12 E–H)

A. Parts
1. **Levator ani muscle**: 3 parts
   a. **Puborectalis**
      i. Originates from posterior surface of pubis and forms **puborectal sling** around junction of rectum and anal canal, kinking anorectal junction anteriorly
      ii. Some of its medial fibers form sphincter vaginae or levator prostatae around vagina or prostate; insert into perineal body or central tendinous point and wall of rectum and anal canal
   b. **Pubococcygeus**
      i. Arises from pubis and anterior portion of arcus tendineus levator ani
      ii. Passes posteriorly to insert into coccyx and anococcygeal raphe between coccyx and anal canal
   c. **Iliococcygeus**
      i. Arises from arcus tendineus levator ani and ischial spine
      ii. Inserts on coccyx and anococcygeal raphe
   d. Innervation: nerve to levator ani (from S3–S4), inferior rectal nerves, and coccygeal plexus
2. **Coccygeus**
   a. Arises from spine of ischium and sacrospinous ligament
   b. Inserts on coccyx and lowest segment of sacrum
   c. Innervation: branches of anterior rami of S3-S5

B. Function
1. Support of pelvic viscera in general; resist increased abdominopelvic cavity pressure; coccygeus also flexes coccyx
2. Puborectal sling: important for urinary and fecal continence

C. Urogenital hiatus: transmits urethra (both sexes) and vagina, between anteromedial fibers of levator ani, to pierce perineal membrane

III. Clinical Considerations

A. Kegel exercises: strengthen pelvic diaphragm and sphincter urethrae muscles; helps in maintenance of urinary and fecal continence as well as being prophylactic for uterine prolapse

B. Obturator hernia: very rare hernia through obturator canal

C. Piriformis syndrome: compression of part or all of sciatic nerve by piriformis muscle; common fibular nerve passes through piriformis in greater than 10% of cases

D. Pelvic floor injury

1. Levator ani and pelvic fascia may be injured (stretched or torn) during childbirth, with pubococcygeus being most frequently torn

2. Childbirth can also change position of urinary bladder neck and urethra, resulting in urinary dribbling when intraabdominal pressure increases (i.e., repeated coughing, straining due to chronic constipation, etc.)

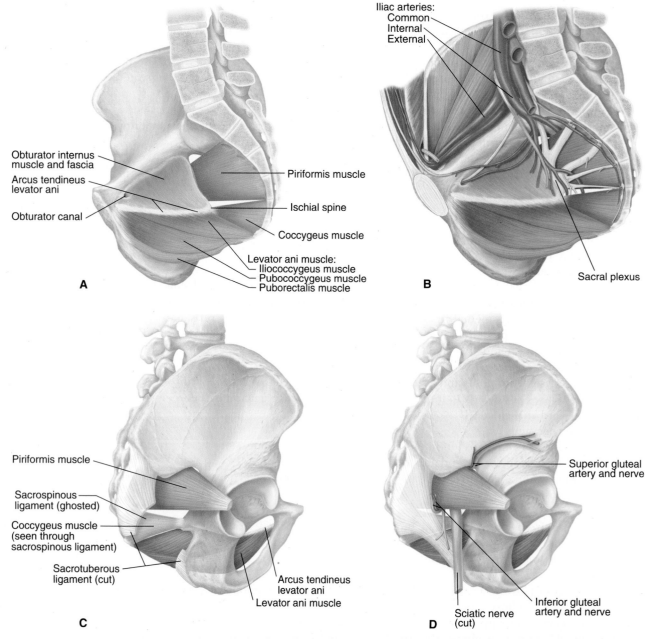

FIG. 3.12A–D. Pelvic Diaphragm and Pelvic Wall. **A.,** Sagittal Section, Medial View. **B.** Neurovascular Relationships, Sagittal Section, Medial View. **C.** Lateral View. **D.** Neurovascular Relationships, Lateral View.

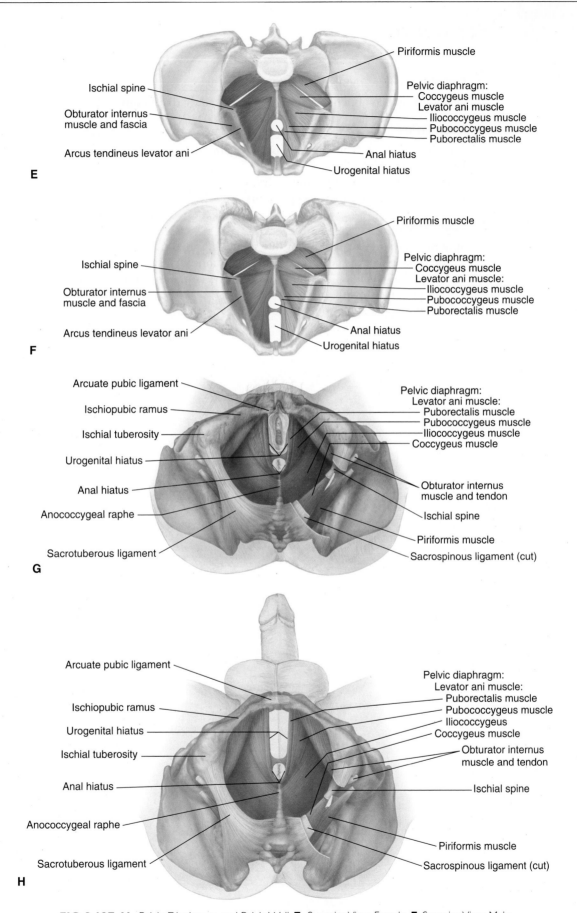

E.

Piriformis muscle

Ischial spine

Obturator internus muscle and fascia

Arcus tendineus levator ani

Pelvic diaphragm:
Coccygeus muscle
Levator ani muscle
Iliococcygeus muscle
Pubococcygeus muscle
Puborectalis muscle

Anal hiatus

Urogenital hiatus

F.

Piriformis muscle

Ischial spine

Obturator internus muscle and fascia

Arcus tendineus levator ani

Pelvic diaphragm:
Coccygeus muscle
Levator ani muscle:
Iliococcygeus muscle
Pubococcygeus muscle
Puborectalis muscle

Anal hiatus

Urogenital hiatus

G.

Arcuate pubic ligament

Ischiopubic ramus

Ischial tuberosity

Urogenital hiatus

Anal hiatus

Anococcygeal raphe

Sacrotuberous ligament

Pelvic diaphragm:
Levator ani muscle:
Puborectalis muscle
Pubococcygeus muscle
Iliococcygeus muscle
Coccygeus muscle

Obturator internus muscle and tendon

Ischial spine

Piriformis muscle

Sacrospinous ligament (cut)

H.

Arcuate pubic ligament

Ischiopubic ramus

Urogenital hiatus

Ischial tuberosity

Anal hiatus

Anococcygeal raphe

Sacrotuberous ligament

Pelvic diaphragm:
Levator ani muscle:
Puborectalis muscle
Pubococcygeus muscle
Iliococcygeus
Coccygeus muscle

Obturator internus muscle and tendon

Ischial spine

Piriformis muscle

Sacrospinous ligament (cut)

FIG. 3.12E–H. Pelvic Diaphragm and Pelvic Wall. **E.** Superior View, Female. **F.** Superior View, Male. **G.** Inferior View, Female. **H.** Inferior View, Male.

Perineum

I. Definition (Fig. 3.13A,B)

A. Diamond-shaped area between thighs below pelvic diaphragm

II. Boundaries

A. Anterior: pubic arch and arcuate pubic ligament
B. Posterior: tip of coccyx
C. Anterolateral: ischiopubic rami (inferior ramus of pubis and ischial ramus)
D. Posterolateral: sacrotuberous ligaments

III. Subdivisions

A. Split into 2 triangular regions by line through ischial tuberosities
   1. **Anal triangle**: faces posteroinferiorly; contains anal canal and anus
   2. **Urogenital triangle**: faces anteroinferiorly; contains vulva (female) and scrotum and root of penis (male)
B. Triangles meet at angle so that diamond-shaped perineum is flexed

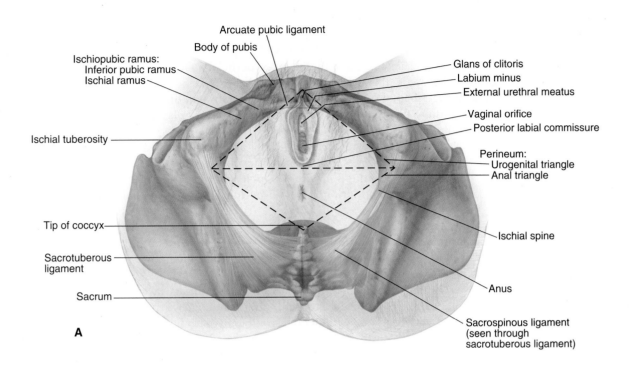

Arcuate pubic ligament
Body of pubis
Ischiopubic ramus:
  Inferior pubic ramus
  Ischial ramus
Ischial tuberosity
Tip of coccyx
Sacrotuberous ligament
Sacrum

Glans of clitoris
Labium minus
External urethral meatus
Vaginal orifice
Posterior labial commissure
Perineum:
  Urogenital triangle
  Anal triangle
Ischial spine
Anus
Sacrospinous ligament (seen through sacrotuberous ligament)

A

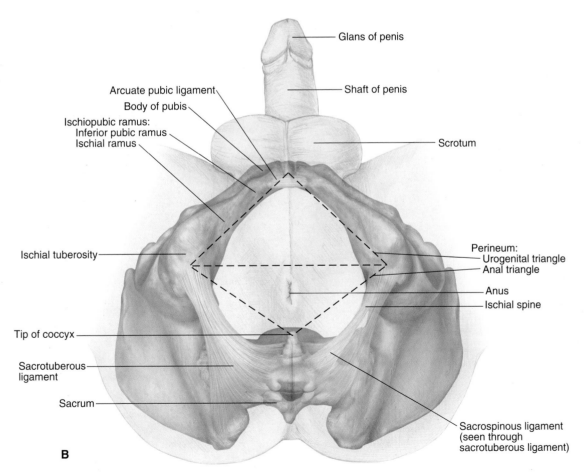

Glans of penis
Shaft of penis
Arcuate pubic ligament
Body of pubis
Ischiopubic ramus:
  Inferior pubic ramus
  Ischial ramus
Ischial tuberosity
Tip of coccyx
Sacrotuberous ligament
Sacrum

Scrotum
Perineum:
  Urogenital triangle
  Anal triangle
Anus
Ischial spine
Sacrospinous ligament (seen through sacrotuberous ligament)

B

FIG. 3.13A,B. Skeleton and Boundaries of the Perineum, Inferior View. **A.** Female. **B.** Male.

IV. Superficial Fascia (Fig. 3.13C,D)

A. 2-layered as on abdomen

B. Superficial fatty layer of superficial fascia

   1. In urogenital triangle: continuous with superficial fatty layer of abdomen (Camper fascia), superficial fascia of thigh, and superficial anal fascia

   2. In anal triangle: fills **ischioanal fossa**

     a. Wedge-shaped space inferior to pelvic diaphragm on either side of anal canal

     b. Contains fat, connective tissue, inferior rectal vessels and nerves

     c. Boundaries

       i. Superomedially: fascia over levator ani and external anal sphincter muscles

       ii. Laterally: fascia over obturator internus muscle and ischial tuberosities

       iii. Posteriorly: gluteus maximus muscle and sacrotuberous ligament

       iv. Anteriorly: posterior edge of perineal membrane and transverse perineus muscles

       v. Inferiorly: skin

     d. Anterior recess: continuation of fossa anteriorly, between sphincter urethrae muscle below, levator ani above, and obturator internus laterally

C. Deep membranous layer (Colles' fascia)

   1. In urogenital triangle: continuous with membranous layer of superficial fascia of abdomen (Scarpa), attached to ischiopubic rami, curves around superficial transverse perineal muscle to fuse with deep fascia; blends with fatty layer to form dartos layer of scrotum (tunica dartos scroti)

   2. In anal triangle: adherent to superficial layer

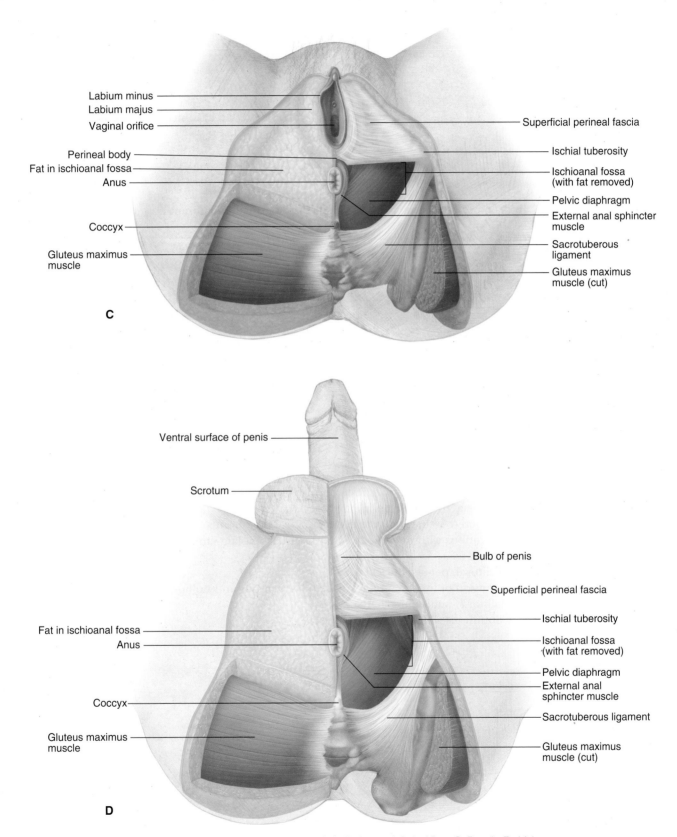

Labium minus

Labium majus

Vaginal orifice

Perineal body

Fat in ischioanal fossa

Anus

Coccyx

Gluteus maximus
muscle

Superficial perineal fascia

Ischial tuberosity

Ischioanal fossa
(with fat removed)

Pelvic diaphragm

External anal sphincter
muscle

Sacrotuberous
ligament

Gluteus maximus
muscle (cut)

C

Ventral surface of penis

Scrotum

Fat in ischioanal fossa

Anus

Coccyx

Gluteus maximus
muscle

Bulb of penis

Superficial perineal fascia

Ischial tuberosity

Ischioanal fossa
(with fat removed)

Pelvic diaphragm

External anal
sphincter muscle

Sacrotuberous ligament

Gluteus maximus
muscle (cut)

D

FIG. 3.13C,D. Superficial Features of the Perineum, Inferior View. **C.** Female. **D.** Male.

V. Muscles of Perineum (Fig. 3.13E,F)

A. All innervated by perineal branch of pudendal nerve

B. In superficial perineal compartment (inferior to perineal membrane)

Muscle	Origin	Insertion	Action
Superficial transverse perineus	Ischial tuberosity	Perineal body or central tendinous point	Fixes perineal body or central tendinous point
Bulbospongiosus	Female: Perineal body and vestibular bulb Male: Central tendinous point and median raphe	Perineal membrane, encircles root of clitoris/penis to attach to dorsal surface of corpus cavernosum	Compresses urethra (male); helps maintain erection
Ischiocavernosus	Ischiopubic ramus and medial surface of ischial tuberosity	Crus of clitoris or penis	Maintains erection

C. In deep perineal compartment (superior to perineal membrane)

Muscle	Origin	Insertion	Action
Deep transverse perineus	Medial surface of ischial ramus	Contralateral muscle and perineal body or central tendinous point	Fixes and stabilizes perineal body or central tendinous point
Sphincter urethrae	Ischiopubic ramus	Extends to neck of bladder encircling urethra and vagina (female) or prostate (male)	Compresses urethra

VI. Deep Fascia of Perineum

A. Obturator fascia: on medial surface of obturator internus muscle on lateral wall of ischioanal fossa

B. Inferior fascia of pelvic diaphragm
   1. Continuous with obturator fascia along arcus tendineus
   2. Forms superomedial boundary of ischioanal (ischiorectal) fossa

C. Deep perineal fascia (Gallaudet)
   1. Investing fascia of superficial perineal muscles (ischiocavernosus, bulbospongiosus, superficial transverse perineus)
   2. Attached to ischiopubic rami and perineal membrane
   3. Continuous with deep abdominal fascia, fascia lata, and deep clitoral/penile (Buck) fascia

D. Deep clitoral/penile (Buck) fascia
   1. Extension of investing fascia of ischiocavernosus and bulbospongiosus muscles at root of clitoris/penis onto shaft
   2. Continuous with deep perineal fascia

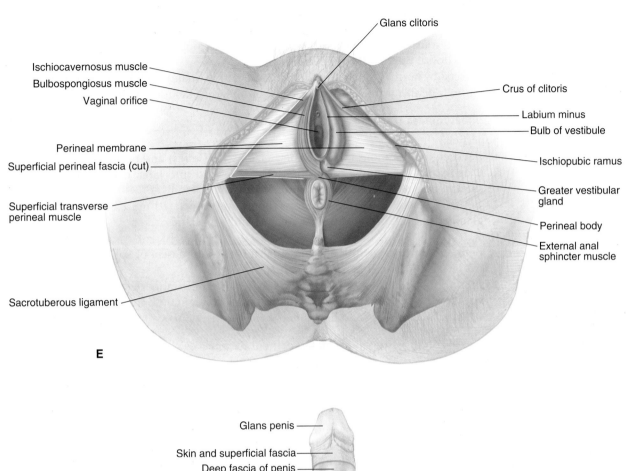

Glans clitoris

Ischiocavernosus muscle

Bulbospongiosus muscle

Vaginal orifice

Crus of clitoris

Labium minus

Bulb of vestibule

Perineal membrane

Ischiopubic ramus

Superficial perineal fascia (cut)

Greater vestibular gland

Superficial transverse perineal muscle

Perineal body

External anal sphincter muscle

Sacrotuberous ligament

E

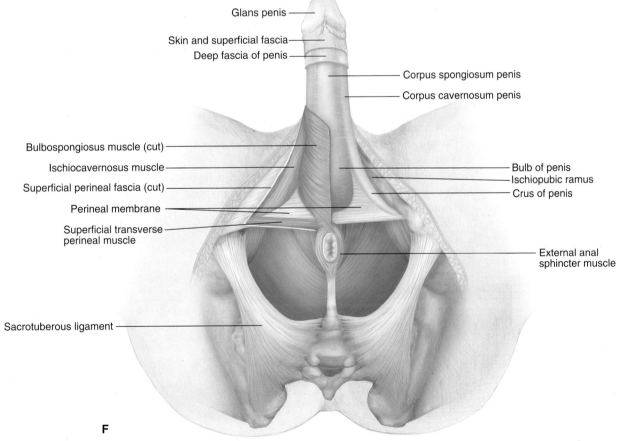

Glans penis

Skin and superficial fascia

Deep fascia of penis

Corpus spongiosum penis

Corpus cavernosum penis

Bulbospongiosus muscle (cut)

Ischiocavernosus muscle

Bulb of penis

Ischiopubic ramus

Superficial perineal fascia (cut)

Crus of penis

Perineal membrane

Superficial transverse perineal muscle

External anal sphincter muscle

Sacrotuberous ligament

F

FIG. 3.13E,F. Muscles of the Perineum, Inferior View. **E.** Female. **F.** Male.

 E. Perineal membrane (Fig. 3.13G,H)

  1. Inferior investing fascia of sphincter urethrae and deep transverse perineus muscles

  2. Attached to both ischiopubic rami, leaving slight space between anterosuperior edge (called **transverse perineal ligament**) and arcuate pubic ligament to permit passage of deep dorsal vein of clitoris/penis

  3. Pierced by urethra, ducts of bulbourethral glands (male), vagina, arteries to bulb, deep clitoral/penile arteries, dorsal arteries and nerves of clitoris/penis

VII. Perineal Spaces (Pouches or Compartments)

 A. Superficial

  1. Between membranous layer of superficial fascia (Colles) and perineal membrane

  2. Closed on 3 sides only; open anteriorly to extend into labia majora/scrotum, along shaft of penis/clitoris, and onto anterior abdominal wall

  3. Contains: crura and bulb of clitoris/penis and associated muscles, greater vestibular glands (female), perineal vessels, nerves, and lymphatics

 B. Deep

  1. Between perineal membrane and superior investing fascia of sphincter urethrae and deep transverse perineus muscles

  2. Contains: membranous urethra, sphincter urethrae and deep transverse perineal muscles, bulbourethral glands (male), part of vagina (female), internal pudendal vessels and branches, and dorsal nerves of clitoris/penis

VIII. Comparison of Female and Male Perineal Structures

 A. Perineal body or **central tendinous point**

  1. Irregular fibromuscular mass in median plane between anal canal and perineal membrane, lying deep to skin posterior to vestibule of vagina or bulb of penis and anterior to anus and anal canal

  2. Contains elastic and collagenous fibers as well as skeletal and smooth muscle

  3. Attachment point of many muscles and fasciae of perineum

  4. More prominent in female and called **perineal body**; **central tendinous point** in male

 B. Corpus spongiosum

  1. **Vestibular bulbs**

   a. Frame vestibule of vagina

   b. Unite at root of clitoris and extend along shaft to end as glans clitoridis

  2. **Bulb of penis**: attached to perineal membrane

   a. Continues into shaft and caps distal ends of corpora cavernosa as glans penis

   b. Traversed by spongy urethra

  3. **Tunica albuginea** of corpus spongiosum: thin in both sexes, which allows distension during ejaculation in male, and, because glans caps more rigid corpora cavernosa, it cushions distal end of clitoris/penis

  4. Bulbospongiosus muscles

   a. Cover vestibular bulbs or bulb of penis

   b. End at root of shaft of clitoris or penis

IX. Clinical Considerations

 A. Episiotomy: surgical incision of perineum and inferior posterior vaginal wall during childbirth to enlarge the vaginal opening and decrease excessive perineal tearing

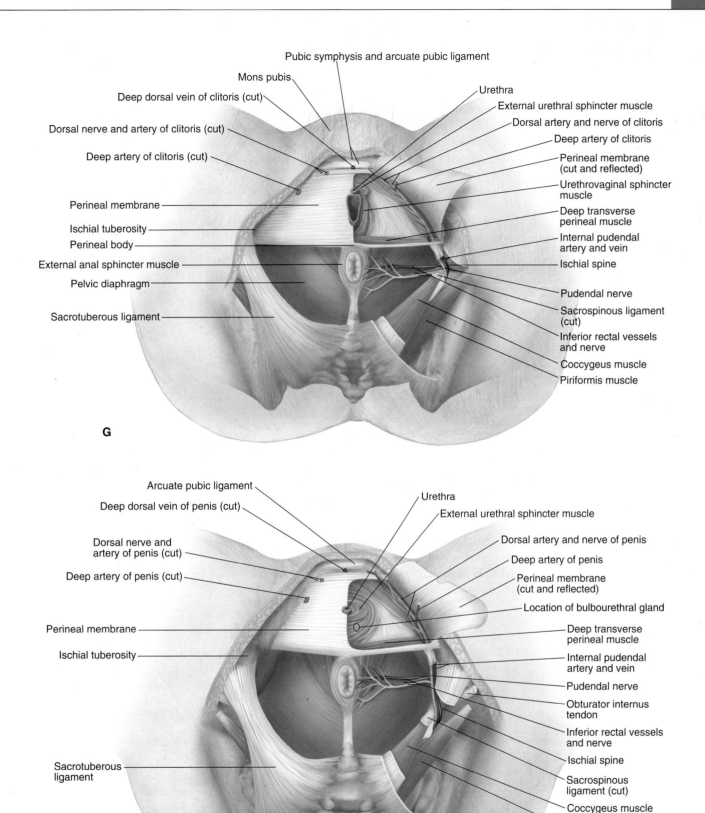

FIG. 3.13G,H. Deep Features of the Perineum, Inferior View. **G.** Female. **H.** Male.

Clitoris, Penis, and Testis

I. Composition of Clitoris and Penis (Fig. 3.14A–D)

A. Corpus cavernosus

1. Cylindrical body of erectile tissue attached by **crus** to each ischiopubic ramus and adjacent perineal membrane
2. Crura are covered by **ischiocavernosus muscles** that constrict crus and help maintain erection
3. Each erectile body consists of core of spongy vascular tissue surrounded by thick, tough fibrous coat, the **tunica albuginea**
4. Paired corpora cavernosa unite at root of clitoris/penis, although septum separates 2 bodies in the shaft
5. Form bulk of shaft of clitoris/penis

B. Corpus spongiosum

1. Medial erectile body(-ies) attached to perineal membrane
   a. Frame vestibule of vagina as **vestibular bulbs**
   b. Fused in male as **bulb of penis**; encloses spongy urethra
2. Tunica albuginea thin and distensible
3. Bulbs covered by **bulbospongiosus muscle**, which encircles root of clitoris/penis and aids maintenance of erection by compression of deep dorsal vein
4. Corpus spongiosum runs distally along ventral surface of clitoris/penis to end as glans, capping distal ends of corpora cavernosa

II. Ligaments

A. Fundiform ligament: sling of membranous layer of superficial fascia (Scarpa fascia) extending to sides and dorsum of clitoris/penis

B. Suspensory ligament of clitoris/penis: deep fascia from linea alba, symphysis pubis, and arcuate pubic ligament

III. Fascia

A. Superficial fascia: continuous with membranous layer of superficial fascia (Scarpa fascia) and dartos of scrotum

B. Deep fascia of clitoris/penis (Buck): investing fascia of muscles of clitoris/penis, extending distally onto shaft at root

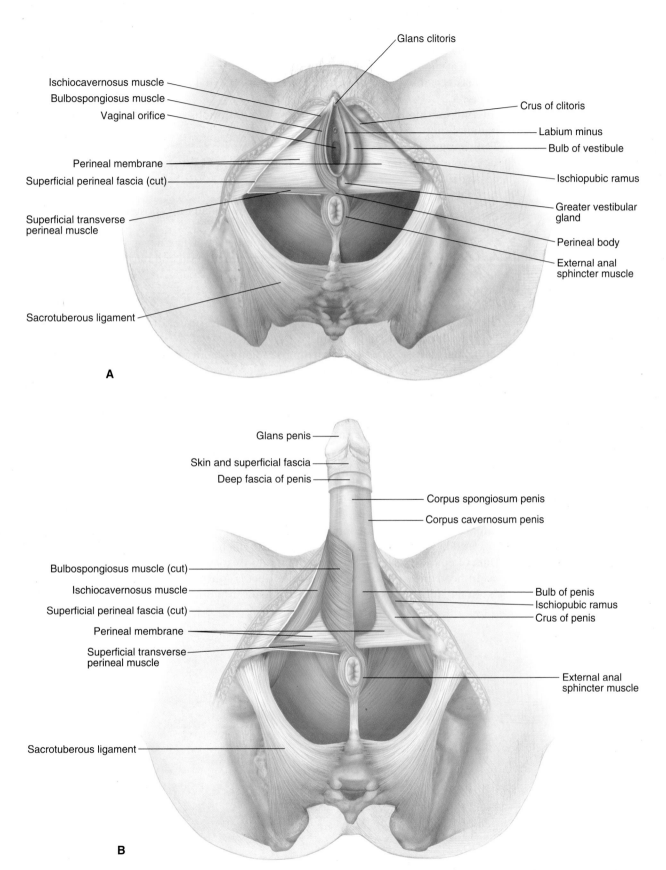

Glans clitoris

Ischiocavernosus muscle

Bulbospongiosus muscle

Vaginal orifice

Crus of clitoris

Labium minus

Bulb of vestibule

Perineal membrane

Superficial perineal fascia (cut)

Ischiopubic ramus

Greater vestibular gland

Superficial transverse perineal muscle

Perineal body

External anal sphincter muscle

Sacrotuberous ligament

A

Glans penis

Skin and superficial fascia

Deep fascia of penis

Corpus spongiosum penis

Corpus cavernosum penis

Bulbospongiosus muscle (cut)

Ischiocavernosus muscle

Superficial perineal fascia (cut)

Bulb of penis

Ischiopubic ramus

Crus of penis

Perineal membrane

Superficial transverse perineal muscle

External anal sphincter muscle

Sacrotuberous ligament

B

FIG. 3.14A,B. Erectile Bodies and Muscles. **A.** Clitoris and Female Vulva, Inferior View. **B.** Penis, Inferior View.

IV. Testis and Epididymis (Fig. 3.14E)

A. Testis coverings

   1. External spermatic fascia: continuous with deep fascia of external abdominal oblique muscle at superficial inguinal ring

   2. Cremasteric muscle and fascia: derived from internal abdominal oblique muscle and its fascia

   3. Internal spermatic fascia: derived from and continuous with transversalis fascia at deep inguinal ring

   4. Tunica vaginalis testis

     a. Serous membrane derived from peritoneum of abdomen (remnant of **processus vaginalis**)

     b. 2 layers

       i. Visceral: covers testis and epididymis anterolaterally; posteriorly reflected onto scrotal lining

       ii. Parietal: lines scrotum within internal spermatic fascia

     c. Cavity of tunica vaginalis testis: space between visceral and parietal layers

B. Testis (Fig. 3.14F)

   1. Structure

     a. Tunica albuginea: dense, fibrous capsule

     b. Mediastinum testis: reflection of capsule along posterior border into interior of testis, forming partial septum

     c. Trabeculae (septa): partial partitions radiating from front and sides of mediastinum; divide testis into numerous conical lobules

     d. Lobules: each contains several highly convoluted seminiferous tubules, which give rise to sperm

     e. Straight tubules (tubuli recti): at apex of lobule, next to mediastinum, seminiferous tubules straighten out, carry sperm to rete testis

     f. Rete testis: network of irregular spaces that transmit sperm across mediastinum to efferent ducts (ductules)

     g. Efferent ductules: lead from rete, penetrate tunica albuginea to enter head of epididymis, where each of the 12–15 ductules becomes highly convoluted

C. Epididymis

   1. Important storehouse for sperm

   2. Covered by visceral layer of tunica vaginalis, which helps bind this structure to testis

   3. Duct of epididymis: efferent ducts open into this

     a. In head and body of epididymis, this duct is convoluted

     b. In tail, it becomes straighter where it leads into ductus deferens

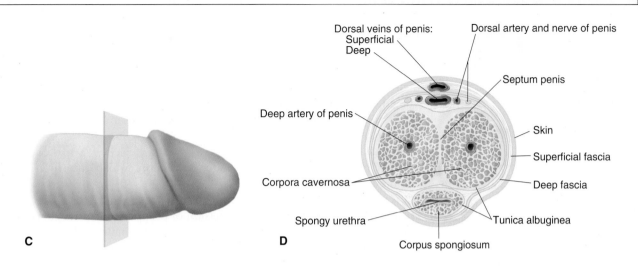

Dorsal veins of penis:
Superficial
Deep

Dorsal artery and nerve of penis

Deep artery of penis

Septum penis

Skin

Superficial fascia

Deep fascia

Corpora cavernosa

Tunica albuginea

Spongy urethra

Corpus spongiosum

C

D

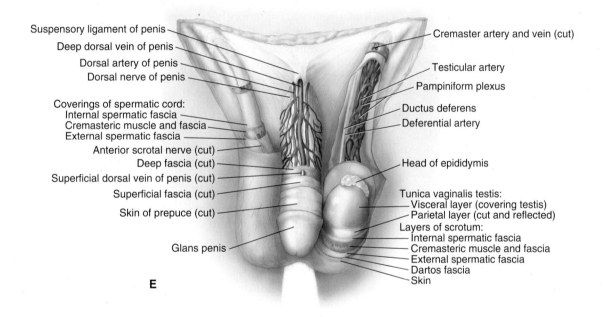

Suspensory ligament of penis

Cremaster artery and vein (cut)

Deep dorsal vein of penis

Dorsal artery of penis

Dorsal nerve of penis

Testicular artery

Pampiniform plexus

Coverings of spermatic cord:
Internal spermatic fascia
Cremasteric muscle and fascia
External spermatic fascia

Ductus deferens

Deferential artery

Anterior scrotal nerve (cut)

Deep fascia (cut)

Superficial dorsal vein of penis (cut)

Superficial fascia (cut)

Head of epididymis

Skin of prepuce (cut)

Tunica vaginalis testis:
Visceral layer (covering testis)
Parietal layer (cut and reflected)

Layers of scrotum:
Internal spermatic fascia
Cremasteric muscle and fascia
External spermatic fascia
Dartos fascia
Skin

Glans penis

E

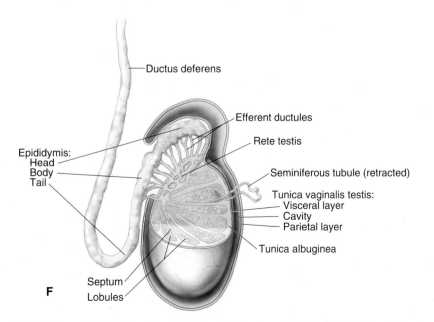

Ductus deferens

Efferent ductules

Rete testis

Epididymis:
Head
Body
Tail

Seminiferous tubule (retracted)

Tunica vaginalis testis:
Visceral layer
Cavity
Parietal layer

Tunica albuginea

Septum

Lobules

F

FIG. 3.14C–F. C. Plane of Section through Penis, Lateral View. **D.** Cross Section through Penis, Anterior View. **E.** Fasciae of the Spermatic Cord and Testis, Anterior View. **F.** Parts of the Testis, Epididymis, and Ductus Deferens, Lateral View.

V. Clinical Considerations

A. **Phimosis**

 1. Prepuce (foreskin) fits tightly over glans and cannot be easily retracted, if at all

 2. Due to modified sebaceous glands in prepuce, oily secretion of cheesy consistency (smegma) can accumulate in preputial sac (between prepuce and glans) and cause irritation

B. **Paraphimosis**

 1. Neck of glans constricted by prepuce retraction, which interferes with vascular and tissue fluid drainage

 2. Glans may enlarge so prepuce cannot cover it

 3. Treated by **circumcision** (surgical excision of prepuce to expose glans)

C. **Hydrocele**: accumulation of fluid in cavity of tunica vaginalis testis

D. **Orchitis**: inflammation of glandular tissue of testis; may occur as complication of mumps and can lead to sterility

E. Testicular trauma

 1. Can lead to testicular contusion, hematoma and pain, pallor, nausea, and anxiety

 2. Significant trauma can result in subfertility and atrophic testes

F. Scrotal masses: evaluate for gynecomastia to rule out Leydig cell tumor

 1. Spermatocele: cystic mass found in epididymis or adjacent to testicle; may be caused by sperm extravasation from infection or trauma

 2. Could be tumor of testes

G. **Undescended testis**

 1. Commonly reside permanently in inguinal canal and cannot be pulled down into scrotum, thus requiring surgery

 2. If left outside scrotum, there is increased risk of cancer and decreased fertility

H. **Vasectomy**

 1. Bilateral ligation of ductus deferens performed to create male sterilization

 2. Does not interfere with secretion of auxiliary genital glands, and testes still function to produce testosterone

I. **Orchiectomy** (castration): testis removal due to malignant tumor

J. Scrotal distention: easily distended with large hernia entering scrotum

K. Penile injuries

 1. Direct blow: can cause vascular injuries and potential impotency due to straddle-like injuries directly below pubic area

 2. Frostbite: inadequate protection in extreme cold weather

 3. Irritation due to trauma to pudendal nerve is common (i.e., bicycle riders)

 4. Can cause priapism, impotence, paresthesia, or ischemic neuropathy

Arteries and Veins of the Pelvis and Perineum

I. Arteries of the Pelvis (Fig. 3.15A,B)

A. **Ovarian artery**
   1. Arises from abdominal aorta at L2 level
   2. Descends on posterior abdominal wall, crossing ureter
   3. Passes over external iliac vessels anterior to ureter
   4. Lies within suspensory ligament of ovary to reach ovary

B. **Internal iliac artery**: terminal branch of common iliac artery; descends from sacroiliac articulation to greater sciatic notch; 2 divisions
   1. Anterior division
      a. **Umbilical artery**
         i. Supplies 3 **superior vesical branches** to bladder and ductus deferens/round ligament
         ii. Becomes **medial umbilical ligament** on inner aspect of anterior abdominal wall
      b. **Obturator artery**: leaves pelvis through obturator canal; may arise from posterior division or inferior epigastric artery (aberrant obturator artery occurs in 30% of cases)
      c. **Uterine artery**: passes anteromedially to reach cervix; crosses over ureter
      d. **Vaginal artery**: passes beneath ureter; provides inferior vesical branches
      e. **Inferior vesical artery**: to fundus of bladder, prostate, and seminal vesicles; branches from vaginal artery in female
      f. **Middle rectal artery**: to rectum
      g. **Internal pudendal artery**: leaves pelvis through greater sciatic foramen, immediately posterior to ischial spine
      h. **Inferior gluteal artery**: curves posteriorly through sacral plexus, then runs between piriformis and coccygeus muscles, through greater sciatic foramen into gluteal region
   2. Posterior division
      a. **Iliolumbar artery**: ascends posterior to external iliac vessels and psoas major muscle; supplies psoas and iliacus muscles
      b. **Lateral sacral arteries**: usually 2
         i. Superior: large, runs medially and enters 1st or 2nd sacral foramen
         ii. Inferior: crosses to sacral foramina; descends and sends branches through foramina
      c. **Superior gluteal artery**: runs posteriorly between lumbosacral trunk and 1st sacral nerve, and leaves pelvis through greater sciatic foramen above piriformis muscle

II. Arteries of the Perineum (Fig. 3.15C,D)

A. **Internal pudendal artery**
   1. Crosses ischial spine, giving off inferior rectal branch
   2. Enters ischioanal fossa through lesser sciatic foramen, passing into pudendal (Alcock) canal, a fascial canal made of obturator internus muscle fascia
   3. Branches given off within anal triangle
      a. **Inferior rectal branches**: cross ischioanal fossa to reach anal canal
      b. **Perineal artery**: enters superficial perineal space to supply ischiocavernosus, bulbospongiosus and superficial transverse perineal muscles and end as **posterior labial/scrotal artery**
      c. From pudendal canal, internal pudendal artery passes through deep transverse perineus and sphincter urethrae muscles
   4. Branches given off within urogenital triangle
      a. **Artery to bulb**: passes medially to supply vestibular bulb/bulb of penis
      b. **Deep artery of clitoris/penis**: penetrates perineal membrane to enter crus of clitoris/penis and run distally in center of erectile tissue

       c. **Dorsal artery of clitoris/penis**: penetrates anterior edge of perineal membrane (transverse perineal ligament) to pass distally on dorsum of clitoris/penis; lies lateral to deep dorsal vein of clitoris/penis, beneath deep fascia of clitoris/penis

    B. Arteries of anterior labium majus/scrotum

      1. **Superficial external pudendal artery**: from femoral; supplies skin of anterior labium majus/scrotum; anastomoses with deep external pudendal artery

      2. **Deep external pudendal artery**: from femoral; anastomoses with superficial external pudendal artery to supply skin of anterior labium majus/scrotum

    C. Arteries of testis and spermatic cord (see Section 3.9 for ovarian arteries)

      1. **Testicular artery**

        a. From abdominal aorta at lower L2 vertebral level (same as ovarian artery)

        b. Passes through deep inguinal ring to become part of spermatic cord

      2. **Deferential artery**: from umbilical artery or superior vesical branch; supplies ductus deferens

      3. **Cremasteric artery**: from inferior epigastric; supplies coverings of spermatic cord

III. Veins of the Pelvis (Fig. 3.15E,F)

    A. Originate in venous plexuses (i.e., vesical, prostatic, vaginal, uterine, and rectal plexuses (Note: rectal plexus drains in part to portal system)

    B. Plexuses are tributary to plexiform veins that correspond to branches of internal iliac artery

    C. **Ovarian vein**

      1. Drains ovary as a plexus, forming venae commitantes of ovarian artery, which ultimately coalesce to form ovarian vein on each side

      2. Terminates in inferior vena cava at level of L2 (on right) or left renal vein (on left)

      3. Communicates with uterine plexus, shares drainage of uterine tube

IV. Veins of the Perineum

    A. **Superficial dorsal vein of clitoris/penis**

      1. Drains skin and superficial fascia

      2. Passes proximally on dorsum of clitoris/penis in midline within superficial fascia

      3. Splits at root of clitoris/penis to drain into superficial external pudendal veins on either side, then to great saphenous veins

    B. **Deep dorsal vein of clitoris/penis**

      1. Drains erectile bodies of clitoris/penis

      2. Passes proximally on dorsum of clitoris/penis in midline deep to deep fascia

      3. At root of clitoris/penis, passes between arcuate pubic ligament and transverse perineal ligament to enter pelvis

      4. Drains into prostatic or vesical venous plexus, then into internal iliac vein

    C. Veins of testis

      1. **Pampiniform plexus** drains testis, form network around testicular artery in order to cool its blood before reaching testis

      2. Veins unite near deep inguinal ring, eventually forming 1 **testicular vein** on each side, which drains to inferior vena cava at level of L2 on right and left renal vein on left

    D. Veins of labium majus/scrotum

      1. **Superficial and deep external pudendal**: drain anterior aspect of labium majus/scrotum

      2. **Posterior labial/scrotal**: drains to perineal then to internal pudendal vein

    E. Other veins of perineum

      1. Veins follow most branches (except dorsal and deep arteries) of internal pudendal artery back to form internal pudendal vein

      2. Drain to internal iliac vein

V. Clinical Considerations

    A. **Varicocele**: condition of enlargement (varicosity) of pampiniform plexus of veins in spermatic cord possibly due to defective venous valves; seen in up to 20% of adult males

    B. **Hematocele of testis**: blood within cavity of tunica vaginalis

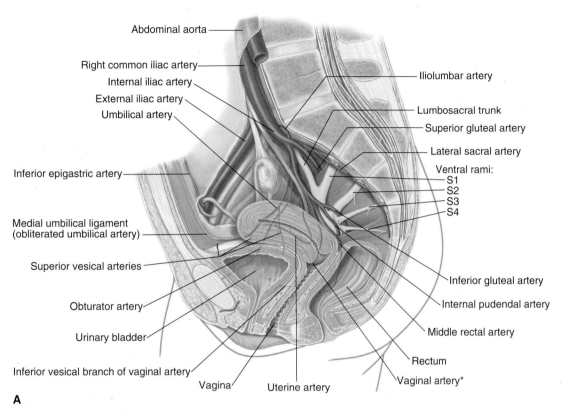

Abdominal aorta

Right common iliac artery

Internal iliac artery

External iliac artery

Umbilical artery

Inferior epigastric artery

Medial umbilical ligament (obliterated umbilical artery)

Superior vesical arteries

Obturator artery

Urinary bladder

Inferior vesical branch of vaginal artery

Vagina

Uterine artery

Iliolumbar artery

Lumbosacral trunk

Superior gluteal artery

Lateral sacral artery

Ventral rami:
S1
S2
S3
S4

Inferior gluteal artery

Internal pudendal artery

Middle rectal artery

Rectum

Vaginal artery*

A

*Vaginal artery arises from uterine artery in 11% of cases

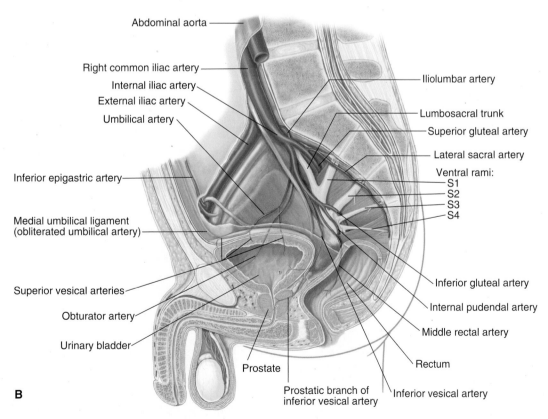

Abdominal aorta

Right common iliac artery

Internal iliac artery

External iliac artery

Umbilical artery

Inferior epigastric artery

Medial umbilical ligament (obliterated umbilical artery)

Superior vesical arteries

Obturator artery

Urinary bladder

Prostate

Prostatic branch of inferior vesical artery

Iliolumbar artery

Lumbosacral trunk

Superior gluteal artery

Lateral sacral artery

Ventral rami:
S1
S2
S3
S4

Inferior gluteal artery

Internal pudendal artery

Middle rectal artery

Rectum

Inferior vesical artery

B

FIG. 3.15A,B. Arteries of the Pelvis, Sagittal Section, Medial View. **A.** Female. **B.** Male.

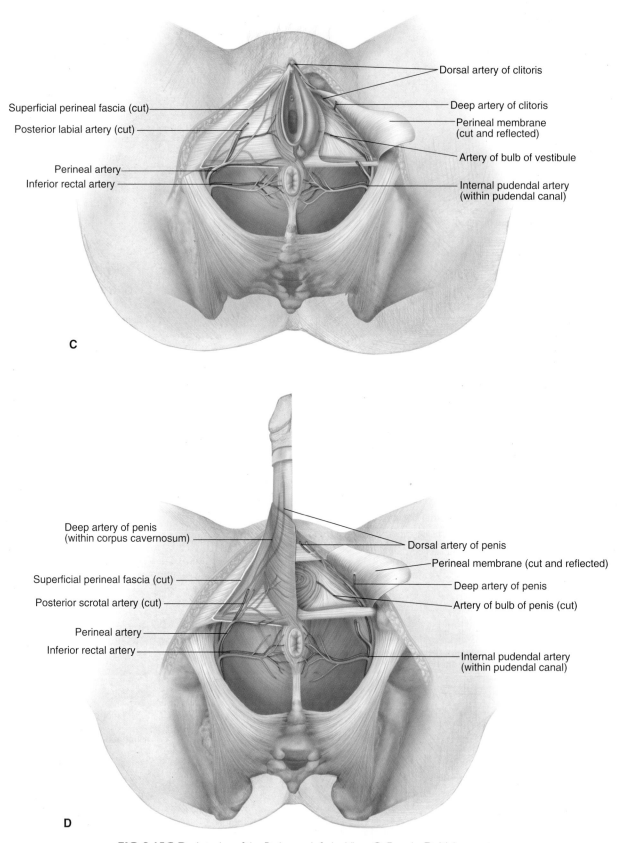

Dorsal artery of clitoris

Deep artery of clitoris

Perineal membrane
(cut and reflected)

Artery of bulb of vestibule

Internal pudendal artery
(within pudendal canal)

Superficial perineal fascia (cut)

Posterior labial artery (cut)

Perineal artery

Inferior rectal artery

C

Deep artery of penis
(within corpus cavernosum)

Dorsal artery of penis

Perineal membrane (cut and reflected)

Deep artery of penis

Artery of bulb of penis (cut)

Superficial perineal fascia (cut)

Posterior scrotal artery (cut)

Perineal artery

Inferior rectal artery

Internal pudendal artery
(within pudendal canal)

D

FIG. 3.15C,D. Arteries of the Perineum, Inferior View. **C.** Female. **D.** Male.

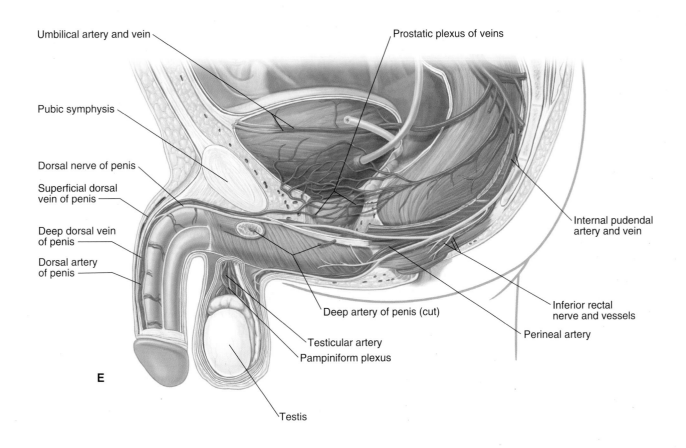

Umbilical artery and vein

Pubic symphysis

Dorsal nerve of penis

Superficial dorsal vein of penis

Deep dorsal vein of penis

Dorsal artery of penis

Prostatic plexus of veins

Internal pudendal artery and vein

Inferior rectal nerve and vessels

Perineal artery

Deep artery of penis (cut)

Testicular artery

Pampiniform plexus

Testis

E

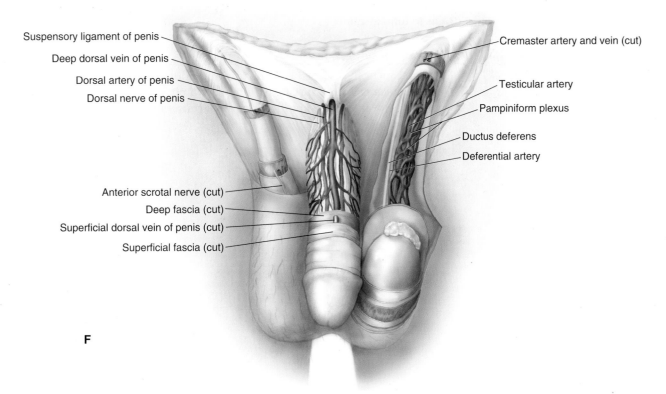

Suspensory ligament of penis

Deep dorsal vein of penis

Dorsal artery of penis

Dorsal nerve of penis

Cremaster artery and vein (cut)

Testicular artery

Pampiniform plexus

Ductus deferens

Deferential artery

Anterior scrotal nerve (cut)

Deep fascia (cut)

Superficial dorsal vein of penis (cut)

Superficial fascia (cut)

F

FIG. 3.15E,F E. Veins of the Male Pelvis and Perineum, Parasagittal View. **F.** Veins of the Male Perineum, Anterior View.

Lymphatics of the Pelvis and Perineum

I. Lymphatics of Pelvic Viscera (Fig. 3.16A,B)

A. Bladder
1. Superior and inferolateral surface drains to **external iliac nodes**
2. Posterior surface drains to both external iliac and **internal iliac nodes**
3. Fundus and neck of bladder drain to internal iliac nodes; some from neck drain into **sacral nodes** and to common iliac nodes

B. Prostate and seminal vesicles: sacral and internal iliac nodes

C. Ovary: vessels following ovarian artery to enter **lumbar nodes**

D. Uterine tube: follows ovarian and uterine drainage

E. Uterus
1. Cervix: to external, internal, and common iliac nodes
2. Body and fundus: mostly follow ovarian drainage to lumbar nodes, some to external iliac and **superficial inguinal nodes** (along round ligament to labia)

F. Vagina
1. Upper, middle, and lower portions drain to external, internal, and common iliac nodes
2. Vestibule drains to superficial inguinal nodes

G. Rectum: through **pararectal nodes** which lie on rectal muscles and sigmoid mesocolon to inferior mesenteric group of preaortic nodes

II. Lymphatics of Perineum

A. Anus: with lymphatics of superficial perineum and scrotum into superficial inguinal nodes

B. Anal canal: accompany middle rectal artery and end in internal iliac nodes around internal iliac vessels; from these to common iliac nodes and then to lateral aortic group

C. External genitalia
1. Most structures drain to superficial inguinal nodes
2. Glans of clitoris/penis: drains to deep inguinal and external iliac nodes
3. Testis: drains to lumbar nodes

III. Clinical Considerations

A. Ovarian cancer may spread to lumbar lymph nodes

B. Testicular cancer may spread to lumbar lymph nodes, whereas cancer of scrotum metastasizes to superficial inguinal lymph nodes

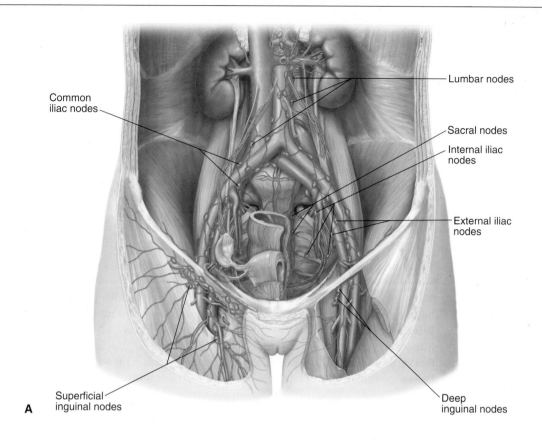

Lumbar nodes

Common
iliac nodes

Sacral nodes

Internal iliac
nodes

External iliac
nodes

Superficial
inguinal nodes

Deep
inguinal nodes

A

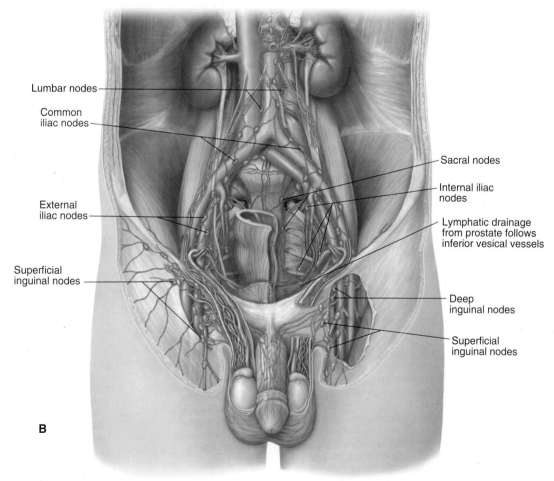

Lumbar nodes

Common
iliac nodes

Sacral nodes

Internal iliac
nodes

External
iliac nodes

Lymphatic drainage
from prostate follows
inferior vesical vessels

Superficial
inguinal nodes

Deep
inguinal nodes

Superficial
inguinal nodes

B

FIG. 3.16A,B. Lymphatics of the Pelvis, Anterior View. **A.** Female. **B.** Male.

Somatic Nerves of the Pelvis and Perineum

I. Sacral Plexus (Fig. 3.17A,B)

A. Source

   1. Anterior rami of L4 to S4; part of L4 and all of L5 unite to form **lumbosacral trunk**, which descends over pelvic brim into true pelvis

   2. Receives gray rami from sacral sympathetic trunk

B. Location

   1. Anterior rami emerge from anterior sacral foramina to lie on anterior surface of piriformis muscle within endopelvic fascia

   2. Internal iliac vessels lie anteriorly, primarily, although sacral plexus is penetrated by several branches

C. Branches

   1. Superior gluteal (L4–L5, S1): follows superior gluteal artery, supplies gluteus medius, gluteus minimus, and tensor fasciae latae muscles

   2. Nerve to quadratus femoris (L4–L5, S1): leaves pelvis through greater sciatic foramen below piriformis muscle, supplies quadratus femoris and inferior gemellus muscles

   3. Inferior gluteal (L5, S1–S2): follows inferior gluteal vessels, supplies gluteus maximus muscle

   4. Nerve to obturator internus (L5, S1–S2): leaves pelvis through greater sciatic foramen below piriformis muscle, supplies superior gemellus, and enters ischioanal fossa through lesser sciatic foramen to supply obturator internus muscle

   5. Sciatic: largest nerve of body

     a. 2 nerves, tibial and common fibular (peroneal) within same sheath

       i. Tibial (L4–L5, S1–S3): supplies all hamstrings except short head of biceps, then enters leg to supply posterior leg and plantar foot

       ii. Common fibular (peroneal) (L4–L5, S1–S2): supplies short head of biceps and enters leg to supply lateral and anterior leg and dorsal foot (Note: occasionally [slightly more than 10%], common fibular passes through or even above piriformis muscle, and may travel distally separate from tibial nerve)

     b. Leaves pelvis through greater sciatic foramen below piriformis muscle, passes inferiorly on obturator internus, gemelli, and quadratus femoris muscles; deep to gluteus maximus muscle

     c. Farther down, it runs on adductor magnus muscle, crossed by long head of biceps muscle; splits above popliteal fossa into its 2 parts

   6. Nerve to piriformis muscle (S1–S2): does not leave pelvis

   7. Posterior femoral cutaneous (S1–S3): leaves pelvis through greater sciatic foramen to reach skin over lower part of gluteus maximus muscle with inferior cluneal branches and then distribute to posterior thigh skin

   8. Perforating cutaneous (S2–S3): pierces sacrotuberous ligament, supplies lower and medial buttock

   9. Pudendal (S2–S4): leaves pelvis through greater sciatic foramen, crosses ischial spine, and enters ischioanal fossa through lesser sciatic foramen

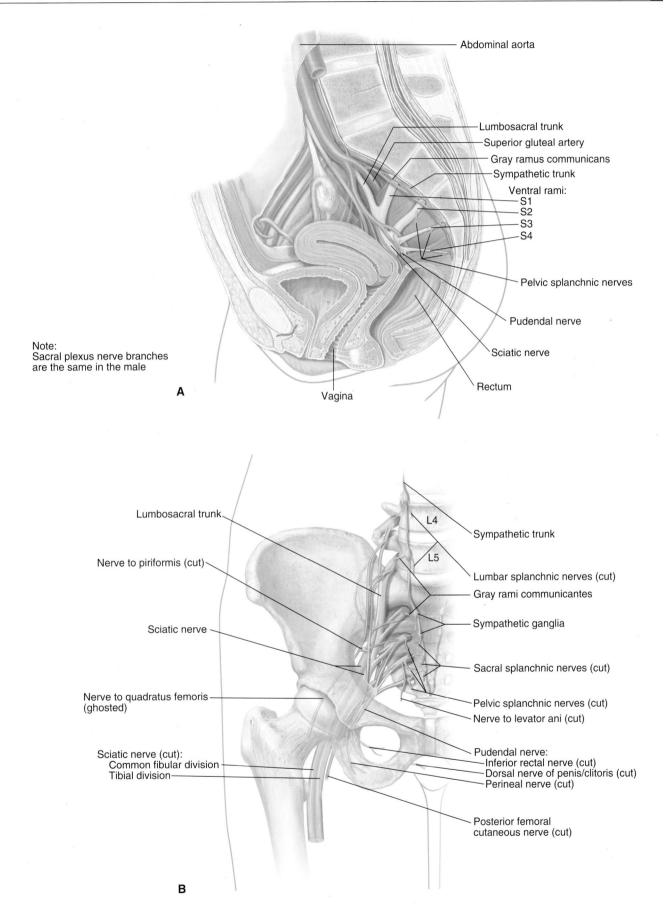

Abdominal aorta

Lumbosacral trunk
Superior gluteal artery
Gray ramus communicans
Sympathetic trunk
Ventral rami:
S1
S2
S3
S4

Pelvic splanchnic nerves

Pudendal nerve

Sciatic nerve

Rectum

Vagina

Note:
Sacral plexus nerve branches
are the same in the male

A

Lumbosacral trunk

Nerve to piriformis (cut)

Sciatic nerve

Nerve to quadratus femoris
(ghosted)

Sciatic nerve (cut):
Common fibular division
Tibial division

L4

L5

Sympathetic trunk

Lumbar splanchnic nerves (cut)
Gray rami communicantes

Sympathetic ganglia

Sacral splanchnic nerves (cut)

Pelvic splanchnic nerves (cut)
Nerve to levator ani (cut)

Pudendal nerve:
Inferior rectal nerve (cut)
Dorsal nerve of penis/clitoris (cut)
Perineal nerve (cut)

Posterior femoral
cutaneous nerve (cut)

B

FIG. 3.17A,B. Sacral Plexus. **A.** Sagittal Section, Medial View. **B.** Anterior View.

II. Nerves of Perineum (Fig. 3.17C,D)

A. Anterior labial/scrotal nerve: from ilioinguinal nerve emerging from superficial inguinal ring to reach skin of labia majora or scrotum anteriorly

B. Perineal branch of posterior femoral cutaneous nerve: to labium majus or posterior scrotum

C. Pudendal

1. From anterior rami of S2–S4, leaves pelvis through greater sciatic foramen, passes around ischial spine, and enters ischioanal fossa and pudendal canal through lesser sciatic foramen

2. Branches

   a. **Inferior rectal nerves:** cross ischioanal fossa to innervate external anal sphincter and skin of anal triangle

   b. **Perineal nerve**

      i. Leaves pudendal canal within anal triangle to swing forward into urogenital triangle

      ii. Branches

         a) **Posterior labial/scrotal branch:** passes superficially to reach skin of this area

         b) **Deep branch:** supplies all muscles of urogenital triangle (ischiocavernosus, bulbospongiosus, superficial and deep transverse perineus, and sphincter urethrae/vaginalis)

   c. **Dorsal nerve of clitoris/penis**

      i. Continuation of pudendal nerve after perineal branch

      ii. Penetrates transverse perineal ligament with dorsal artery to reach root of clitoris/penis lateral to dorsal artery

      iii. Passes distally to supply skin of clitoris/penis

      iv. Important in maintaining erection

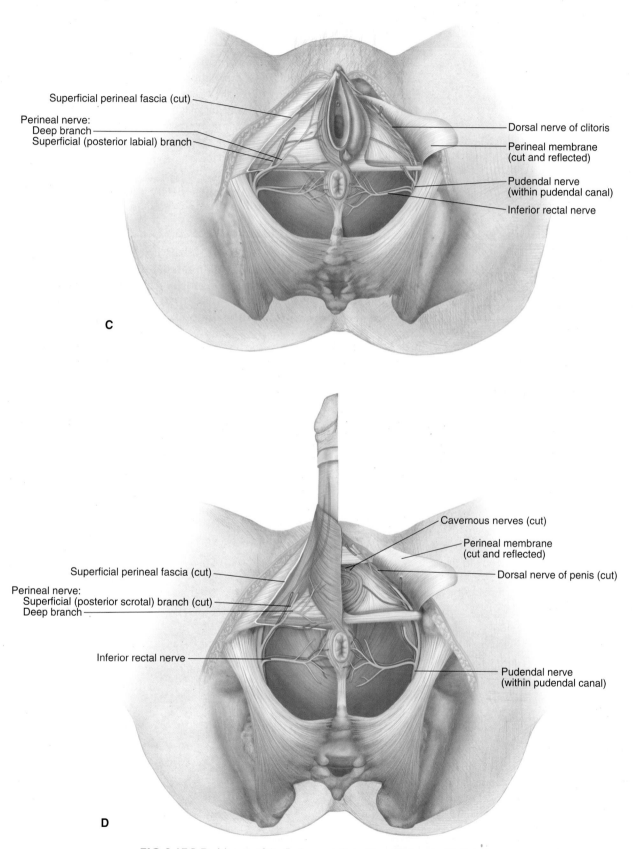

Superficial perineal fascia (cut)

Perineal nerve:
Deep branch
Superficial (posterior labial) branch

Dorsal nerve of clitoris

Perineal membrane
(cut and reflected)

Pudendal nerve
(within pudendal canal)

Inferior rectal nerve

C

Cavernous nerves (cut)

Perineal membrane
(cut and reflected)

Superficial perineal fascia (cut)

Dorsal nerve of penis (cut)

Perineal nerve:
Superficial (posterior scrotal) branch (cut)
Deep branch

Inferior rectal nerve

Pudendal nerve
(within pudendal canal)

D

FIG. 3.17C,D. Nerves of the Perineum, Inferior View. **C.** Female. **D.** Male.

III. Clinical Considerations (Fig. 3.17E,F)

A. **Pudendal nerve block**
  1. Peripheral nerve block giving anesthesia over S2–S4 dermatomes (most of perineum and inferior 1/4 vagina)
  2. Does not block pain from upper birth canal (uterine cervix and superior vagina so mother can still feel contractions)
  3. Particularly useful during childbirth
  4. Can anesthetize external genitalia by placing needle through vagina into area of ischial spine (palpated by finger in vagina)

B. **Epidural anesthesia**
  1. Needle introduced into epidural space
  2. Needle does not puncture dural sac
  3. Anesthetic injected into fat surrounding dural sac
  4. Spinal nerves anesthetized within dural sleeves

C. **Spinal anesthesia**
  1. Anesthetic agents injected into subarachnoid space
  2. Needle punctures dural sac between lumbar vertebrae
  3. Anesthetic mixes with cerebrospinal fluid to anesthetize nerve roots

D. **Caudal anesthesia**: epidural anesthesia performed by inserting needle through sacral hiatus

E. **Ilioinguinal nerve block**: to abolish sensation from anterior part of perineum

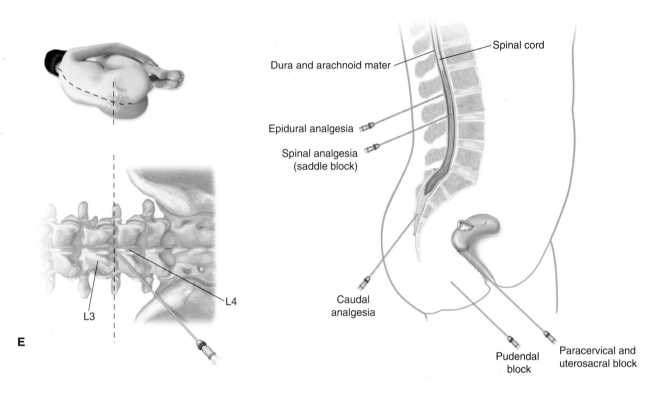

Spinal cord

Dura and arachnoid mater

Epidural analgesia

Spinal analgesia
(saddle block)

Caudal
analgesia

L3

L4

E

Pudendal
block

Paracervical and
uterosacral block

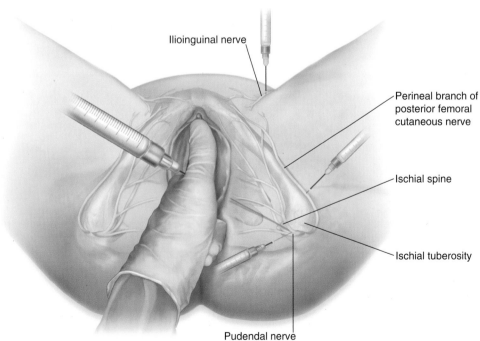

Ilioinguinal nerve

Perineal branch of
posterior femoral
cutaneous nerve

Ischial spine

Ischial tuberosity

Pudendal nerve

F

FIG. 3.17E,F **E.** Anesthesia of the Female Pelvis and Perineum, Posterior and Sagittal Views. **F.** Anesthesia of the Female Perineum, Pudendal Nerve Block, Inferior View.

Autonomic Nerves of the Pelvis and Perineum

I. Sympathetic Supply (Fig. 3.18A,B)

A. **Sacral sympathetic trunk**
  1. Continuous with lumbar sympathetic trunk across pelvic brim (pelvic inlet) at sacral ala
  2. Lies on sacrum medial to sacral foramina
  3. Ends anterior to coccyx by uniting with contralateral trunk to form ganglion impar, lowest sympathetic ganglion

B. **Sacral sympathetic ganglia**
  1. 4–5, with frequent fusions; lowest ganglion, the coccygeal, of each side fuses in midline as **ganglion impar**
  2. Branches
      a. **Gray rami communicantes**: to all sacral and coccygeal nerves
      b. **Sacral splanchnic nerves**: slender branches that pass anteriorly into inferior hypogastric plexus

C. **Superior hypogastric plexus**
  1. Caudal continuation of intermesenteric plexus over aortic bifurcation
  2. Receives lower 2–3 lumbar splanchnic nerves
  3. Passes over common iliac arteries to enter pelvis and aggregate as **hypogastric nerves**, which reach lateral surface of rectum and spread out as **inferior hypogastric plexus**

D. Functions
  1. Supplies pelvic vascular smooth muscle
  2. Passes into sacral plexus to supply vascular smooth muscle, sweat glands, and arrector pili muscles of lower limb
  3. Inhibit micturition: innervates internal sphincter, inhibits detrusor muscle
  4. Emission and ejaculation: innervates smooth muscle of ductus deferens, seminal vesicle, and ejaculatory duct

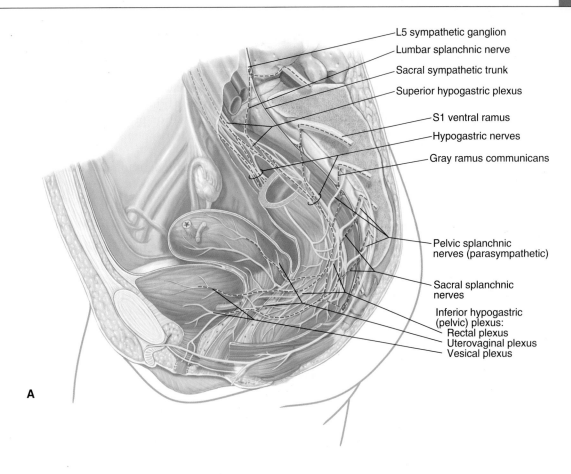

L5 sympathetic ganglion
Lumbar splanchnic nerve
Sacral sympathetic trunk
Superior hypogastric plexus
S1 ventral ramus
Hypogastric nerves
Gray ramus communicans
Pelvic splanchnic nerves (parasympathetic)
Sacral splanchnic nerves
Inferior hypogastric (pelvic) plexus:
Rectal plexus
Uterovaginal plexus
Vesical plexus

A

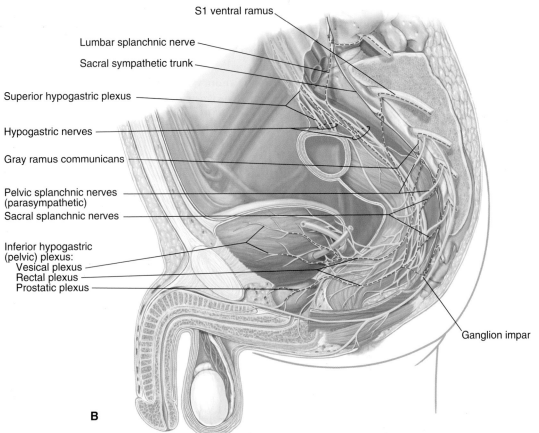

S1 ventral ramus
Lumbar splanchnic nerve
Sacral sympathetic trunk
Superior hypogastric plexus
Hypogastric nerves
Gray ramus communicans
Pelvic splanchnic nerves (parasympathetic)
Sacral splanchnic nerves
Inferior hypogastric (pelvic) plexus:
Vesical plexus
Rectal plexus
Prostatic plexus
Ganglion impar

B

FIG. 3.18A,B. Sympathetics of the Pelvis, Parasagittal Section, Medial View. **A.** Female. **B.** Male.

II. Parasympathetic Supply (Fig. 3.18C,D)

A. Pelvic splanchnic nerves
1. From anterior rami of S2–S4
2. Pass into inferior hypogastric plexus to reach pelvic organs
3. Some fibers pass superiorly over left pelvic brim to reach descending and sigmoid colon
4. **Cavernous nerves**: some fibers of vaginal or prostatic plexus pass through perineal membrane to reach erectile bodies of clitoris/penis

B. Functions
1. Defecation: innervate smooth muscle of hindgut to provide motility
2. Micturition: innervates detrusor muscle of bladder
3. Erection: inhibits vasoconstriction of deep arteries of penis/clitoris

III. Autonomic Plexuses of Pelvis

A. Inferior hypogastric plexus: lateral to rectum, but often used as name for entire collection of pelvic plexuses

B. Rectal plexus: subsidiary plexus to supply rectum and anal canal

C. Uterovaginal plexus: supplies uterus, uterine tube, vagina; provides cavernous nerves

D. Prostatic plexus: for prostate, ampulla of ductus deferens, seminal vesicles; provides cavernous nerves

E. Cavernous nerves: autonomic fibers (from inferior hypogastric plexuses) to erectile bodies; necessary for erection

F. Vesical plexus: for bladder and pelvic ureters

G. Ovarian/testicular plexus
1. Contains sympathetic fibers from T10 and parasympathetic fibers from vagus
2. Travels from renal and intermesenteric plexus with gonadal vessels
   a. Ovarian plexus travels over pelvic brim/inlet to reach ovary
   b. Testicular plexus travels through deep inguinal ring to become part of spermatic cord

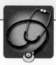

IV. Clinical Considerations

A. Resection of superior hypogastric plexus may alleviate urinary retention resulting from lesions of spinal cord

B. Nerve sparing in abdominal aortic aneurysm grafting: care is taken to preserve sympathetic fibers of superior hypogastric plexus to prevent retrograde ejaculation

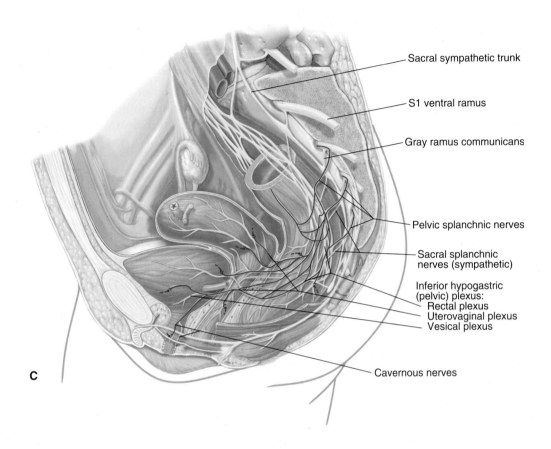

Sacral sympathetic trunk

S1 ventral ramus

Gray ramus communicans

Pelvic splanchnic nerves

Sacral splanchnic nerves (sympathetic)

Inferior hypogastric (pelvic) plexus:
Rectal plexus
Uterovaginal plexus
Vesical plexus

Cavernous nerves

C

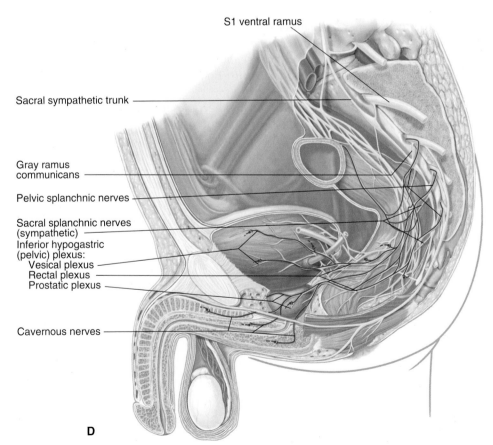

S1 ventral ramus

Sacral sympathetic trunk

Gray ramus communicans

Pelvic splanchnic nerves

Sacral splanchnic nerves (sympathetic)

Inferior hypogastric (pelvic) plexus:
Vesical plexus
Rectal plexus
Prostatic plexus

Cavernous nerves

D

FIG. 3.18C,D. Parasympathetics of the Pelvis, Parasagittal Section, Medial View. **C.** Female. **D.** Male.

Micturition

I. Urination (Micturition) Reflex (Fig. 3.19A–C)

A. Normally controlled by voluntary contraction of sphincter urethrae muscle (voluntary, striated muscle) and by inhibition of reflex due to impulses from brainstem and cerebral cortex via corticospinal tracts to S2–S4 cord segments

B. Voluntary control is normally developed by age 2–3 years; in younger children, micturition is simple reflex action and occurs when bladder distends

II. Essential Events of Micturition

A. Urinary bladder distends and wall thins as it fills with urine
   1. Urethral walls are brought close together due to circularly arranged elastic fibers around urethra at neck of bladder, associated with sphincter urethrae muscle
   2. Aided by elongation of urethra due to combined downward movement caused by contraction of sphincter urethrae muscle and an upward movement caused by pubovesical portion of levator ani muscle (both voluntary)

B. As bladder distends, stretch receptors in bladder wall are stimulated
   1. Afferent impulses travel via pelvic splanchnic nerves to micturition reflex center in sacral spinal cord (S2–S4)
   2. Need to urinate sensed as urgent (uncomfortable feeling) when bladder contains 300 mL of urine; bladder can hold 600 mL, but desire to urinate is usually experienced when it has 150 mL

C. Parasympathetic efferent impulses leave cord
   1. Presynaptic fibers
      a. Pelvic splanchnic nerves (from S2–S4)
      b. Pass through inferior hypogastric plexus and vesical plexus to reach bladder
   2. Postsynaptic fibers
      a. Presynaptic fibers enter bladder wall where they synapse with postsynaptic neurons
      b. Innervate detrusor (smooth) muscle; bladder contracts rhythmically

D. Internal (vesical, controlled by sympathetics) and external (urethral, somatic via pudendal nerve, S2–S4) sphincters are relaxed and reflex further facilitated by impulses from pons and hypothalamus
   1. During micturition, urethra is shortened and becomes funnel shaped due to relaxation of pubovesical part of levator ani and contraction of detrusor muscle
   2. After urine enters first part of urethra, sphincter urethrae muscle is relaxed, and there is further shortening of urethra; micturition occurs as urine is expelled through urethra
   3. In males, any urine remaining in spongy urethra is ejected by contraction of bulbospongiosus muscle

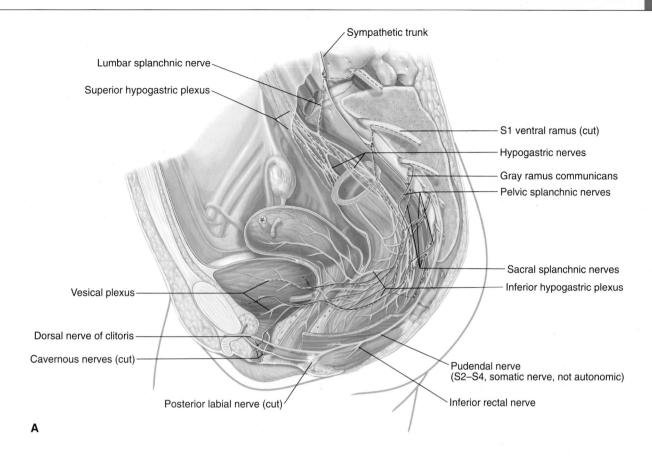

Sympathetic trunk

Lumbar splanchnic nerve

Superior hypogastric plexus

S1 ventral ramus (cut)

Hypogastric nerves

Gray ramus communicans

Pelvic splanchnic nerves

Sacral splanchnic nerves

Inferior hypogastric plexus

Vesical plexus

Dorsal nerve of clitoris

Cavernous nerves (cut)

Pudendal nerve
(S2–S4, somatic nerve, not autonomic)

Posterior labial nerve (cut)

Inferior rectal nerve

A

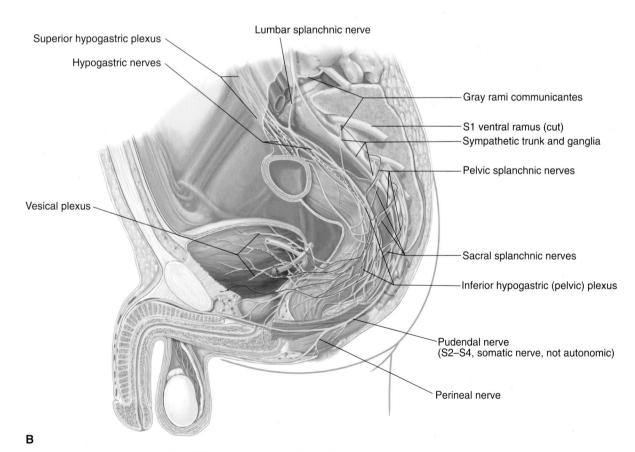

Superior hypogastric plexus

Lumbar splanchnic nerve

Hypogastric nerves

Gray rami communicantes

S1 ventral ramus (cut)

Sympathetic trunk and ganglia

Pelvic splanchnic nerves

Vesical plexus

Sacral splanchnic nerves

Inferior hypogastric (pelvic) plexus

Pudendal nerve
(S2–S4, somatic nerve, not autonomic)

Perineal nerve

B

FIG. 3.19A,B. Mechanism of Micturition. **A.** Female. **B.** Male.

III. Essential Nerve Responses

A. Via vesical plexus, which contains both sympathetic and parasympathetic fibers; continuous with inferior hypogastric plexus

B. Parasympathetic innervation

1. Presynaptic fibers begin as pelvic splanchnic nerves (S2–S4) and pass through inferior hypogastric plexuses to reach bladder, where they synapse with postsynaptic neurons

2. Postsynaptic fibers are motor to detrusor muscle and inhibitory to internal sphincter

C. Sympathetic innervation

1. Presynaptic fibers from T11–L2 pass to sympathetic trunk ganglia Ll–L2 and synapse

2. Postsynaptic fibers pass via superior hypogastric plexus to supply motor fibers to muscles of ureter, trigone, and urethral crest

   a. Fibers to bladder inhibit contraction of detrusor muscle and stimulate contraction of internal sphincter

   b. Also carry sensory nerves from bladder, which are visceral and transmit pain sensation (e.g., due to overdistension)

D. Somatic innervation: pudendal nerve (S2–S4) is motor to sphincter urethrae (voluntary, striated) muscle

E. Although bladder emptying is controlled by reflex, it can be initiated voluntarily and stopped at will due to cerebral control of external sphincter and certain muscles of pelvic diaphragm

IV. Clinical Considerations: Spinal Cord Transection

A. During spinal shock after injury, the bladder is flaccid and unresponsive and becomes overfilled, with urine dribbling through the sphincters (overflow incontinence)

B. If spinal cord is damaged above sacral region, typical micturition reflex may exist, but there is no conscious control over onset and duration of reflex

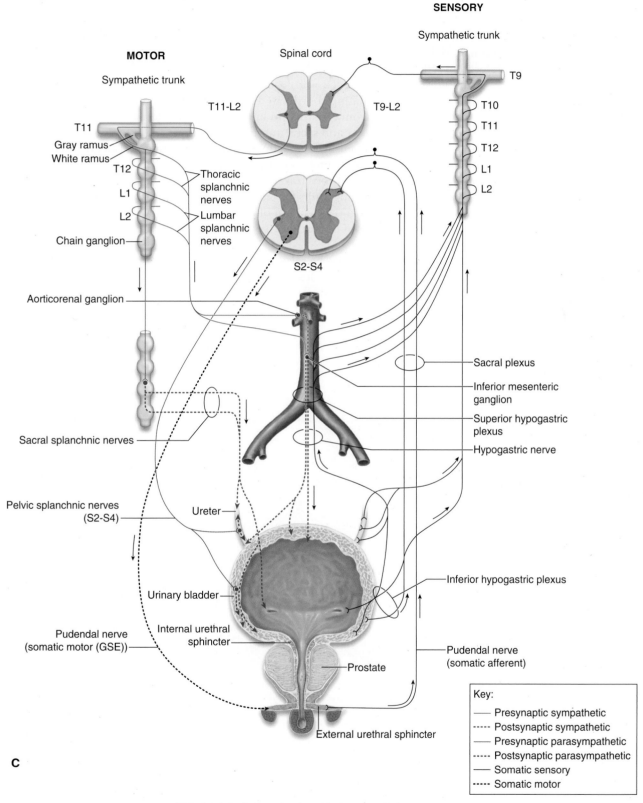

SENSORY

Sympathetic trunk

Spinal cord

MOTOR

Sympathetic trunk

T11-L2

T9-L2

T9

T11

T10

Gray ramus

T11

White ramus

T12

T12

L1

L1

L2

L2

Thoracic splanchnic nerves

Lumbar splanchnic nerves

Chain ganglion

S2-S4

Aorticorenal ganglion

Sacral plexus

Inferior mesenteric ganglion

Superior hypogastric plexus

Hypogastric nerve

Sacral splanchnic nerves

Pelvic splanchnic nerves (S2-S4)

Ureter

Inferior hypogastric plexus

Urinary bladder

Pudendal nerve (somatic motor (GSE))

Internal urethral sphincter

Prostate

Pudendal nerve (somatic afferent)

External urethral sphincter

Key:
— Presynaptic sympathetic
···· Postsynaptic sympathetic
— Presynaptic parasympathetic
···· Postsynaptic parasympathetic
— Somatic sensory
···· Somatic motor

C

FIG. 3.19C. Schematic of the Mechanism of Micturition, Male.

Defecation

I. Process of Defecation (Fig. 3.20A,B)

A. Initiation: mass peristaltic movements passing down descending and sigmoid colon push fecal material from colon into rectum

B. **Defecation reflex**

   1. Resulting distention of rectal wall leading to sense of "fullness" stimulates pressure-sensitive receptors, initiating coordinated reflex for defecation (emptying of rectum)

      a. Visceral afferents from rectum and anal canal (down to pectinate line) return to spinal cord via lumbar and sacral autonomic fibers

      b. Somatic afferents from below pectinate line follow pudendal nerve back to cord and provide sensation from lower end of anal canal

   2. Motor impulses from spinal cord travel along parasympathetic pelvic splanchnic nerves (S2–S4) back to descending and sigmoid colon, rectum and anus and are responsible for increased peristalsis and relaxation of internal anal sphincter muscle

   3. Contraction of longitudinal muscle of rectum shortens rectum and further increases pressure inside it

   4. Intraabdominal pressure may be raised by descent of diaphragm, closure of glottis, and voluntary contractions of muscles of anterior abdominal wall; all of the above aid by increasing pressure inside abdomen, which pushes walls of sigmoid colon and rectum inward

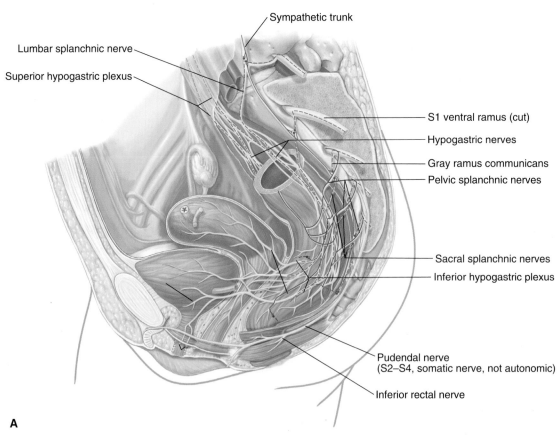

FIG. 3.20A. Mechanism of Defecation, Female, Parasagittal Section, Medial View.

A

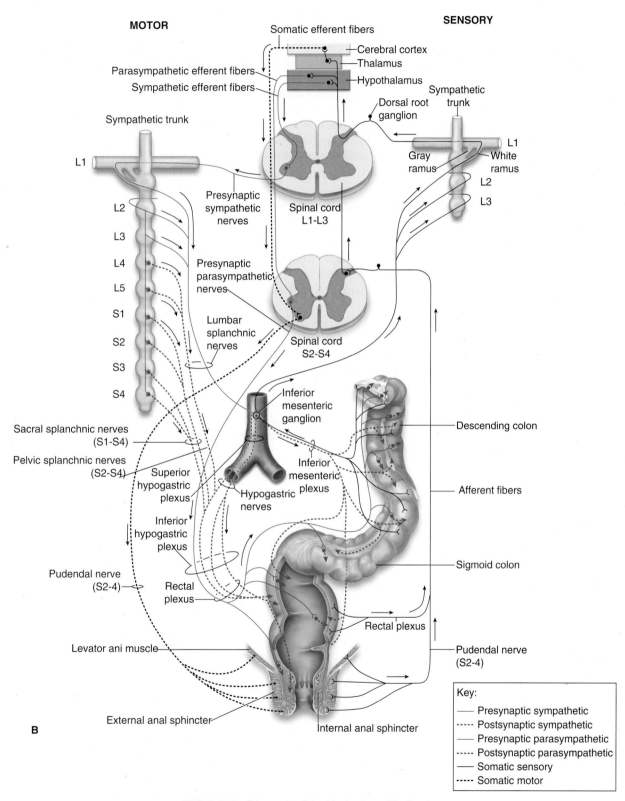

MOTOR

SENSORY

Somatic efferent fibers

Cerebral cortex
Thalamus
Hypothalamus

Parasympathetic efferent fibers
Sympathetic efferent fibers

Sympathetic trunk

Dorsal root ganglion

Sympathetic trunk

L1

Gray ramus
White ramus

L1

L2
L3

Presynaptic sympathetic nerves

Spinal cord L1-L3

Sympathetic trunk

L1

L2

L3

L4

L5

S1

S2

S3

S4

Presynaptic parasympathetic nerves

Lumbar splanchnic nerves

Spinal cord S2-S4

Inferior mesenteric ganglion

Descending colon

Sacral splanchnic nerves (S1-S4)

Pelvic splanchnic nerves (S2-S4)

Superior hypogastric plexus

Inferior mesenteric plexus

Afferent fibers

Hypogastric nerves

Inferior hypogastric plexus

Sigmoid colon

Rectal plexus

Pudendal nerve (S2-4)

Rectal plexus

Rectal plexus

Pudendal nerve (S2-4)

Levator ani muscle

External anal sphincter

Internal anal sphincter

B

Key:
— Presynaptic sympathetic
···· Postsynaptic sympathetic
— Presynaptic parasympathetic
···· Postsynaptic parasympathetic
— Somatic sensory
···· Somatic motor

FIG. 3.20B. Schematic of the Mechanism of Defecation.

5. External pressure applied to colon and waves of peristalsis force internal anal sphincter to open, expelling feces through anus
   a. If voluntary muscles of external anal sphincter and puborectalis portion of levator ani muscles are relaxed, defecation takes place; if they are voluntarily constricted, defecation can be delayed
   b. If defecation does not take place, feces back up into sigmoid colon until next wave of mass peristalsis again stimulates pressure receptors to initiate reflex
6. Depending on looseness of submucous coat, mucous membrane of lower part of anal canal is extruded through anus ahead of fecal mass
   a. When defecation is over, mucosa returns to anal canal by tone of longitudinal fibers of anal walls and contraction and upward pull of puborectalis muscle
   b. Empty lumen of anal canal is now closed by tonic contractions of anal sphincters
7. At rest, sympathetic nerves (from upper lumbar segments) to rectum and anal canal cause decrease in peristalsis and maintenance of tone of internal anal sphincter muscle

II. Clinical Considerations

A. In infants, defecation reflex results in automatic emptying of rectum without voluntary control of external anal sphincter
B. In some cases of spinal cord injury, reflex is abolished, and defecation requires supportive measures
C. **Diarrhea**: frequent defecation of liquid feces due to increased intestinal motility
   1. Intestinal contents pass through small intestine too quickly, and feces pass through large intestine too quickly with little time for absorption
   2. Can lead to dehydration and electrolyte imbalance
D. **Constipation**: infrequent or difficult defecation
   1. Can be due to decreased motility of intestines with feces in colon for long periods of time with much water absorption, making feces dry and hard
   2. Can be due to poor bowel habits, colon spasms, lack of diet bulk, too little water intake, lack of exercise, or even emotional problems

Mechanisms of Human Sexual Response

I. Sexual Response (Fig. 3.21A,B)

A. 4 stages: excitement, plateau, orgasm, and resolution

B. **Excitement stage**: vascular phenomenon

  1. Tactile and psychic stimuli result in a great number of afferent stimuli to central nervous system (CNS)

    a. Efferent impulses pass down spinal cord to parasympathetic outflow (pelvic splanchnic nerves, S2–S4) where reflexes are integrated

    b. Presynaptic fibers enter inferior hypogastric plexuses and synapse on postsynaptic neurons, which distribute to erectile tissue of clitoris/penis (arterioles of corpora cavernosa and spongiosum)

    c. Normally, constant sympathetic stimuli to arterioles of penis/clitoris maintain partial constriction of smooth muscle in arteriole walls allowing for an even flow of blood through organ

  2. Marked vasodilation of arterioles now occurs, producing increase in blood flow through blood spaces of erectile tissue, which become engorged and compress venous drainage against the surrounding fascia

    a. Blood volume entering arterioles is greater than that leaving veins and maintains internal pressure; thus, clitoris/penis enlarges in length and diameter and becomes erect

    b. Vestibular bulbs also enlarge

  3. Normally, parasympathetic centers are more important, but erection can come from sympathetic centers (T1–L2) in spinal cord (e.g., in case of spinal cord injury)

  4. Conscious thought not required for erection; stimulation can cause reflex response

  5. Parasympathetic impulses cause mucous glands in spongy urethra and bulbourethral glands to secrete mucus to lubricate urethra: vagina elongates and produces a watery (mucous) fluid by exudation, and vestibular glands secrete fluid to lubricate vaginal vestibule (to provide lubrication of penis during intercourse)

C. **Plateau stage**

  1. Maintenance of excitement stage needs continual sexual stimulation (afferent pathways) via activated tactile receptors in glans clitoris/penis and skin of shaft that reach cord via pudendal nerves

  2. Friction during coitus helps transmit sensory impulses to CNS

D. **Orgasm**

  1. In contrast to erection, involves sympathetic innervation of accessory reproductive organs

  2. In males, occurs in 2 stages

    a. **Emission**: movement of sperm from epididymis to ejaculatory ducts and into urethra and secretion of accessory glands to form semen

      i. Friction on glans penis along with other afferent nerve impulses causes discharge along sympathetic nerve fibers to smooth muscle of duct system (epididymis, ductus deferens, seminal vesicle, ejaculatory ducts and prostate)

      ii. With contraction of smooth muscle, spermatozoa and secretions from seminal vesicle and prostate discharged into prostatic urethra

        a) Bulbourethral gland fluid and penile urethral gland mucus added in proximal spongy urethra just before ejaculation to form final semen

        b) Accumulation of semen produces afferent impulses via pudendal nerve to cord to further help coordinate somatic and sympathetic output

    b. **Ejaculation**: immediately follows emission and is propulsion of semen out of urethra at time of orgasm

      i. Semen is propelled through urethra by vigorous contraction of urethral smooth muscle (parasympathetic efferents from S2–S4) and bulbospongiosus and other perineal muscles (efferent somatic impulses via the pudendal nerve)

      ii. During ejaculation, sphincter at base of bladder is closed so sperm can neither enter bladder nor can urine be expelled from it (sympathetic control)

      iii. In females, vaginal, uterine, and perineal muscles contract rhythmically to trigger orgasm after tactile stimulation of female genitals during sexual intercourse

         a) Orgasm occurs in females without emission or ejaculation

         b) Because system functions as a unit, orgasm involves other body areas influenced by sympathetic system, resulting in an increase in muscle tension throughout body, increased heart rate, rise in blood pressure, and an increased respiratory rate

E. Resolution stage

    1. After ejaculation or cessation of sexual stimulation, sympathetic impulses cause vasoconstriction of clitoral/penile arterioles in erectile tissue, reducing blood inflow

    2. Venous return becomes normal, blood leaves erectile tissue, and organ becomes flaccid

    3. Following ejaculation, males experience a latent period (minutes to hours) before another erection and ejaculation can be triggered; females, however, are often receptive to further stimulation immediately and can experience successive orgasms

II. Clinical Considerations

    A. Erectile dysfunction: inability to obtain an erection (impotence)

      1. May be due to lesions of prostatic plexus or cavernous nerves or reduced testosterone secretion

      2. Nerve fibers may fail to stimulate erectile tissue or blood vessels, or there may be insufficient response to autonomic stimulation

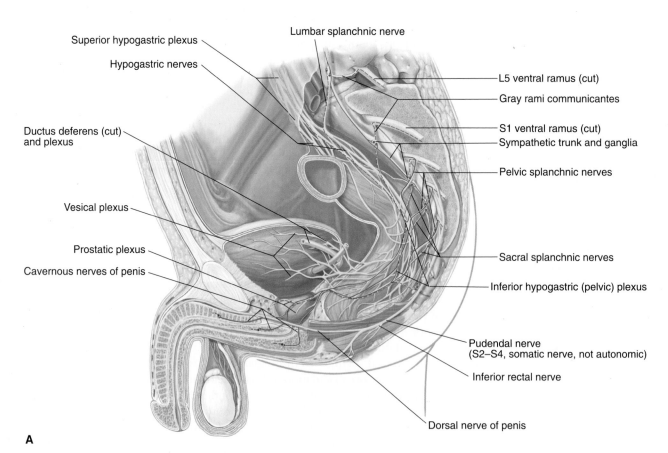

FIG. 3.21A. Mechanism of Sexual Response, Male, Parasagittal Section, Medial View.

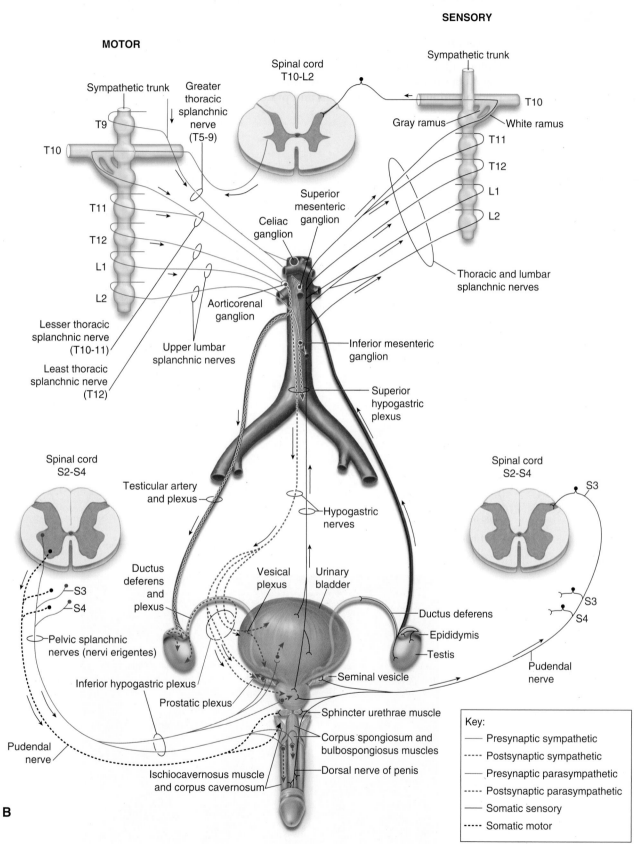

FIG. 3.21B. Schematic of the Mechanism of Sexual Response, Male.

Cross-sectional Anatomy of the Pelvis

I. Female Pelvis (Fig. 3.22A–C)

A. Urinary bladder lies posterior to pubic symphysis

B. Vagina lies between bladder and rectum

C. Levator ani muscles, puborectalis and pubococcygeus, frame pelvic viscera

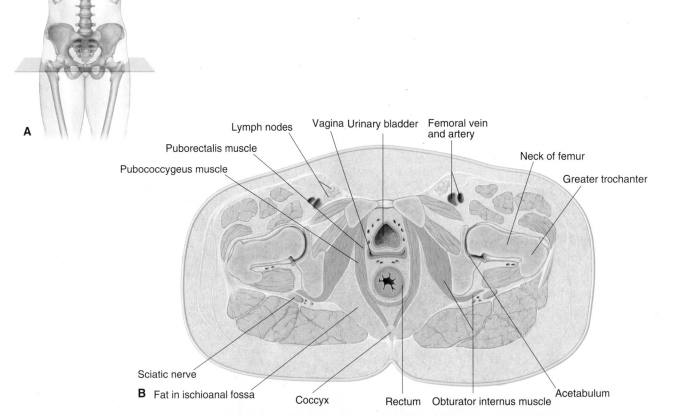

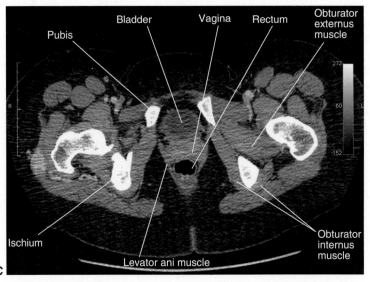

FIG. 3.22A–C. Female Pelvis. **A.** Plane of Section. **B.** Cross Section. **C.** Computed Tomography Scan.

II. Male Pelvis (Fig. 3.22D–F)

A. Prostate lies posterior to pubic symphysis

B. Rectum lies behind prostate

C. Pelvic diaphragm (levator ani muscles) frames pelvic viscera

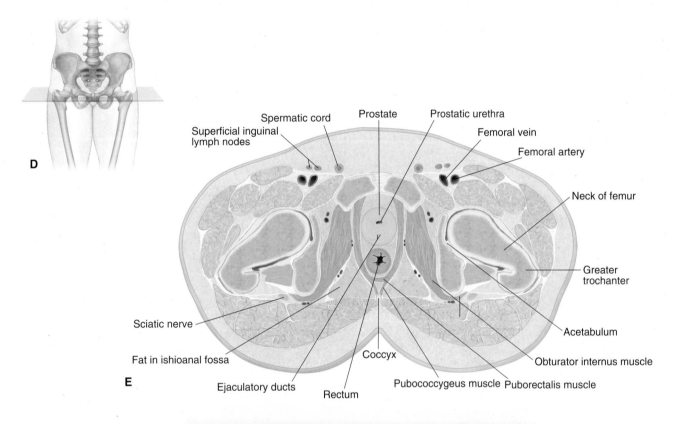

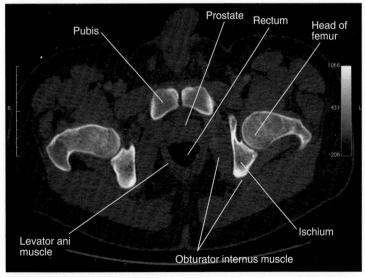

FIG. 3.22D–F. Male Pelvis. **D.** Plane of Section. **E.** Cross Section. **F.** Computed Tomography Scan.

Note: Page numbers in *italics* refer to figures